THORNTON'S MEDICAL BOOKS, LIBRARIES AND COLLECTORS

Thornton's Medical Books, Libraries and Collectors

A Study of Bibliography and the Book Trade in Relation to the Medical Sciences

third, revised edition

edited by Alain Besson

Published by
Gower Publishing Company Limited
Gower House
Croft Road
Aldershot
Hants GU11 3HR
England

Gower Publishing Company
Old Post Road
Brookfield
Vermont 05036
USA

British Library Cataloguing in Publication Data
Thornton, John L.
  Thornton's Medical books, libraries and collectors. – 3rd,
  rev. ed.
  1. Medicine. Information sources
  I. Title   II. Besson, Alain   III. Thornton, John L.
  Medical books, libraries and collectors.
  610′.7

  ISBN 0 566 05481 7

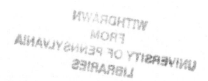

Printed in Great Britain by
Billing & Sons Ltd, Worcester

Contents

Foreword

This book originated in a title suggested to me in 1938 by R.A. Peddie (1870–1951), a partner in the firm of Grafton & Co. I drafted several chapters before I was called up to serve in the Forces from 1942 to 1946. On my return to civilian life I started again from scratch, and the book was finally published in 1949, with an introduction by Sir Geoffrey Keynes. He aptly described the work as a 'semi-readable book'. A second edition appeared in 1966, but it was already evident that the subject was becoming too vast for revision by one person. Since then the increasing interest in the history of medicine and the expansion of literature on the subject have made such a task even more impossible. My retirement as Librarian of St Bartholomew's Hospital Medical College in 1978 and subsequent events emphasized that I could take no part in revising the book, and I was pleased to hand the work over to others.

I was glad that the editor, Alain Besson, had mustered a team of experts which includes many of my friends and former colleagues. Having read their respective contributions, I congratulate them all on the result of their labours.

John L. Thornton

Wembley,
April 1989

Introduction

When John L. Thornton first published his *Medical books, libraries and collectors* in 1949, his chief objective was 'to record the chief writings of every prominent medical author' and to chart the growth and development of ancillary subjects such as periodicals, bibliographies and libraries. This third edition is in keeping with the author's original intention, and the basic structure of the first two editions has been retained.

Following Mr Thornton's retirement, it was felt that this wide-ranging work could be usefully revised and updated by a team rather than an individual, and each member of the team was given responsibility for one chapter. The resulting collective effort has given fresh impetus to the book. For instance, the opening chapter on 'Medical Books Before the Invention of Printing', now focuses on the production and transmission of medical manuscripts in the West, instead of giving shallow treatment to the entire field of manuscript studies. Members of the team also contributed to the selection of new illustrations for this edition.

Selectivity is of the essence in a book of this nature, and the real difficulty is not to decide what to include but to decide what to omit. This selection process is necessarily subjective, but the more pressing limitations of space have also exacted their toll: even if a universally-recognized list of all the major libraries of the world could be drawn, not all of them could be included in the concluding chapter on 'Medical Libraries of Today'.

Two chapters in the previous edition have not been retained here. The history of general publishing houses is no longer the *desideratum* it once was, and publishing has not been allocated a separate chapter in this edition. The decision not to devote a separate chapter to the rise of medical societies was reached, after much deliberation, for the simple reason that to deal with the subject adequately would call for more than a single chapter. In this respect, the previous editions of this book are not superseded, and this is especially the case with the list of societies published as an appendix to the first edition. The relevance of societies to the authors mentioned in the book, and to the formation of libraries and the growth of periodical literature, is discussed in individual chapters in this edition.

Regrettably it has not proved possible to open a new chapter devoted to post-nineteenth century bibliographical developments, although the twentieth century is featured towards the end of the chapter on 'Medical Books of the Nineteenth Century', as well as in the chapters on 'The Growth of

Medical Periodical Literature', 'Medical Bibliographies and Bibliographers', 'Private Medical Libraries' and 'Medical Libraries of Today'.

Thanks to the expertise of the contributors to the book, editorial intervention has been kept to a minimum, and it is with pleasure that I record my gratitude to all of them.

Alain Besson

London,
September 1989

Extract from the preface to the first edition

Medical bibliography is a vast field upon which comparatively little research has been undertaken. Medical men interested in bibliography are too rare, while bibliographers embarking upon the subject of medicine are usually confined to medical librarians, and these are also in the minority. This volume makes no pretence to be an exhaustive treatise upon the subject, but is rather an introductory history of the production, distribution and storage of medical literature from the earliest times. Books have been published (and many more could be written) upon the subjects of several of the chapters between these covers, and my objective has been the recording of knowledge accessible only at the expense of much research, rather than the presentation of new material.

The history of medicine is a fascinating subject that has received the attention of several prominent authorities, and is here only recorded further to illustrate the background of bibliographical development. Historical periods have been ignored in some cases, and quite prominent figures probably omitted from the story, my chief object being the recording of material valuable from the bibliographical viewpoint. A person unconnected with the production, distribution or storage of medical literature would probably be ignored, but I have endeavoured to record the chief writings of every prominent medical author, with the more important printed editions of his works, referring those interested to sources providing fuller details. It is, of course, impossible to note every book or edition published during the periods covered by the respective chapters, but an attempt has been made to record the most important authorities and their works, as frameworks upon which the medical literature of those times depended. For more complete details readers are referred to the literature listed in the Bibliography.

There is room for much bibliographical investigation in the field of medicine, and each chapter could readily be worked into a complete volume, while many of the writers dealt with are possible subjects for more intensive investigation. In recording what has already been accomplished in medical bibliography, I hope I have revealed the numerous gaps to would-be bibliographers.

My chief difficulty has been to decide what to omit when selecting possible material, and this was partially overcome by planning simultaneously a volume devoted to Science, which is so frequently intermingled with medicine, particularly during the early periods. That volume is being compiled with the co-operation of a librarian having extensive experience with scientific material.[1]

---

[1] This was published as Thornton, John L. and R. I. J. Tully, *Scientific books, libraries and collectors* (1954); second, revised edition, 1962; third, revised edition, 1971 (Supplement, 1976).

List of contributors

Peter Murray Jones, Fellow and Librarian, King's College, Cambridge

Dennis E. Rhodes, The British library

Yvonne Hibbott, Librarian, St Thomas's Campus, United Medical and Dental Schools of Guy's and St Thomas's Hospitals, London

Christine R. English, formerly Wellcome Institute for the History of Medicine, London

Patricia C. Want, Librarian, Royal College of Obstetricians and Gynaecologists, London

Geoffrey Davenport, Librarian, Royal College of Physicians of London

Leslie T. Morton, formerly Librarian, National Institute for Medical Research, London

John Symons, Assistant Wellcome Institute for the History of Medicine, London

Alain Besson, Assistant Librarian, St Bartholomew's Hospital Medical College

Roy B. Tabor, Regional Librarian, Wessex Regional Library Information Service

Illustrations

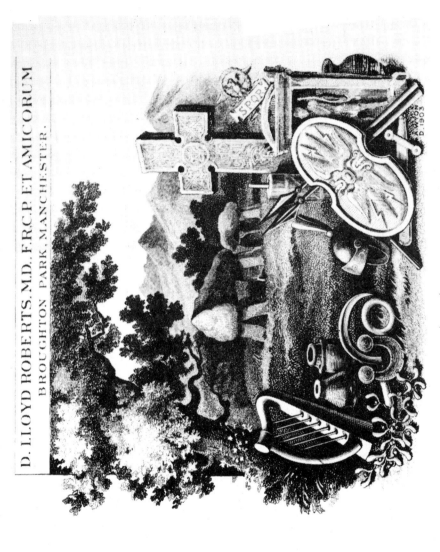

Plate 1   Bookplate made for the collection of the Manchester physician David Lloyd Roberts (1835–1920). This bookplate is now among the H. M. Barlow Collection of Bookplates in the Library of the Royal College of Physicians of London.

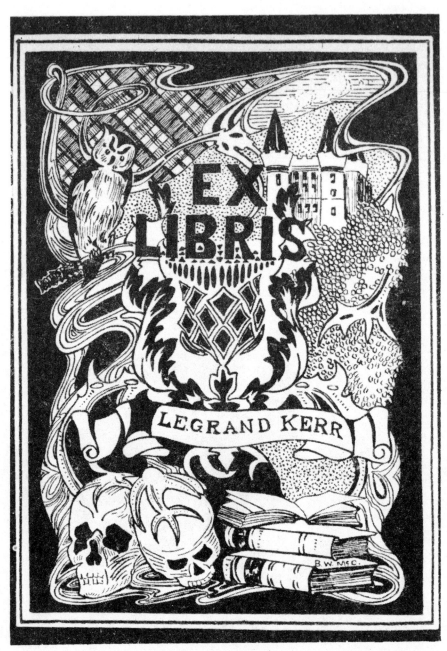

Plate 2   Bookplate, as used for the collection of the American physician LeGrand Kerr (1870–1956). Like the ex-libris reproduced on Plate 1, this is now among the H. M. Barlow Collection of Bookplates in the Royal College of Physicians of London.

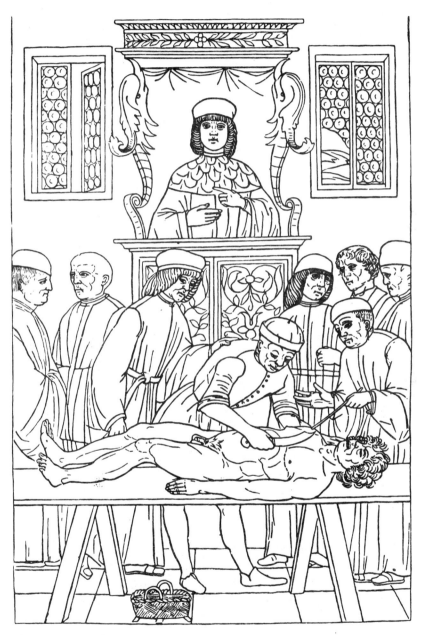

Plate 3   One of the earliest anatomical woodcuts (from Johannes de Ketham, Fascilus medicinae 1491).

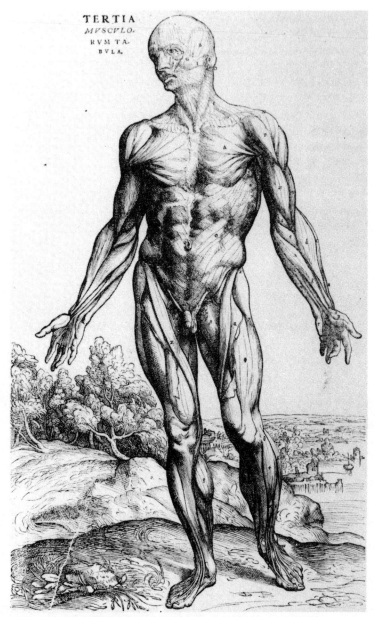

Plate 4   An outstanding woodcut of the sixteenth century (from Andreas Vesalius, De humani corporis fabrica, *Basle, 1543).*

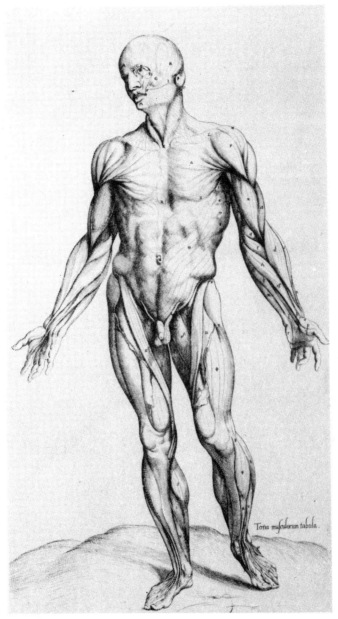

Totius musculorum tabula.

Plate 5   Copperplate from Thor as Geminus, Compendiosa totius anatomie delineatio, *1545. The Compendiosa was a landmark in the
transition from woodcut (Plate 4) to copperplate engraving.*

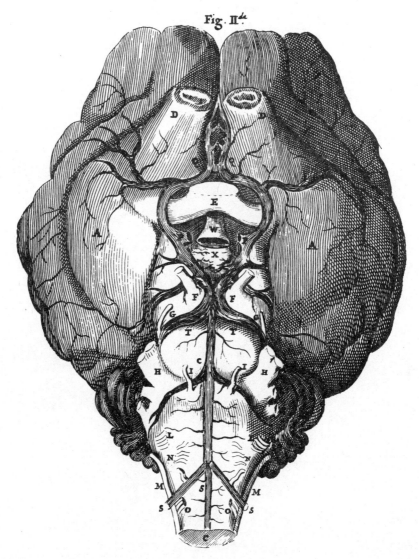

Fig. II.

Plate 6   Engraving of drawing by Sir Christopher Wren, showing the 'circle of Willis' (from Thomas Willis, Cerebri anatome, nervorumque descriptio et usus, *London, 1664).*

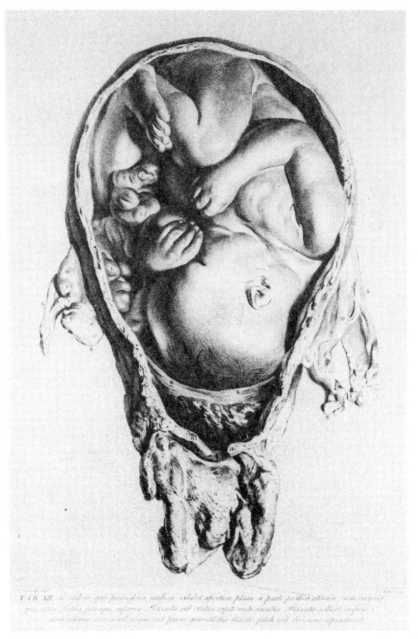

Plate 7   *Engraving of drawing by Jan van Rymsdyk (from William Hunter,*
Anatomia uteri humani gravidi, *Birmingham, 1774).*

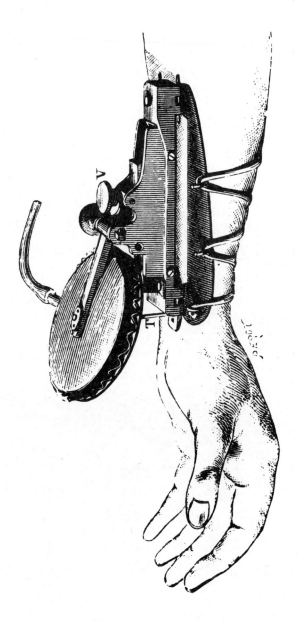

Fig. 114. Sphygmographe à transmission envoyant la pulsation artérie le a un levier inscripteur situé à distance.

Plate 8 Scientific aid to physiological and clinical investigation in the nineteenth century (from Etienne Jules Marey, La circulation du sang à l'état physiologique et dans les maladies, Paris, 1881).

Abbreviations

Titles of journals have been given in a form which can readily be reconstructed, and the following are frequently cited references that have been more severely abbreviated.

Bib-Osler	*Bibliotheca Osleriana: a catalogue of books illustrating the history of medicine and science* (1929).
DSB	*Dictionary of scientific biography*, C. C. Gillipsie, editor-in-chief (New York, [1970–80]).
Duff	Duff, E. Gordon, *Fifteenth-century English books* (1917).
Garrison–Morton	Morton, Leslie T. (comp.), *Garrison and Morton's Medical bibliography: an annotated check-list of texts illustrating the history of medicine*, 2nd edn (1954).
Goff	Goff, Frederick R. (ed.), *Incunabula in American libraries: third census* (1964); Supplement, 1972.
Index-Catalogue	*Index-Catalogue of the Library of the Surgeon-General's Office, United States Army, Washington.*
Osler	Osler, Sir William, *Incunabula medica* (1923).
STC	Pollard, A. W. and G. R. Redgrave (comps), *A short-title catalogue of books printed in England, Scotland and Ireland and of English books printed abroad 1475–1640*, 2nd edn, revised and enlarged, 2 vols (1976–86).
Thornton–Tully	Thornton, John L. and R. I. J. Tully, *Scientific books, libraries and collectors*, 3rd rev. edn (1971); Supplement, 1976.
Wing	Wing, Donald (comp.), *Short-title catalogue of books printed in England, Scotland, Ireland, Wales and British America and of English books printed in other countries 1641–1700*, 2nd edn, revised and enlarged, 2 vols (1972–82).

1 Medical books before the invention of printing

Peter Murray Jones

> There is a dead medical literature, and there is a live one. The dead is not all
> ancient, the live is not all modern. There is none, modern or ancient, which, if it
> has no living value for the student, will not teach him something by its autopsy.
> (Oliver Wendell Holmes)

This chapter has two aims: to provide a sketch of the history of the
medical book before the invention of printing; and to provide a guide to
the bibliography of medical authors and texts in the Middle Ages. No
familiarity with the medical culture of the manuscript era is assumed, and
in fact this chapter is intended to be of most use to those without such
knowledge – to those who wish to pursue a theme in medical history back
beyond the era of the printed book, or who wish simply to gain some idea
of the conditions under which medical information was transmitted
through the Middle Ages.

Focussing on the history of the manuscript book means of course that
this chapter will make no attempt to survey the history of medical learning
in all its aspects, still less to tell the story of medicine in ancient and
medieval society. These are vast and underexplored areas of research, and
a single chapter could not do justice to them at all. Concentration on the
much more limited topic may at least make the chapter useful as an
introduction to some unique, and often forgotten, features of medical
culture in the Middle Ages.

It is easy for us to underestimate the significance of books written by
hand for medicine in earlier periods. Modern western medicine is dependent on technology and drugs, but even more on information. The information comes in electronic and other forms which have tended increasingly to replace print as a medium of communication. It has become hard
for us to imagine an era in which scribal copying and recopying was the
vehicle of communication, still harder to appreciate the extent to which
medicine was dependent on the manuscript book. For ancient and medieval medicine was *livresque*, to use a French term for which there is no good
English equivalent. The written word was not just the form in which
medical knowledge was transmitted, but since experiment and observation
did not have the role they have today, it was the very substance of
medicine for the educated person. Reading and writing were also activities
invested with special significance by reason of their association with the
sacred word, and so even the copying of books had an authority and

dignity which was scriptural rather than merely scribal. Much of what we now know of ancient medicine has survived only because of this respect for the written word which outweighed mere consideration for the usefulness of the information it represented. So an account of the circumstances of medical book production in the manuscript era will not simply be an excursion down bibliographical byways, but an introduction to the central activity on which medical theory and practice both depended.

The production of medical manuscripts

This section will sketch the development of medical manuscript production in the west over a period of time from the earliest examples known, around the beginning of the sixth century AD, to the sixteenth century, when the printed book was replacing manuscript production as the standard vehicle for the circulation of texts. It deals only with the codex, the book in volume form as we know it today. Earlier equivalents, some of which, like the papyrus roll, survived to compete with the codex form, are excluded from consideration. This helps to make a more coherent tale, and, so far as the Christian and Islamic traditions are concerned, does not really mean excluding any major sources for our knowledge of early medicine. What we know of Greek medicine through the survival of papyri in the sands of Egypt is relatively insignificant compared to what has survived in codex form. But it does preclude any discussion of the significance of the written word for Egyptian medicine or for other near-eastern cultures which used wax or clay tablets to transmit medical knowledge. There are many ways in which Greek medicine is linked to what used to be called 'primitive' medicine, to be sure, but the advent of the codex, even more than that of the papyrus roll, marks a decisive break between medical cultures. Chinese and Indian medical cultures are also excluded because their development had few recognizable bibliographical points of contact with western medicine, though there is a superficial resemblance between the western codex and some of the manuscript productions of the east which long preceded it.

Bearing in mind these considerable exclusions, medical book production in the Middle Ages can conveniently be discussed under four headings, representing four successive types of book, none of which simply replaced its predecessor, but instead comfortably coexisted with it: pre-Salernitan; Salernitan (the south Italian medical school of Salerno flourished first in the late eleventh century); scholastic; laicized/vernacular. Before discussing each of these in turn, yet another disclaimer must be made. The most important source of medical texts for the medieval Latin west from the Salernitan period onwards was translation from Arabic manuscripts, for the Islamic world was the guardian of the medical tradition it had taken over from the Greeks, and Arab authors had in turn made their own contribution to this heritage, on which all subsequent

Latin writing on medicine depended. Not enough has yet been written in western languages about the history of the book in the Arab world in the critical period from the seventh to the eleventh centuries AD to fit into this sketch satisfactorily, but the significance of Arabic manuscripts should not be forgotten.

Pre-Salernitan

Medical books before the period of the translations associated with Constantine the African in the late eleventh century share certain important characteristics. The medical knowledge they contain had survived the fall of the western Roman empire only in scraps preserved by good fortune, and the texts found in these early manuscripts are often fragmentary and unreliably attributed. Accidents of survival determined the nature of the corpus of medical writing, and prevented the assimilation of medical ideas into coherent or systematic form. Many of these early texts were translated from the Greek in the fifth to the seventh centuries AD, and in their Latin dress continued to be influential for centuries afterwards.

The best way to get an idea of the sort of texts which went to make up a medical manuscript of this first stage is to look at one fairly typical example. British Library Sloane MS. 2839 was probably written in England, and dates from about 1100. It begins with illustrations of cautery scenes, accompanied by very brief captions and the title *Liber cirurgicum cauterium Appollonii et galeni de artis medicine*. After some recipes, a longer tract called *Tereoperica* follows, prefaced by a list of contents and the pseudo-Hippocratic *Epistola perhereseon*. The *Tereoperica* is also found in a ninth-century manuscript, but it is very hard to say anything more definite about it. It follows the usual head-to-toe order of ailments in such compilations, and may well have originally been put together in the late antique period.

In the middle of this compilation, which takes up some 107 folios in the manuscript, occur a number of shorter tracts, many of them pseudonymous. We find the pseudo-Hippocratic letters *De quattuor humoribus* and *Ad Antigonum*, the pseudo-Galenic letter *De febribus*, and an *Epistula de anima* in the form of a dispute between Plato and Aristotle. The other short pieces are dietetic calendars, a list of Egyptian or inauspicious days, and two short tracts on blood-letting. The way in which these smaller tracts simply interrupt the longer work, and their spurious attribution to great authorities, reflect the indifference of the time towards purely bibliographic issues of authorship, title and internal consistency. One consequence of the apparently seamless web of text in this manuscript has been a later misbinding, so that folios 107–12 are out of order. Augusto Beccaria, whose catalogue of such early medical writings is an authoritative guide to this literature[12] was well aware of the possibility of yet more independent tracts lurking within the main text, to say nothing of stray recipes (he talks of 'uno zibaldone di testi'). In fact there are additional recipes on fol. 107 recto and verso of this manuscript, and perhaps another short tract beginning *maleficium datum idem venenum aut medulla* (fols 107v, 111r, 111v), which are not mentioned in his model description of the manuscript.

Besides pseudo-Hippocratic and pseudo-Galenic writings, the genuine text of the Hippocratic Aphorisms, and a later Byzantine commentary on it, were amongst the most widely found of these early writings. Much of what was known of the medical writings of antiquity was first refracted through the work of Byzantine excerpters and compilers. Prominent among these were Oribasius (AD 325–403), author of an encyclopaedia of medicine entitled *Synagoge*, and Aetius of Amida, in Mesopotamia (*fl. c.* AD 502–75), whose *Tetrabiblion* contains quotations from Oribasius, Soranus and others. Parts of these compendious Greek works were then translated into Latin from the fifth to the seventh centuries AD, often in Ravenna and South Italy, and thus experienced yet another process of refraction at the hands of the translators before their first appearance in extant codices of the eight, or ninth century AD.

Another typical complex of works found in pre-Salernitan medical books is that associated with the pseudo-Apuleius herbal. A group of such texts is so commonly found as to be almost standard – a pseudo-Hippocratic letter to Maecenas; Antonius Musa, *De herba vettonica* (betony); Sextus Placitus, *Liber medicinae ex animalibus*; and pseudo-Dioscorides, *Liber medicinae ex herbis feminis*. The centrepiece of the group is normally the pseudo-Apuleius *Herbarius*, and the guiding idea behind this grouping of texts may have been an attempt to bring together writings on *materia medica* for therapeutic purposes. Very little is known of the authors, the circumstances in which these writings were composed, or about their first circulation in manuscript form.

Almost without exception such early manuscripts were actually written by monastic scribes, and most can be assumed to have had no medical responsibilities or particular interest in the subject matter. They copied what they found in the exemplar before them, and added little or nothing to the textual inheritance. There is little evidence that such manuscripts were used for teaching purposes in the monasteries or cathedral schools, and it seems more probable that they were used, if at all, as reference sources for the infirmary.

Salernitan
A much wider selection of texts begins to be found in manuscripts from the late eleventh century, as the first fruits of the translations from the Arabic of Constantine the African. Constantine (*fl.* 1065–85) was born at Carthage in North Africa, and is reported to have visited South Italy, learned of the lack of a Latin medical literature there, and returned with a

supply of medical texts in Arabic. He evidently joined the Benedictine community at Monte Cassino, and must have spent much of his time there working on translations. In the course of time the new works came to influence teaching at the south Italian school of Salerno, which was to become the dominant centre of medical teaching until the thirteenth century. Many of the new texts were credited to Constantine, and Constantine himself claimed Hippocrates and Galen as his authorities, but all his works are translations from the Arabic. Thus the work known as the *Pantegni* is an adaptation of Haly Abbas ('Ali ibn al-'Abbas, died 994) *Kitab al-maliki*. Constantine's technique as a translator was very free, and he felt able to leave out whole passages and paraphrase where he saw fit. The effect of this was to simplify and avoid difficult questions raised by his authorities, but the efforts of the Constantinian school of translation did make available for the first time in the medieval west a rudimentary corpus of Galenic medicine. This included the first works of *theorica*, introducing physiology and the theory of the elements, humours, and qualities, as well as the *practica* which had dominated medical writing hitherto.

Another set of translations from the Greek contributed vitally to the teaching of the Salernitan school. This set included short tracts on urine and pulse attributed to Theophilus Protospatharius (*fl*. reign of Heraclios, 610–41) and Philaretus (in fact this Greek text circulated in pseudo-Galenic form too); an alphabetical version of Dioscorides' herbal, and the *Practica* of Alexander of Tralles. Alexander (born in Lydia in the first half of the sixth century) differed from other Byzantine medical authors, like Oribasius and Aetius, in that his handbook was not just an anthology, but reflected his own experience to some extent, as well as his reading of earlier Greek authorities. His works were frequently translated into Latin and Arabic. The eleventh-century poem *De viribus herbarum* by Odo de Meung (Macer) is also based on Greek sources, and was to have a remarkable influence on therapeutics for the remainder of the Middle Ages. Nothing is known of the author, save the attribution to him of the poem in one manuscript.

In the twelfth century the medical teachers at Salerno managed to contribute a number of works of their own, based on their assimilation of the new Galenic medicine. The dissemination of Salernitan medicine throughout western Europe led others to emulate their writings, notably in Italy and France. Some works were to remain standard texts for the remainder of our period, particularly those to do with surgery and the art of the apothecary. One such is the *Chirurgia* of Roger Frugardi of Parma, another the *Antidotarium Nicolai*. Roger's surgery was assembled with the help of his pupils in 1180; we suspect that the school was north Italian rather than Salernitan, but know little more about it except the name of his most famous pupil and editor, Guido d'Arezzo. This work became the standard surgery of the thirteenth century, and so became associated with the school of Salerno. The *Antidotarium Nicolai* did originate at the school of Salerno, and was in effect a collection of lists of ingredients for named medicaments authorised by the professors there by royal sanction. It circulated in the thirteenth century, but nothing is known of the Nicolaus who may have put it together from earlier sources.

The earliest books which include the new Salernitan texts were written in the distinctive Beneventan script of South Italy, but they rapidly achieved a wider circulation and copies proliferated in local scripts. But the most significant legacy of Salerno to medical learning was the emergence of a medical curriculum which established a small group of teaching texts as the core of medical education. This assemblage of texts was known as the *articella*, and its components usually included the *Isagoge* of Johannitius (an introduction – *al - Madkhal fi'l - tibb* – to the Galenic system of medicine in the form of short questions and answers by Hunayn ibn Ishaq al-'Ibadi Abu Zayd, AD 808–73), the *Aphorisms* and *Prognostics* of Hippocrates, and the two short works on urine and the pulse of Byzantine origin, mentioned above. Later the *Tegni* or *Ars Parva* of Galen, and the *De regimine acutorum morborum* of Hippocrates with a commentary by Galen were added. This combination of texts is by some distance the most frequently found in western medical manuscripts – by the late fifteenth century in the library of the monastery of St Augustine in Canterbury, for instance, as many as 10 manuscripts contained the *articella*, out of a total of 102 medical books in all. Originating in Salerno in the last part of the twelfth or early thirteenth century, the *articella* was rapidly introduced wherever medicine was taught in the burgeoning European university system. It spawned a large number of commentaries in the same way as the set texts of other faculties.

Another form of medical literature which seems to have sprung out of the Salernitan educational environment was the putting together of *quaestiones* or *problemata* on medical topics. Typically a number of such questions are posed and then answered in pithy fashion by a short paragraph of text. The questions deal as much with matters like the differences between the sexes as with matters of medical practice, and are found in both verse and prose form. The questions and answers are usually anonymous, but are drawn from a variety of medical works by the masters of Salerno, or their near contemporaries further north, in Italy, in France and in England.

Scholastic
In the twelfth century the Constantinian translations from the Arabic were supplemented with others, both from Greek and Arabic. The centres for new translations from the Greek seem to have been Salerno and Sicily, and the best known name amongst these translators is that of Burgundio of Pisa, who translated as many as ten of Galen's works into Latin.

Burgundio (died 1193) was a judge and diplomat, who must have been an indefatigable translator, including within his interests, law, medicine and literature. By contrast the centre of Arabic translation moved away from Italy to Spain, and in particular to Toledo, where Gerard of Cremona (*c.* 1114–87) was responsible for translations of the *Almansor* of Rhases (al-Razi), the surgery of Abulcasis (Abu'l-Qasim al-Zahrawi) and the *Canon* of Avicenna (Ibn Sina), all three of which became central to western medicine. These new translations, whether from Greek or Arabic, are much more literal than the Constantinian, proceeding generally *de verbo ad verbum*. Characteristically they are much longer than the medical texts in circulation hitherto, reflecting the encyclopedic nature of the Arabic originals as well as the fidelity of the translations. For the first time in the west a substantial corpus of Galenic medicine came into existence – a Galen in Arab dress, admittedly, but nevertheless impressive enough to provide a truly philosophic medicine, a proper *scientia*. This applied to pharmacology, as much as to *theorica* and *practica*: the *Grabadin* and *Practica* of pseudo-Mesue and the *Liber aggregatus* of Serapion put the compounding of medicinal simples on a theoretical basis for the first time, going well beyond the simple regulative lore of the *Antidotarium Nicolai*.

From the thirteenth century onwards the monastery is no longer the most likely place for a medical manuscript to have been written. As medicine established itself at the Italian and French universities, and translations introduced a new Galen to put alongside the new Aristotle, most manuscripts were written to the order of the stationers' shops which sprang up in the university environment. But the burgeoning of the book trade in the university towns catered not only for the needs of the poor scholar and his master, but for a growing band of bibliophiles, who wanted books which were well written, and above all, finely illuminated. It may seem surprising that medical books should be given this treatment, alongside the histories, romances and bibles, but it is true nevertheless. Such bibliophiles took their lead from courtly and aristocratic circles, and one form of medical literature which proved to have a particular attraction for such circles was advice on diet and regimen. Such works as *Li livres dou santé* of Aldobrandino da Siena (known only as a thirteenth-century Tuscan, who may have been physician to the king of France) distilled the advice of Galen and the Arabs, Avicenna in particular, in an accessible form for a non-professional audience. It is the first medical work known to have been composed in French rather than Latin, as befits a book written at the request of Beatrix de Savoie, countess of Provence, to be taken with her on a journey she made in 1256 to visit her daughters (respectively queens of France, England and Germany, and countess of Anjou). The surviving copies of this work are very often illuminated and were obviously made for customers almost as grand as the countess.

The course of scholastic medicine north and south of the Alps diverged,

even though both types took their origin from the same sources in translation from Greek or Arabic. Broadly speaking, north of the Alps the
philosophic implications of medical scholasticism held sway, distancing
medicine from the more practical concerns of surgeons and apothecaries.
For medical books this means that the commentary form tended to
dominate the productions of the medical faculty, as it did those of the
faculties of arts, law and, of course, theology. Towards the turn of the
fourteenth century, at the important medical school of Montpellier, there
seems to have been an attempt to extend to the interpretation of the
medical canon the same principles of quantification and analysis which
were already being applied to the natural philosophy of Aristotle. The best
known exponent of such principles was Arnald of Villanova, in whom
medical scholasticism reached its apogee. Arnald (1240–1311) was a Cata-
lan, who took up medicine as a student master in the newly established
studium generale at Montpellier by 1291. He wrote on theological and
mystical topics, and may have owed his safety to his success as physician
to the Aragonese court. In his commentaries and translations of Galenic
works we can discern the ambition to make Galen sustain the same weight
of interpretation in the schools as did Aristotle himself, and great effort
was devoted to the reconciliation of the views of both on the physiology of
the human body.

By contrast, in Italy the same Galenic medicine, entering the universities
through the same channels, generated a much more practically-oriented
medical literature. Anatomy, for instance, was pursued by the Italians
with far more commitment than north of the Alps, and dissections were
being carried out for teaching purposes in Bologna a century before they
were taken up in Paris. The *Anatomia* of Mundinus (Mondino de'Luzzi,
who taught at Bologna, 1290–1326, and conducted autopsies on two
women in 1315), which was to guide the practice of dissection until
Vesalius, and even afterwards, was composed in 1316 or 1317, and had a
far greater currency in Italy than elsewhere. Practical medicine also gave
birth in Italy to a wholly new form of medical literature, the *consilia*,
purporting to be professional medical advice written down in response to
the request of an individual patient. The earliest are associated with the
circle of Taddeo Alderotti (died 1295, one of the founders of medical
study at Bologna, and a civic physician) in the early fourteenth century,
and their form may have been influenced by that of the legal *consilia* which
proliferated at Bologna in the late thirteenth century. Medical *consilia* are
in fact hard to tie in closely with clinical situations, but they do differ
sharply from the commentary form in their concern for specific directions
for treatment of particular conditions, and in recommending recipes. The
consilia are found in Italian manuscripts of the fourteenth and fifteenth
centuries, but never seem to have become popular elsewhere.

In the later Middle Ages, especially the fourteenth and fifteenth centuries, scholasticism assumed its definitive form, at least so far as the written manuscript was concerned. One manifestation was the writing of further commentaries on the acknowledged medical classics, and in this Italian doctors took the lead. Jacopo da Forli (otherwise known as Jacopo Dondi, of the famous clock-making family) wrote a popular commentary on the Aphorisms of Hippocrates, Gentile da Foligno (died 1348) one on the *Canon* of Avicenna (Ibn Sina). In fact the *Canon* became by far the favourite vehicle for this commentating; Leonardo da Bettipaglia and Dino del Garbo (a pupil of Taddeo Alderotti, who composed his commentary between 1313 and 1325) also tried their hand, with notable success, at least to judge by the number of copies that circulated. Such long and systematic works as those of Avicenna, as opposed to more original and unusual texts, lent themselves very well to scholastic commentary.

Compendia of medicine were another favourite vehicle of late scholastic writing, and perhaps the most successful of the European compendia was the *Lilium medicinae* of Bernard of Gordon, though the *Thesaurus pauperum* of Petrus Hispanus (*c.* 1220–77, later Pope John XXI) may rival it for the palm. Bernard (*c.* 1258–*c.* 1330) taught at Montpellier, and became dean of the *studium generale* in 1293, writing the *Lilium* in 1303–5. There were many others which won more local fame, but which shared the same virtue of bringing within the compass of one work judicious summaries of authorities on all the topics of medical scholasticism. Related closely to such compendia were the medical dictionaries, which were really just alphabetisations of similar content. However such works as the *Liber pandectarum medicinae* of Matteo Silvatico also introduced early humanist attempts to grapple with the philological and philosophical issues raised by differences in medical terminology. The best known of such works was the *Conciliator* of Pietro d'Abano, which wrestled with the differences on medical matters between the two greatest authorities, Aristotle and Galen.

When medical books first came to be printed, the most popular product of medical scholasticism was the surgery, which of course contained a good deal of practical medicine related to specific conditions, as well as manual surgery. Following Roger of Parma there is an almost continuous line of succession connecting authors of such surgeries. Apart from Roland of Parma and the glosses of the Four Masters, which all belong to the 'Salernitan' school, the first important surgery after Roger was that written by William de Congenis. He taught at Montpellier, having previously been physician and surgeon to Simon de Montfort, and died in 1218. At Bologna the mantle of Roger was assumed by Bruno Longoburgo, in whose work the surgery of Albucasis was used extensively for the first time. Theodoric, the son of another famous surgeon Hugh of Lucca, came to Bologna in 1214 when his father was appointed surgeon to the city, and, despite becoming a Dominican and later Bishop of Cervia in

1266, continued to practise himself, and wrote a *Chirurgia Magna*. Another city surgeon, this time to Verona, was William of Saliceto, who composed his surgery in 1275 and related many cases from his own experience. William's teaching was carried into France by Lanfranc of Milan, one of his pupils driven from Milan by the Visconti. He was invited to give lectures in Paris, and as a result completed his own *Chirurgia Magna* in 1296. His contemporary Henri de Mondeville gave lectures at Montpellier, and became surgeon to Philippe le Bel. Between 1306 and 1312 he composed two books of his surgery before joining the service of Charles de Valois, brother to the king of France. His book was never finished but summarizes the opinions of almost all the significant Latin authorities. Finally we may mention the last in this line of surgical authors, Guy de Chauliac, surgeon to the popes at Avignon, whose own work, composed in the 1360s, achieved a greater circulation than any of them, despite its lack of originality. All the names mentioned above are liable to be found in manuscripts of practical medicine written anywhere in Europe, and this popularity carried them forward into the age of print.

Laicized and vernacular

In Anglo-Saxon and German-speaking countries translation of medical texts from the Latin took place much earlier than in the areas of the romance languages, and indeed there is evidence that in eleventh-century England and Thuringia native-speaking authors were already composing independent works that must be regarded as adaptations of the common heritage of Greco-Latin medicine rather than as simple translations. By comparison, as we have seen above, the first such writings in French arrive in the thirteenth century, and the proliferation of practical writings with advice on health, the preparation of drugs and treatment comes after 1300. Nevertheless all vernacular medical writing in western Europe built upon the foundations of the international corpus of Latin medicine, and it is a mistake to believe that vernacular medicine as it survives in manuscript is evidence for a folk tradition of medicine distinct from the learned medicine of élites. Even the considerable number of charms and magic spells which appear in vernacular writings at all periods should not lead us to suppose that the Greco-Arab-Latin heritage had been contaminated from outside. A high proportion of such material can be traced back to Latin sources, and behind them to Greek; there is no need to suppose the influence of wise-women and soothsayers on the written tradition.

Instead of hypothesizing the contamination of Latin medicine by folk elements, we should recognize the extent to which, particularly in the fourteenth and fifteenth centuries, learned medicine was adapted to the health requirements of the lay reader. While the transmission of medical learning depended on the monastic or academic Latin speaking and writing community, others outside that community wished to have the practical benefits of medical knowledge for their own use in the surgery, barber-shop or household. The extension of lay literacy in the later Middle Ages was at least as much effect as cause here. There was every incentive to acquire a minimal reading ability in one's native language when it gave access to practical knowledge of all sorts, but especially medical knowledge (to judge by the large numbers of vernacular medical writings which survive). Translators of Latin medical texts into the vernacular must have been far more numerous than original medical authors, and certainly far more significant in terms of spreading the medical gospel.

For the outstanding characteristic of this vernacular and laicized medicine was its practical and utilitarian bias. What the lay readership required were rules to maintain and restore health, directions for making drug compounds from simples, diagnostic and prognostic tools which could be applied directly and readily understood, and calendrical information which would determine the proper times for preventative measures and therapy. By comparing such vernacular writings with the Latin originals from which they were derived it is easy to see how this practical bias dictated what was translated and adapted, and what was not. The theoretical considerations which played such an important role in scholastic medicine, the natural philosophical context, and the descriptive element in learned writings were all left out for the sake of the prescriptive and practical. Many of the vernacular versions of Latin medical texts should really be regarded as compilations based on, or edited from, the Latin, because of the freedom with which the originals were treated.

So far as medical manuscripts are concerned, the effect was not only to create a new class of vernacular texts, sometimes found in the same manuscripts as Latin, and sometimes on their own, but to change the way manuscripts were put together. Many of the practically-oriented texts were very short by comparison with the typical scholastic production, and the *mise en page* was much less formal. Instead of text surrounded by commentary, or set in neat columns, very many of the newer non-scholastic texts were written more like the modern book page (but without footnotes). In appearance such texts are more likely to have been written in semi-current or bastardized hands than in full *textura*, and in many cases to have been written by far less professional scribes than was the case with manuscripts produced for monastic or university use. The shortness of the texts meant that a number might be written in one gathering of parchment or paper, and it is quite possible to find dozens of texts assembled within one manuscript book. Sometimes these books consist of no more than apparently random assemblages of such texts, mixing medical with calendrical, cookery, veterinary, and other such materials. But other manuscripts are more properly regarded as sorts of compendia, put together deliberately in such a way as to make the whole more than simply the sum of its parts. A medical compendium may follow a head to toe order of ailments, or it may assemble texts in such a way as to deal with regimen, diet, diagnosis, prognosis and treatment between the covers of one book. Especially in German-speaking areas, many vernacular medical texts are found in manuscripts written for the master or mistress of the household, manuscripts which bring together short texts on husbandry, both animal and vegetable, cookery and dyeing, and other household tasks, as well as medicine.

By the fifteenth century it is not uncommon to find these short medical texts being translated from the vernacular back into Latin, and even within the learned environment of university medicine, practical and technical information seems to have been more highly valued than dialectic and philosophical synthesis. Although we have to make allowance for the fact that fifteenth-century manuscripts are more likely to have survived the accidents of time than fourteenth, and fourteenth than thirteenth, it is obvious that the later Middle Ages saw an enormous proliferation of medical manuscripts, and that production outside the academic environment accounted for the greater part of this increase.

One genre of medical literature in the later Middle Ages was very much a new phenomenon, though related both to scholastic medicine and to the laicized and vernacular sort. The Great Pestilence which moved across Europe in 1347–50 (now known as the Black Death) spawned the new genre, that of plague tracts, or *Pestschriften*. These were writings which encapsulated both rules of regimen for avoiding the plague, and recommendations for treatment. Both these types of prescription were based on scholastic thought rather than any new ideas which might have evolved specifically in response to the crisis. Many of the best known of them were written by university physicians or surgeons, and others were credited to such figures spuriously. They witness the prestige of scholastic medicine and, surprisingly perhaps, that prestige never seems to have been seriously dented by experience of the recurrent epidemics of plague in the fourteenth and for much of the fifteenth century. But in form these writings have more in common with the short texts of laicized and vernacular medicine, and a number were indeed translated into vernacular languages. They contain succinct rules and prescriptions rather than theory, and very often a text with a new title turns out to be a rehash of an older text, but credited to a new authority.

One feature of far more medieval medical manuscripts than might at first seem likely is the presence of illustration. Given the necessity of producing each manuscript laboriously by hand, illustration might seem to be a luxury which could be ill afforded in terms of the extra labour involved, and the difficulty of mere copyists reproducing the designs of their models. Text after all is readily copied, and meant to be so – this is not the case with hand-made illustrations. Yet something like two-thirds of surviving medical manuscripts do in fact have illustration, and a much higher proportion of non-scholastic texts are illustrated in some way.

There are at least two good reasons to explain why medical texts were so commonly illustrated. One is that, in the period in which the bulk of manuscripts were produced within monasteries, medical texts like all others were thought to require illustration and embellishment because these glorify the author and the word. In a way, that argument only pushes the question back still further, since the models inherited by the monks from the late antique period were themselves frequently illustrated. We can guess that illustration of medical texts in late antiquity was already common, since a number of pictures found in medieval manuscripts betray the stylistic influence of the art of an earlier era. For instance, the figures marked with cautery points or in the three surgical operations of couching of cataract, extirpation of nasal polyps, and excision of haemorrhoids, first found in late eleventh- and twelfth-century manuscripts, show by their posture and dress that they come originally from much older pictorial traditions.

The threefold effect of new translations of medical texts, scholasticism and manuscript production outside the monasteries had at first an inhibiting effect on illustration. Although there are more medical illustrations in Islamic manuscripts than is often supposed, given the reluctance to employ naturalistic techniques and to depict the human form, translation was more a matter of borrowing texts than pictures from the Arab world. Similarly the coming of medical schools which stimulated the production of texts for teaching purposes offered less incentive to the production of illustrations. A variety of diagrams which summarized philosophical views on the elements, humours and qualities, or served prognostic purposes, are found in the earliest surviving manuscripts, but there does not seem to have been any attempt to harness these to the purposes of scholasticism in the medical schools. The thirteenth century, in which the European universities established themselves, and great medical schools flourished at Bologna, Paris and Montpellier, saw an end to older traditions of illustration, but few new developments, save in the specialized area of books produced for bibliophiles.

But if scholasticism was a climate hostile to the development of medical illustration, the same could not be said of laicized and popular medicine. At some point in the fourteenth century a new canon of medical subjects seems to have established itself with remarkable consistency right across Europe. The canon was a more limited one perhaps than the more eclectic type of medical illustration which flourished in an earlier period. The most popular subject was that of the circle or table of urine glasses, in which twenty-one different colours, and sometimes additional features, corresponding to different symptoms, were picked out within outline drawings of the glasses. Other popular types include the vein-man, on which veins proper for blood-letting are depicted on the human body, and the wound-man, on whom various injuries and ailments are graphically represented. The zodiac-man illustrates the signs of the zodiac which correspond to the parts of the human body. Tables of surgical instruments are also found within texts or as separate illustrations.

In general these sorts of illustration are remarkable because very often the text is really an adjunct of the illustration, rather than vice versa. The text serves to clarify and expand on what is represented in the illustration, and the texts themselves are short and prescriptive. Sometimes a group of such texts and illustrations are found gathered within a folded parchment, which, when sewn, could be worn at the girdle, and this enabled the practitioner to carry a digest of medical information which he could consult when away from the study or shop. In this context medical illustration serves a highly practical purpose, rather than being simply the adornment of a book. It is a mistake to assume that medical illustration in the later Middle Ages is merely an incidental feature of the medical book.

One special class of illustrated medical manuscripts is that of the herbal. Primarily the herbal is a medical rather than botanical thing, and the description of plants or other materia medica is not essential to it. Thus the vast majority of herbal texts are unillustrated, and contain lists of materia medica with notes of their suitability as simples or as ingredients in compounds which might be used to treat patients. It might be supposed that, given the much more widespread knowledge of plants and their habitats that seems to have prevailed in the Middle Ages, and the notorious liability of plant illustrations to deteriorate through copying, that the practical usefulness of an illustrated herbal would be much reduced. Yet the earliest known of the herbal texts are usually accompanied by illustrations, and this seems to have been true, by inference, of the age of Dioscorides, Galen and Pliny. Similarities may be recognized between methods of depicting plants in the sixth century AD and those of the sixteenth century. The plants illustrated in the pseudo-Apuleius herbal which dominated the field among early manuscript herbals are recognizably the same plants as those shown in the early printed herbals.

In the course of the thirteenth century a new generation of herbals grew up alongside the pseudo-Apuleius group, and eventually came to surpass them in popularity. This new generation built on material taken from translation from the Arabic, including new medicinal simples and recipes. Probably because this new material was translated, early manuscripts do not appear to have been illustrated. The earliest known example of an illustrated manuscript of the *Tractatus de herbis* comes from the first half of the fourteenth century, and was made in Apulia in southern Italy. There may have been contact at this time with illustrated Arabic sources, as there was in the field of illustrated romances. In any case, there was a clear break with the tradition established by earlier herbals, with new subjects, and old subjects treated in a different way.

By around 1400 we find the first illustrated herbals which attempt to impose naturalistic values on plant portraits. In the great Carrara herbal written for Francesco Carrara II, Lord of Padua, by a monk called Jacopo Filippo, we can see examples of particular paintings which are evidently founded on observation of particular plants, with all their individuality and imperfections. Paradoxically such herbals, which are very much books for bibliophiles rather than practising medical men, may have suited the purpose of plant recognition rather less well than more stylized types of herbal. The collector of plants wants to compare specimens with a picture which captures the essential characteristics of the species, not with a portrait of an individual plant. In any case such herbals, made in Italy and in France for special clients, should not be taken as representative of the herbal in general in the fifteenth century. Most herbals remained unillustrated, and of those that were illustrated, the most part were much cruder affairs, which relied on the copying of models which were stylized and schematic in the first place.

What happened to the medical book with the coming of printing? Did medical manuscripts disappear from currency? If such manuscripts were still produced, what difference did the new technology make to older patterns of production? These are questions very hard to answer, given present knowledge of book production in the first century after the introduction of printing. What we can see from looking at the texts and illustrations which appear in the printed incunabula, is that the first printed medical books were not only very like manuscripts in appearance, but also drew on manuscript models as sources. Content and format of manuscripts and printed books were so similar that it is sometimes quite difficult to tell them apart without close examination. The technical boundary was often blurred by the appearance of hand illumination within printed books, as well as all the other devices that scribes had used to divide up and lay out texts, and by the appearance within manuscripts of texts copied from printed books or of inserted single woodcuts. In short, while printed books increased the circulation of medical writings they did not for a long time make any difference to conventions of book production which had a much older history.

Nor does there seem to have been any great shock to the manuscript book trade at first. At least as many medical manuscripts seem to have been written in the second half of the fifteenth century as in the first, to judge by their survival in such numbers in collections like that of Sir Hans Sloane in the British Library or Sir Kenelm Digby in the Bodleian Library. English book production was no different from that of Italy or Germany in this respect, though the manuscript had less competition than in the cradles of printing. It seems that it took the mass production of medical books in centres like Strasbourg and Venice in the first quarter of the sixteenth century to disrupt the production of manuscripts. This new generation of printed books was aimed at a much broader market than most incunabular book production, and for the first time the lay consumers of practical medical handbooks had the opportunity to purchase printed books at a price which competed successfully with that of manuscripts, and which offered the same mixture of texts and illustration (now in crude woodcuts rather than coloured sketches). We can surmize that because of this competition the production of manuscripts, except in the form of the private copy of a borrowed printed book, began to dry up. Certainly far fewer examples have survived from this period than from the previous one, and by the mid-sixteenth century there can have been no commissions for the writing of such books by professional scribes.

In a much more limited way, the production of luxury manuscript books continued into the sixteenth century, but for private patrons whose interests were those of bibliophiles rather than consumers of medical information. In the fields of technical and academic writing, authors now wrote manuscripts to be circulated among friends and critics, and eventually, if reception was favourable, to be published. A considerable number of commentaries and lectures by sixteenth-century physicians and humanists do survive in manuscript, though very little work has been done in the way of lists of such material, let alone editions or critical works. However the impact of such writings by comparison with those that found their way into print was very much muted. The long reign of the manuscript medical book was over.

Bibliographical guide to authors and texts
The first section of this chapter has owed a great deal to the studies of two scholars in particular who have directed their attention to the history of the medical book in the Middle Ages. Gerhard Baader has contributed a number of studies on the wider theme of medical learning which throw much light on the transmission of medical knowledge, but one article in particular might be singled out for special mention here.[6] This study of transmission in the light of the two cultures of manuscript and printed book is fundamental to the approach of this chapter, and should be read by any scholar wishing to pursue the subject further.

Linda Voigts's studies, though restricted in scope to Old and Middle English, are no less valuable than Professor Baader's. One essay which we have had the privilege of consulting in advance of publication will be especially relevant to the themes of this chapter.[103] It provides an overall survey of the history of the medical book in England in the critical period between 1375 and 1500. Perhaps the most significant contribution of this study is to show that there is indeed such an identifiable construct as the medical book, definable in terms of the texts it contains and its physical make-up. In the light of this construct Professor Voigts is able to highlight the comparative poverty of the medical book in its first appearances in print. Neither of these two pioneering scholars should however be held in any way responsible for errors or omissions in the coverage of this chapter.

The second part of this chapter is devoted to a discussion of the literature available to those interested in particular medical authors, texts or topics in the Middle Ages. This can at best be but a selective guide, and one in which the emphasis will be less on the bibliography of secondary studies on ancient and medieval medical literature as a whole than on the production of medical books. If the reader wishes to get a broad grasp of the nature of medieval medical theory, a good English language guide is the chapter by Charles Talbot in a general survey of medieval science, which also has some very relevant additional material in the chapters on the transmission of learning, the philosophical background, the university setting, and on natural history[65] So far as the bibliography of medical literature is concerned, there are already some extremely useful aids to research in this area. The standard history of European literature in the Middle Ages by Max Manitius puts medical writing in the context of all types of literary production.[67] For secondary literature on medieval medical learning specifically, two essays by Siraisi[91,92] and one by Durling[36] are very good reviews of current trends in research, and contain into the bargain a number of important bibliographical references. Margaret Pelling's chapter in *Information sources in the history of science and medicine*[26] is also useful in this respect, as is C. B. Schmitt's on the universities. Less well-informed though still useful is Claudia Kren.[58] The *Einleitung* by Baader and Keil to *Medizin in mittelalterlichen Abendland*,[8] a collection of reprinted essays which are in themselves a useful handbook to medical history for this period, summarizes in convenient chronological form both the history of scholarship in this area and the broad development of medical literature from the early Middle Ages onwards, as described in the preceding section of this chapter. This perspective can be supplemented by the bibliography of articles published, mostly in German monographs and periodicals, in the years 1950 to 1980.[9]

Other general bibliographical tools include the standard bibliographies of medical history, which contain entries under authors, subjects and places, for the medieval period, as for others. Those produced by the National Library of Medicine (annual, cumulated every five years[15]) and by the Wellcome Institute in London (quarterly[28]) are the principal ones, but the *Isis* annual bibliographies of the history of science[50] also contain sections on medicine. Section 22 of the *Bulletin Signalétique (Histoire des Sciences et des Techniques)*, appearing quarterly,[19] is also useful, and particularly helpful is the section specifically devoted to 'Sciences, Techniques, Métiers' of *L'Année Philologique*.[4] The relatively new *Medioevo latino*[70] promises well too. Other serial bibliographies of potential use are indicated, with brief notes, in Rouse.[81] But least known, and certainly more useful than any other for the bibliography of ancient medical authors, is the *Newsletter of the Society of Ancient Medicine and Pharmacy*.[94] The bibliographical section of this *Newsletter* started as a supplement to Helmut Leitner's bibliography,[63] but has expanded to include not only veterinary medicine (excluded by Leitner) but medieval authors too. Unfortunately the *Newsletter* has appeared occasionally rather than regularly, being the work of Professor John Scarborough alone, but it may be hoped that its continuance will be assured.

Some catalogues of large modern medical libraries are still very useful bibliographical tools for ancient and medieval medical authors. The Wellcome Historical Medical Library Subject Catalogue of the History of Medicine and Related Sciences[105] is one such (despite its apparent limitation to subjects); and the Index to the Catalogue of the Library of the Surgeon-General's department[97] is another. For an English reader, it will be essential to consult the card indexes and updated catalogues at the Wellcome Library as well as the printed versions. The Library consistently pursues English and foreign works which will be unavailable elsewhere, even at the British Library.

The range of authors who wrote on medical and allied subjects in ancient and medieval times, and whose works survive in manuscript, is vast. In very many cases we know nothing of them save the works they wrote, and those only in copies. The first step for many researchers will be to try to find out more about an author identified only by a name. A very useful starting-point for such researches is Sarton.[82] Though its references are by now very much dated, it has not been replaced or bettered. It is basically a series of bio-bibliographical essays on individual authors, arranged by century. Unfortunately it ends at the fourteenth century, and thus leaves out the century for which most authors and texts survive. The fifteenth century is covered, however, by Thorndike,[99] which also deals with the earlier centuries. Despite appearances, this is basically a bio-bibliographical work too and, like Sarton, has never been replaced or brought up to date, which limits, but does not vitiate its usefulness. The indexes are the essential starting-point. Hirsch[46] is also occasionally of help with medieval doctors. Especially as regards the eleventh and twelfth centuries, Haskins[44] is still vital for medieval scientific authors in the context of the revival and transmission of learning.

The most important medical authors whose works first circulated in manuscript are included in the *Dictionary of Scientific Biography*.[30] The entries are by different authorities, which means that the depth of bibliographical coverage tends to differ from case to case, but as a whole this work is a reliable guide to manuscripts and recent scholarship for the very limited number of early medical authors it can include. A much more specialized guide to medieval medical authors can be found in the *Verfasserlexikon*,[31] which has now reached the letter P. The coverage is not limited to German authors, but naturally it is particularly helpful on the bibliography of this prolific group. For French authors, Wickersheimer[106] brought up to date by Jacquart,[51] is a very comprehensive guide to what is known about their biographies and bibliographies. The English equivalent is Talbot and Hammond,[98] for which a supplementary database is being created at the Wellcome Institute in London by Dr Faye Getz. This work and Wickersheimer/Jacquart is based on extensive research in public and university records, as well as on findings in manuscripts. Talbot and Hammond have one limitation, in that they do not include apothecaries, although this will not be true of the supplement. A surprising number of authors of medical works can also be traced in the indexes to Migne's great collection of patristic writings.[72] Many, indeed most, of the medical authors of the Middle Ages were monks or secular clerics, and would therefore qualify for inclusion in the Latin series.

It is a sad truth that most texts found in medieval manuscripts do not come with a statement of authorship, and that much hard work must often be done to identify the author of these texts. The best way of classifying such texts is to establish the incipit, that is to say the words which begin the text, which can then be compared with lists of such incipits which have been published. The problem here is that establishing the incipit is not always easy, particularly when the text has a prologue or other introductory matter. Even the title of the text, or of the first subheading of the text, can be confusing when they are taken as the incipit. The incipit should consist of a number of words which begin the text proper, excluding such introductory matter, although sometimes it can be quite difficult to sort out which is which. Luckily the standard reference work for scientific and medical incipits, Thorndike and Kibre,[100] includes a good number of incipits for the prologues of works, although the cross-referencing from prologue to text is not always perfect. Nevertheless Thorndike and Kibre, with its addenda and corrigenda, is undoubtedly the single most necessary and useful reference work for the history of medical texts in manuscript. It is arranged alphabetically in order of incipit, and in each case will give a printed source where one is known for the text, or list a few manuscripts in which the text is found. Beware of assuming that all manuscripts in which it is found are listed, because this is not the case, as the Introduction makes clear.

The other main limitation of Thorndike and Kibre is that it deals only with Latin incipits, which means that vernacular texts cannot be identified in the same way. However Professor Linda Voigts and Dr Patricia Kurtz are at present engaged in compiling an equivalent to Thorndike and Kibre for Anglo-Saxon and Middle English scientific and medical texts, in the form of a database which will eventually be available in hard copy. The continuing series of the *Index of Middle English Prose*[48] also contains important lists of incipits and explicits of medical texts in the libraries it covers. It should also be noted that other more general lists of incipits are available, i.e. lists not restricted to scientific and medical texts.[45] Many printed catalogues of individual large libraries (see below) contain further lists of incipits, and sometimes libraries will be found to have lists of incipits on index cards, or in registers. One such specialized list is part of the Singer Index to British scientific manuscripts.[87] Many medical texts circulated in verse form in the Middle Ages, whether written in Latin or the vernacular. More often than not of course such verses were anonymous, distilling as they did *doctrina* in a more easily memorizable form. For this reason, any researcher dealing with a verse text should consult Walther[104] and, for Middle English, the *Index of Middle English Verse*.[18]

Another device for identifying a text which does not have an author statement at the beginning is the colophon. Before the invention of printing, and indeed for most incunabular book production, statements of authorship were commonly in the form of colophons. At the end of the text comes a sentence or two which gives the author and title of the text, together with information about the writing of the particular manuscript in which it is found. The standard reference source for colophons is the work of the Bénédictins du Bouveret.[13] There will be found references to the scribes of manuscripts, which may provide clues to the place of writing or date of a manuscript if a match can be established. Colophons are certainly the most important source for the dating of manuscripts, and may therefore help to establish a *terminus ante quem* or *post quo* for a text.

There are two major series of facsimiles and commentary which will be of immense use to the student of any branch of medieval literature. The first and earliest in time is that edited by Lowe.[66] There are samples in facsimile from every known codex or fragment written in bookhand (as opposed to cursive and charter scripts) from the earliest period to *c*. 800 AD. Each volume is described and a bibliography provided. The twelve volumes published are arranged geographically by country, city and library in which the manuscript is found. The last volume contains a supplement which includes a supplementary bibliography for the first eleven volumes, an index of authors and a list of manuscripts by library in all twelve volumes, as well as a brief index of provenances. The Comité international de paléographie has mounted a project which serves as a continuation of Lowe's work, bringing it from 800 AD to *c*. 1500, and adding to the entries on earlier manuscripts where appropriate. The Manuscrits Datés project[68] depends on the initiative of scholars in different countries, and the conventions and standards of particular volumes vary quite widely. Nevertheless they are extremely useful in their concentration on evidence of date and location, not least for comparison with undated manuscripts. The following countries have made considerable progress with their share of the enterprise: Austria, Belgium, France, Great Britain, Holland, Italy, Sweden and Switzerland. The parts are conveniently listed in Boyle[16] nos. 313–40. This last work is generally invaluable as a guide to matters of interest to any student of medieval books, whatever their subject matter, and medical historians who neglect such matters in favour of looking only for catalogues and bibliographies devoted to medicine, will pay the price of exploring only a tiny fraction of the bibliographical aids listed in Boyle's work.

Two early collections of texts important for the history of medieval medicine should be mentioned here. De Renzi[77] brings together a range of early medical texts which achieved a wide circulation throughout the Middle Ages, as the *prisca scientia* of Salerno. This includes the famous poem *Schola Salernitana*, whose advice on regimen and diet was to have an influence on popular medical thinking far outlasting the medieval period. Lawn[62] has illuminated the history of Latin medical problem literature originating in Salerno, in both verse and prose. In a series of studies early in this century, Karl Sudhoff and his pupils at Leipzig edited a number of texts in Latin and the vernacular in the series of *Studien*[95] and the periodical *Archiv*.[5] Later this journal became *Sudhoffs Archiv*, and is still the premier journal of German medical history.

Many medieval medical texts are commentaries on authors, or translations of authors, rather than simply the works of authors. An invaluable guide to commentaries and translations of a few of the most significant classical medical authors in the Middle Ages is provided by the *Catalogus translationum et commentariorum*.[27] Volume IV, for instance, includes bibliographical essays on Dioscorides, Paul of Aegina, and Pliny the Elder. In the cases of Hippocrates,[55] Galen[7,34,75] and Avicenna,[2,79] there are distinct series which deal with the Latin tradition of these authors, which, though not yet very far advanced in the cases of Galen and Avicenna, will help researchers attempting to find their way through the enormous numbers of Latin texts which were associated, sometimes spuriously, with these authors. Galen presents particularly intractable problems, and the best guide to the huge Galenic corpus is still the early nineteenth-century work of Karl Gottlob Kuhn.[61] This is now available in microform, with a valuable introduction by Nutton.[74] Some help may also be had from Kotrc and Walters,[57] although it does not replace the 'Bemerkungen' by Schubring, prefaced to the reprint of Kuhn's Galen.[61]

Many researchers will wish to establish the whereabouts of extant manuscripts of the works associated with the ancient medical authors, and here Diels[32] is still very useful, though obviously seriously outdated. It provides listings for most of the better known Greek medical authors of the classical period, and should be corrected and supplemented by Durling's articles.[33] The continuous bibliography of Galenic and pseudo-Galenic writings to be found in Leitner[63] is superseded up to 1983 by Fichtner.[37]

The series *Corpus medicorum graecorum* has recently been revived after a long interval, and is particularly helpful for Galenic works important in the Renaissance.[24] Similarly the volumes of *Corpus medicorum latinorum*[25] can be used for a select handful of the best known medical authors.

Any systematic search for manuscripts of a particular work will have to involve the inspection of catalogues of the libraries in which these books can now be found. A starting-point for such research is Kristeller.[60] The potential scope of such searches is vast, and all but the most persevering will find it necessary to search so far and no further. For manuscripts in English libraries, the series undertaken by Ker,[54] and still to be completed, provides excellent descriptions of texts found in libraries not separately catalogued. When the index volume is completed, it will be possible to identify medical authors and texts without reading each separate volume cover to cover. A useful clearing house for information about manuscripts and texts is the Institut de Recherche et d'Histoire des Textes in Paris. Microfiche editions have recently appeared of their indexes[49] which will be useful to researchers in medical history, as in many other subject areas.

The major national libraries must in any case be searched through printed catalogues or by direct enquiry to the staff of manuscripts departments. Many finding aids are not available in printed form, but in card indexes or handwritten registers, and can be consulted in person or through staff channels. What can be done through these means is illustrated best by another continuing work of Kristeller.[59] This does in fact cover manuscripts of the period between 1300 and 1600, and is not restricted to humanistic manuscripts narrowly defined. Durling[36] has catered to medical interest by providing a subject guide to vol. III of Kristeller's *Iter Italicum*.[59]

There are also specialist catalogues of medical manuscripts, or of scientific manuscripts including medicine. The earlier manuscripts are best served in this respect, two catalogues of medical manuscripts in particular being outstanding. Augosto Beccaria's[12] was a pioneer work and is still the best means of understanding the nature of early medieval medicine, as well as providing unsurpassed descriptions of particular manuscripts. Wickersheimer[107] is a worthy companion to Beccaria. Both these works are limited to manuscripts written before 1100. The least known of the major European countries with medieval medical books is Spain, and here Beaujouan[10,11] is fundamental. A number of the very rich Italian libraries are provided with specialist medical catalogues: the Biblioteca del Seminario Vescovile di Padova,[14] the Biblioteca di Lucca[21] and above all the Vatican Library.[71,84] Venice has a catalogue of Greek medical manuscripts in three of its great libraries.[38] Agrimi has also published a catalogue of scientific items for Lombardy[1] and Gabriel[39] deals with the Ambrosiana Library, Milan. Among the German libraries, Würzburg has a specialist medical catalogue.[85] Calcoen's catalogue of the scientific manuscripts conserved in the Bibliothèque Royale in Brussels contains many entries for medical manuscripts.[20] Central European libraries, though very rich in some cases, are not so well served with specialist catalogues, though an exception must be made for Grmek.[42]

In the British Isles there is Moorat's catalogue of the important collection of the Wellcome Medical Library,[73] which is to be supplemented by Dr Faye Getz. A mine of information on scientific manuscripts, including all medicine and related subjects, is to be found in the card indexes of Singer.[87] Some of the information is outdated, and some was based on descriptions of manuscripts not seen by the compiler, but it is always worth consulting. Robbins[80] is the best guide to material in the English language.

Languages other than Latin often have their own catalogues which will be of use to the researcher in pursuit of medical texts and authors. Greek codices have their own guide to libraries and catalogues in Richard.[78] Greek papyri also have their own guides, by Kollesch[56] and Marganne[69] – this last restricted to medicine. Anglo-Saxon is fortunate in that surviving manuscripts have been catalogued by Ker,[52] and it is not difficult to identify a number of medical texts from his catalogue and its supplements. Most libraries maintain separate catalogues of Latin and vernacular texts, and both types may have to be searched in pursuit of a particular textual quarry.

Medicine in the Middle Ages can of course be regarded as an agglomeration of different subject areas, and the individual researcher may look for bibliographical guidance. Some of these areas are better served in this respect than others. Anatomy, for instance, has been investigated by those who wished to trace the lineaments of pre-Vesalian knowledge of human anatomy, and Corner[23] and Lind[64] have made useful compilations of early texts. These are by no means exhaustive, but those interested in this area have much more to guide them before plunging into the manuscripts themselves than, for example, have those who want to know more of medieval or ancient surgery. Between these two poles there are a number of other areas in which the reader can be referred to useful works. These include alchemy[22,43,88,108] and astrology,[83] whose relationship to medicine was much more direct than might at first occur to a modern student. Much the same applies to the penumbra of medieval science which we might wish now to call magical or divinatory, but which played a significant role in determining medical practice of diagnosis and therapeutics. The relationship of physiognomy to medicine is less direct, but writings on physiognomy are often found within longer medical compilations, or in association with medical texts, for the art of divining character from the face was not thought of as essentially different from the Hippocratic art of diagnosis.

Other sorts of specialized texts are more obviously related to those we find comprehended within modern medicine. Diagnosis was just as critical to medieval physicians as to modern, and diagnostic writings can be identified separately, though of course they are often found in the introductory parts of scholastic treatises. The same applies to pharmaceutical and pharmacological texts, often associated with antidotaries or recipe collections.[86] The materia medica themselves, particularly herbs, but also minerals, oils and waters, animal products, and more exotic substances, were also dealt with independently of the theory and practice of medicine. Herbals of one sort or another form a very considerable corpus of literature, and have sometimes been treated by modern bibliographers as forerunners of later botanical science (e.g. Frank J. Anderson[3]), though their connection with medicine was fundamental in the Middle Ages.

Veterinary medicine was very obviously a matter of crucial importance to those whose means of subsistence and welfare depended so absolutely on animal husbandry. It is not surprising therefore that veterinary medicine formed a literature of its own, though in its theoretical underpinnings, and in much of its procedure, it was very closely related to human medicine (see Poulle-Drieux[76]). But it did have a vocabulary of diseases of its own, which is hardly the case for gynaecological writings. Another genre of medical literature which deserves notice is that of *Pestschriften* or plague literature, which was stimulated into independent existence by the Black Death, though the very many small tracts that came into being in the fourteenth and fifteenth centuries[17,89,96] had little to offer in the way of preventative or therapeutic medicine that was not already to be found in academic writings, or recipe collections.

What has survived in manuscript from the Middle Ages is of course only a tiny fraction of what was actually in circulation during the period. Some idea of the scope and amount of the circulating literature of medicine can be gathered from looking at lists of books owned by individuals or institutions at the time. Derolez[29] is a good place to begin to learn what resources are available to the student who wishes to know more about medieval libraries. There is in addition a very outdated though still useful survey, country by country, of catalogues of medieval libraries, and of notices of books in wills, in print and in manuscript, by Gottlieb.[41] Various countries, including Austria, Belgium, Germany with Switzerland, and Great Britain, have attempted since to provide particular lists of these sources but with only limited success so far in the last case. Institutional libraries are by far the best documented bookowners, including those of colleges and monasteries. The mendicant orders seem also to have been very interested in medical books, and Humphreys has dealt with the medical books of the friars.[47] Ker[53] provides a list of the books known to have survived from medieval institutional libraries, and gives references to original lists of books which were once owned by such libraries.

Gneuss[40] has a useful list of books written or owned in Anglo-Saxon England.

The book lists of individual owners are much harder to trace, and most of what we know about which books were owned by medical men and women in the Middle Ages is based on bio-bibliographical sources mentioned above.[51,98,106] It would be extremely helpful if this information could be gathered together into one database, but at the moment it is only possible to draw conclusions about individuals, and not categories of medical personnel.

Notes

1. Agrimi, Jole, *Tecnica e scienza nella cultura medievale. Inventario dei manoscritti relativi alla scienza e alia tecnica medievale (saec. xi–xv) (Biblioteca di Lombardia,* Florence, 1976).
2. Alverny, Marie Thérèse d' 'Avicenna Latinus', *Archives d'Histoire Doctrinale et Littéraire du Moyen Age,* 36 (1961) pp.281–316.
3. Anderson, Frank J. *An illustrated history of the herbals* (New York, 1977).
4. *L'Année Philologique,* 'Bibliographie critique et analytique de l'antiquité gréco-latine', (1924–). 1– See particularly the section, 'Sciences, Techniques, Métiers'.
5. *Archiv für Geschichte der Medizin,* (1908–). 1 –Continued from 1928 as *Sudhoffs Archiv.*
6. Baader, G., 'Handschrift und Frühdruck als Überlieferungs-instrumente der Wissenschaften', *Berichten zur Wissenschafts-Geschichte,* 3 (1980) pp.7–22.
7. Baader, G., 'Galen in mittelalterlichen Abendland', in V. Nutton (ed.), *Galen: problems and prospects* (London, 1981).
8. Baader, G. and G. Keil, *Medizin im mittelalterlichen Abendland,* Wege der Forschung, 363 (Darmstadt, 1982).
9. Baader, G. and G. Keil, *Medizinhistorische Mittelalterforschung. Eine Auswahlbibliographie der Jahre 1950–1980,* Würzburger medizin historische Forschungen, 25, 1982.
10. Beaujouan, Guy, *Manuscrits scientifiques médiévaux de l'Université de Salamanque et de ses 'colegios mayores',* Bibliothèque de l'école des hautes études hispaniques, 32 (Bordeaux, 1962).
11. Beaujouan, Guy, 'Manuscrits médicaux du moyen âge conservés en Espagne', *Mélanges de la Casa de Velasquez,* 8 (1972) pp.161–221.
12. Beccaria, Augosto, *I codici di medicina del periodo presalernitano, secoli IX, X, e XI* (Rome, 1956).
13. Bénédictins du Bouveret, *Colophons de manuscrits occidentaux des origines au XVIe siècle,* 6 vols (Fribourg, 1965–82).
14. Bertolario, B., *Manoscritti di medicina esistenti nella Biblioteca del Seminario Vescovile di Padova* (Padua, 1961).
15. *Bibliography of the History of Medicine* (1964–) National Library of Medicine (Bethesda, Md) 1–.
16. Boyle, Leonard E., *Medieval Latin paleography: a bibliographical introduction* (Toronto, 1984).
17. Braekman, W. L. and G. Dogaer (1972) 'Laatmiddelnederlandse pestvoorschriften', *Verslagen en Mededelingen van de Koninklijke Academie voor Nederlandse Taal- en Letterkunde,* N.S., (1972) pp.98–122.
18. Brown, Carleton and Rossel Hope, Robbins, *The index of Middle English verse* (New York). See also R. H. Robbins, and John L. Cutler (1965) *Supplement to the index of Middle English verse* (Lexington, 1943).
19. *Bulletin Signalétique. Histoire des sciences et des techniques.* (1947–) A quarterly review of periodical literature. See especially sections *Médecine; chirurgie; pharmacie. Histoire de la médecine* (Paris) 1–. Before 1969 published as *Bulletin Analytique.*
20. Calcoen, Roger, *Inventaire des manuscrits scientifiques de la Bibliothèque Royale de Belgique,* 3 vols (Brussels, 1965–75).

21. Ceccarelli, U., and R. Manara, *Manoscritti medici e incunaboli della Biblioteca di Lucca* (Pisa, 1964).
22. Corbett, James A., *Catalogue des manuscrits alchimiques latins*, 2 vols (Brussels, 1939, 1951).
23. Corner, G. W., *Anatomical texts of the earlier middle ages: a study in the transmission of culture* (Washington, 1927).
24. *Corpus medicorum Graecorum* (1908–) (Leipzig) 1– .
25. *Corpus medicorum Latinorum* (1915–28) (Leipzig); (1964–) (Berlin) 1.
26. Corsi, P. and P. Weindling (eds) *Information sources in the history of science and medicine* (London, 1983).
27. Cranz, F. E. and P. O. Kristeller, *Catalogus translationum et commentariorum: medieval and renaissance Latin translations and commentaries*, vol. 4 (Washington, 1980).
28. *Current work in the history of medicine. An international bibliography of references received* ... (1954–) 1–. Wellcome Institute for the History of Medicine, London, quarterly.
29. Derolez, Albert, *Les catalogues de bibliothèques*, Typologie des sources du moyen âge occidental, 31 (Turnhout, 1979).
30. *Dictionary of Scientific Biography*, ed. C. C. Gillispie, 16 vols (New York, 1970–80).
31. *Die deutsche Literatur des Mittelalters, Verfasserlexikon* (1933–55) ed. W. Stammler, and K. Langosch 5 vols (Berlin); revised, ed. K. Ruh *et al.*, 1– (Berlin) 1978– .
32. Diels, Hermann (1905–7) *Die Handschriften der antiken Ärzte*, 2 vols (Leipzig), repr. 1970.
33. Durling, R. J. (1967, 1981) 'Corrigenda and addenda to Diels' Galenica, 2 parts', *Traditio*, 23, (1967), pp.461–76; 37 (1981) pp.373–81.
34. Durling, R. J. (1976) *Burgundio of Pisa's translation of Galen's Peri Kraseon, 'De complexionibus'*, Galenus Latinus, 1 (Berlin).
35. Durling, R. J., 'Medico-historical research in medieval and renaissance manuscripts' in P. M. Teigen (ed.), *Books, manuscripts, and the history of medicine: essays on the fiftieth anniversary of the Osler Library* (New York, 1982) pp.31–43.
36. Durling, R. J. 'A guide to the medical manuscripts mentioned in Kristeller's "Iter Italicum" III', *Traditio*, 41 (1985) pp.341–65.
37. Fichtner, Gerhard, *Corpus Galenicum: Verzeichnis der galenischen und pseudogalenischen Schriften* (Tübingen, 1983).
38. Formentin, Mariarosa, *I codici greci di medicina nelle tre Venezie*, Universita di Padova studi bizantini e neogreci, 10 (Padua, 1978).
39. Gabriel, Astrik L., *A summary catalogue of microfilms of one thousand scientific manuscripts in the Ambrosiana Library, Milan* (Notre Dame, 1968).
40. Gneuss, H., 'A preliminary list of manuscripts written or owned in England up to 1100', *Anglo Saxon England*, 9 (1981) pp.1–60.
41. Gottlieb, Theodor, *Ueber mittelalterliche Bibliotheken* (Leipzig, 1890).
42. Grmek, M. D., *Recueil d'anciens manuscrits relatifs à la médecine, aux mathématiques, à la physique, à l'astronomie, à la chimie et aux sciences naturelles, conservés en Croatie et en Slovénie* (Zagreb, 1963).
43. Halleux, Robert, *Les textes alchimiques*, Typologie des sources du moyen âge occidental, 32 (Turnhout, 1979).
44. Haskins, Charles H., *Studies in the history of mediaeval science* (Cambridge, Mass., 1927); repr. New York, 1960.
45. Hauréau, J. B., *Initia operum scriptorum Latinorum medii potissimum aevi ex codicibus manuscriptis et libris impressis alphabetice digessit*, 8 vols (Turnhout, 1973–4).
46. Hirsch, A. (ed.) *Biographisches Lexikon der hervorragenden Ärzte aller Zeiten und Volker*, 2nd edn (1929–35) 5 vols (Berlin); repr. with additions, 1970.
47. Humphreys, K., 'The medical books of the mediaeval friars', *Libri*, 3 (1954) pp.95–103.
48. *Index of Middle English prose* (1977–) general ed. A.S.G. Edwards, Handlist 1-.
49. Institut de Recherche et d'Histoire des Textes (1987) *Répertoire bio-bibliographique des auteurs latins, patristiques et mediévaux*, Microfiche edition (Paris). See also the *Répertoire des fins de textes latins classiques et médiévaux* (Paris, 1987).

50. *Isis critical bibliography, 1913–1965* (1971–84) ed. M. Whitrow, 6 vols; *1966–1975*, ed. J. Neu, 2 vols so far (1980, 1985).

51. Jacquart, Danielle, *Dictionnaire biographique des médecins en France au moyen âge. Supplément* (Geneva, 1979).

52. Ker, N. R., *Catalogue of manuscripts containing Anglo-Saxon* (Oxford, 1957).

53. Ker, N. R. (ed.) *Medieval libraries of Great Britain; a list of surviving books*, 2nd edn (London, 1964). Supplement to the 2nd edn (1987) ed. A. G. Watson (London).

54. Ker, N. R., *Medieval Manuscripts in British Libraries*, 3 vols so far (Oxford, 1969–83).

55. Kibre, Pearl, 'Hippocrates Latinus: repertorium of Hippocratic writings in the Latin middle ages. In 8 parts', *Traditio*, (1975–82) 31–8. See also Agrimi, Jole, 'L'Hippocrates Latinus nella tradizione manoscritta e nella cultura altomedievale', in I. Mazzini and F. Fusco (eds), *I testi di medicina latini antichi* (Rome, 1985).

56. Kollesch, Jutta, 'Papyri mit medizinischen, naturwissenschaftlichen und mathematischen Texten', *Archiv für Papyrusforschung*, 26 (1978) pp. 141–8.

57. Kotrc, R. F. and K. R. Walters, 'A bibliography of the Galenic corpus: a newly researched list and arrangement of the titles of the treatises extant in Greek, Latin, and Arabic', *Transactions and Studies of the College of Physicians of Philadelphia*, N.S. 1 (1979) pp.236–304.

58. Kren, Claudia, *Medieval science and technology. A selected, annotated bibliography* (New York, 1985).

59. Kristeller, Paul Oskar, *Iter Italicum. A finding list of uncatalogued or incompletely catalogued humanistic manuscripts of the renaissance in Italian and other libraries*, 3 vols so far (London/Leiden, 1963–83).

60. Kristeller, Paul Oskar, *Latin manuscript books before 1600. A list of the printed catalogues and unpublished inventories of extant collections*, 3rd edn (New York, 1965). See also no. 27 above, and additions in *Scriptorium*.

61. Kuhn, K. G., *Galen: opera omnia* (Oxford Microform Publications Ltd., 1977). See also 74 below. Also see the Leipzig edition of 1821–33, 20 vols in 22, and the Hildesheim reprint of 1965.

62. Lawn, Brian, *The Salernitan questions. An introduction to the history of medieval and renaissance problem literature* (Oxford, 1963). Translated with additions as *I quesiti salernitani* (Rome, 1969). See also *The prose Salernitan questions* ed. B. Lawn, (London, 1979).

63. Leitner, Helmut, *Bibliography to the ancient medical authors* (Bern, 1973). Supplemented by the *Society for Ancient Medicine and Pharmacy Newsletter* (see no. 94 below).

64. Lind, L. R., *Studies in pre-Vesalian anatomy. Biography. Translations. Documents*, Memoirs of the American Philosophical Society, 104 (Philadelphia, 1975).

65. Lindberg, David C. (ed.), *Science in the middle ages* (Chicago, 1978).

66. Lowe, E. A. (ed.), *Codices latini antiquiores: a paleographical guide to Latin manuscripts prior to the ninth century*, 12 vols (Oxford, 1934–72).

67. Manitius, Max, *Geschichte der lateinischen Literatur des Mittelalters*, 3 vols (Munich, 1911–31). Reprinted in 3 vols (Munich, 1965–73).

68. *Manuscrits datés*. For details see no. 16 above, nos. 313–40.

69. Marganne, Marie Hélène, *Inventaire analytique des papyrus grecs de médecine* (Geneva, 1981).

70. *Medioevo Latino. Bollettino bibliografico nella cultura europa dal secolo VI al XIII*, 1-(1980–).

71. Micheloni, P., *La medicina nei primi tremila codici del Fondo Vaticano* (Rome, 1950).

72. Migne, J. P. (ed.) *Patrologia cursus completus ... series Latina*, 1844–65 and *Supplementum*, 1958–. See also *Clavis patrum latinorum*, ed. E. Dekkers (Steenbrugge, 1961).

73. Moorat, S. A. J., *Catalogue of western manuscripts on medicine and science in the Wellcome Historical Medical Library*, vol. 1 (1962) *Manuscripts written before 1650 AD* (London). This catalogue is in process of revision by Dr Faye Getz.

74. Nutton, Vivian, *Karl Gottlob Kuhn and his edition of the works of Galen: a bibliography* (Oxford, 1976). See no. 61 above.

75. Nutton, Vivian, 'A forgotten manuscript of Galenus Latinus', in K. Treu *et al.* (eds), *Studia codicologica* (Berlin, 1977).

76. Poulle-Drieux, Y., *L'hippiatrie dans l'occident latin du XIIIE au XVE siècle. Médecine humaine et vétérinaire à la fin du moyen âge* (Paris) (1966) pp.9–168.
77. Renzi, Salvatore de (ed.) *Collectio salernitana ossia documenti inediti, e trattati di medicina appartenenti alla scuola medica salernitana*, 5 vols (Naples). See also P. Giacosa (1901) *Magistri salernitani nondum editi* (Turin, 1952–9).
78. Richard, Marcel, *Répertoire des bibliothèques et des catalogues de manuscrits grecs*, 2nd edn (Paris) (1958). *Supplément*, 1964.
79. Richler, Benjamin, 'Manuscripts of Avicenna's Kanon in Hebrew translation: a revised and up-to-date list', *Korath*, 8 (1982) pp.145–68.
80. Robbins, Rossel Hope, 'Medical manuscripts in Middle English', *Speculum*, 45 (1970) pp.393–415.
81. Rouse, Richard H., *Serial bibliographies for medieval studies* (Berkeley, 1969).
82. Sarton, George, *Introduction to the history of science*, 3 vols (Washington, 1927–48).
83. Saxl, F. *et al.*, *Verzeichnis astrologischer und mythologischer illustrierter Handschriften des Lateinischer Mittelalters*, 4 vols (Heidelberg and London, 1915–66).
84. Schuba, Ludwig, *Die medizinischen Handschriften der Codices Palatini Latini in der Vatikanischen Bibliothek* (Wiesbaden, 1981).
85. Schwarz, I., *Die medizinischen Handschriften der kgl. Universitäts-Bibliothek Würzburg* (Würzburg, 1907).
86. Sigerist, Henry E., *Studien und Texte zur frühmittelalterlichen Rezeptliteratur*, Studien zur Geschichte der Medizin, 13 (Leipzig, 1923). Repr., Liechtenstein, 1977.
87. Singer, D. W., 'Survey of medical manuscripts in the British Isles dating before the sixteenth century', *Proceedings of the Royal Society of Medicine*, History of medicine section, 12 (1918–19) pp.96–107. See also R. H. Robbins 'A note on the Singer survey …', *Chaucer Review*, 4 (1970) pp.66–70. The card indexes on which the survey was based are kept in the Department of Manuscripts in the British Library, with copies in the Warburg Institute, London, and Columbia University, New York.
88. Singer, D. W. and A. Anderson, *Catalogue of Latin and vernacular alchemical manuscripts in Great Britain and Ireland dating from before the XVIth century*, 3 vols (Brussels, 1928–31). See also no. 22 above.
89. Singer, D. W. and A. Anderson, *Catalogue of Latin and vernacular plague tracts in Great Britain and Eire in manuscripts written before the sixteenth century* (Paris and London, 1950).
90. Siraisi, Nancy G., *Taddeo Alderotti and his pupils: two generations of Italian medical learning* (Princeton, 1981).
91. Siraisi, Nancy G., 'Some recent work on western European medical learning, ca.1200–ca.1500', *History of Universities*, 2 (1982) pp.225–38.
92. Siraisi, Nancy G., 'Some current trends in the study of renaissance medicine', *Renaissance Quarterly*, 37 (1984) pp.585–600.
93. Siraisi, Nancy G., *Avicenna in Renaissance Italy: the Canon and medical teaching in Italian universities after 1500* (Princeton, 1987).
94. *Society for Ancient Medicine and Pharmacy Newsletter* (1976–) (formerly Society of Ancient Medicine Newsletter), 1-. Contains lists of items supplementary to no. 63 above.
95. *Studien zur Geschichte der Medizin*, 1–22 (Leipzig, 1907–34).
96. Sudhoff, Karl, 'Pestschriften aus den ersten 150 Jahren nach der Epidemie des "schwarzen Todes" 1348', *Archiv für Geschichte der Medizin*, 5 (1911) pp.36–87.
97. *Index-catalogue of the Library of the Surgeon-General's Office, U.S. Army*, Authors and subjects, 62 vols (Washington, 1880–1961). Succeeded by the catalogues of the National Library of Medicine.
98. Talbot, C. H., and E. A. Hammond, *The medical practitioners of mediaeval England* (London, 1965).
99. Thorndike, Lynn, *A history of magic and experimental science*, 6 vols (New York, 1923–41).
100. Thorndike, Lynn and P. Kibre, *A catalogue of incipits of mediaeval scientific writings in Latin*, 2nd edn (Cambridge, Mass., 1963). See also *Scriptorium* 19 (1965) pp.273–8; and *Speculum* 40 (1965) pp.116–22; ibid. 43 (1968) pp.78–114, for corrections and additions.

101. Voigts, Linda E., 'Editing Middle English medical texts: needs and issues', in T. H. Levere (ed.) *Editing texts in the history of science and medicine* (New York, 1982) pp.39–68.
102. Voigts, Linda E., 'Medical prose', in A. S. G. Edwards (ed.), *Middle English prose: a critical guide to major authors and genres* (New Brunswick, 1984).
103. Voigts, Linda E., 'Scientific and medical books', in J. Griffiths (ed.), *Book production and publishing in Britain, 1375–1475* (Cambridge, 1989).
104. Walther, Hans, *Carmina medii aevi posterioris latina, Pars I: Initia carminum ac versuum ... Pars II: Proverbia sententiaeque ...*, 6 vols (Göttingen, 1959, 1963–9).
105. Wellcome Institute for the History of Medicine, *Subject catalogue of the history of medicine and related sciences*, 18 vols (Munich, 1980).
106. Wickersheimer, Ernest, *Dictionnaire biographique des médecins en France au moyen âge*, 2 vols (Paris, 1936).
107. Wickersheimer, Ernest, *Les manuscrits latins de médecine du haut moyen âge dans les bibliothèques de France* (Paris, 1966).
108. Wilson, W. J., 'Catalogue of Latin and vernacular alchemical manuscripts in the United States and Canada', *Osiris*, 6 (Bruges, 1939).

2 Medical incunabula

Dennis E. Rhodes

Books of the early presses have a flavour all their own, less personal perhaps than that roused by manuscripts, but of even greater intensity as illustrating the origin and evolution of the art which, more than any other, has set free the human mind.

(Sir William Osler)

The years immediately following the invention of printing brought a spate of semi-popular works on medicine in the form of purgation calendars, or broadsides, many of which bore astronomical figures or zodiacal men. A total of 46 of these appeared before 1480, and about 100 before the end of the century. The first piece of medical printing was one of these, being the Mainz Kalendar issued in 1457, which gives approximate dates for bleeding and purging. The unique copy of this, of which the top half only was discovered in 1803, is in the Bibliothèque Nationale, and is printed with the Gutenberg types used for the Thirty-six Line Bible. These calendars are all very rare, and are chiefly in German collections.[1]

'Pestblätter' were also common in the fifteenth century, 41 having been collected by Paul Heitz and W. S. Schreiber.[2] This material has also been studied by Arnold Carl Klebs and Eugénie Droz in *Remèdes contre la peste. Fac-similés, notes et liste bibliographique des incunables sur la peste*, Paris, 1925 (also issued with title in English), which provides a list of the editions of 130 plague tracts, with facsimiles of five of them. This was augmented in 1926 by A. C. Klebs and Karl Sudhoff, *Die ersten gedruckten Pestschriften*, Munich, which provides fuller details of individual items and contains facsimiles. Henry R. Viets and James F. Ballard have provided details of the 29 plague tracts contained in the Boston Medical Library, with appropriate illustrations.[3] Dorothea Waley Singer has reproduced the 1371 French version of John of Burgundy's treatise, which is dated 1365, and represents the earliest of plague tracts, being the parent of a host of descendants. The same article provides details of many of these.[4] A Portuguese pest-tract printed in Lisbon, probably in 1496, was the *Regimento proveytoso contra ha pestenença*.[5]

Another item of printing apart from actual books are the 'graphic incunabula' of anatomy. These consist of pictorial representations of dissections, and include all pre-Vesalian illustrations, such as Johannes de Ketham's *Fasciculus medicinae*, one of the most remarkable examples, first printed in Venice in 1491, of which there were 33 editions (see Plate 3). Charles Singer edited an English translation, Milan, 1925, and the Italian translation by Sebastiano Manilio Romano, Venice, 1493, was printed in facsimile in 1963. These illustrations were often very primitive, not being based on actual dissections. F. H. Garrison has contributed a study of the subject.[6]

The title of the earliest printed medical book is generally ascribed to Rabanus Maurus, *De sermonum proprietate, seu de universo* [the R-Printer (Adolf Rusch), Strasbourg, 1467?], although in fact this book is a general encyclopaedia, Book 18, Chapter 5 only being devoted to medicine.[7] Rabanus Maurus (?776–856 AD) was Archbishop of Mainz, and his book was printed with the first roman type to be cast. This was succeeded by the following nine volumes, according to Osler's *Incunabula medica*:[8] Rodericus Zamorensis, *Speculum vitae humanae*, Sweynheym and Pannartz, Rome, 1468; Caius Plinius Secundus, *Historia naturalis*, Johannes de Spira, Venice, 1469; another edition of this, edited by Johannes Andreae, Sweynheym and Pannartz, Rome, 1470; Gulielmus de Saliceto, *De salute corporis* [Holland, *c.*1470]; another edition of this; Albucasis, *Liber servitoris*, translated by Simon Januensis, Nicolas Jenson, Venice, 1471; Nicolaus Salernitanus, *Antidotarium ...*, Nicolas Jenson, Venice, 1471; Joannes Mesue, Junior, *Opera*, Clemens Patavinus, Venice, 1471; another edition of this, with the Additiones of Petrus de Abano [Padua] 9 June 1471.

The first medical work printed in German is *Regimen sanitatis Deutsch (Von der Ordnung der Gesundheit)*, Augsburg, 23 April 1472, printed by Johann Bämler. This must not be confused with the *Regimen sanitatis Salernitanum* first printed at Augsburg in 1475 by Bämler, of which many translations and about 250 editions were subsequently published. *La ciroxia vulgarmente fata*, by Gulielmus de Saliceto, of Bologna, is believed to be the first printed work on surgery, as well as the first printed medical book in Italian. It was printed at Venice in 1474, by Filippo di Pietro. The first French medical printed book is the *Chirurgia magna* of Guy de Chauliac (1300–68), of which a translation was published at Lyons in 1478. A third important surgical book was the *Cirurgia* of Hieronymus Brunschwig, printed at Strasbourg by Johann Grüninger in 1497. This volume is noteworthy for its beautiful woodcuts, and was reproduced in facsimile in 1911.

It is relevant here to ask who was Mundinus, since his name occurs in various catalogues of early printed books. His work entit!ed *Anothomia* (Anatomy, the Greek word not properly understood by the Italian printers) was first printed at Pavia by Antonius de Carcano in 1478 (copy in British Library), and there is a rare second edition printed at Bologna by Johannes de Noerdlingen and Henricus de Harlem in 1482, of which there is no copy recorded in the British Library or in America; but there is one copy in the Royal Society of Medicine, London, and there are four copies in Italian libraries. Further editions followed at Padua in 1484, Venice 1493, 1494 and 1498, and Leipzig 1493. The author was Mondino (or Raimondino) dei Liucci (or Liuzzi), born of an old Florentine family at Bologna about 1270. As a professor of medicine at the University of Bologna, he was the first to teach the necessity of dissecting corpses in medical training. He completed the writing of his *Anatomia* in 1316, and died in 1326. The work was eventually published in 40 editions; there was a commentary on it by Berengario da Carpi; and it figures in most editions of the *Fasciculus medicinae* of Johannes de Ketham.

The earliest printed work devoted to paediatrics is Paolo Bagellardi's *De infantium aegritudinibus et remediis* [Padua, 1472], printed by Bartholomaeus de Valdezoccho and Martinus de Septem Arboribus. Another incunable on disorders of pregnant women and diseases of children is Cornelius Roelans, of Mechlin in Belgium, *De aegritudinibus infantium*, Louvain, Jan Veldener [not before 16 February 1486]. It is a curious fact that all recorded copies of this work lack the first 77 leaves, and no-one seems to know why. Very recently six of the missing leaves have been discovered as end-papers in various British libraries. It seems that they were discarded by the printer, but found their way accidentally to Britain to be used by binders as waste. The text of them deals with ailments in women before childbirth, so that it was natural that the part which has survived *in toto*, from fol. 78 to the end, should deal with illnesses of infants.[9]

The *Regimen sanitatis* of the famous medical School of Salerno (the Schola Salernitana), which has already been mentioned above, was published with the commentary of Arnoldus de Villanova and printed, probably by Bernardinus Benalius at Venice about 1495, and at least three other undated Venetian editions followed up to about 1505.

The first printed work on ophthalmology is represented by Benvenuto Grassi's *De oculis eorumque aegritudinibus et curis* [Ferrara, 1471].[10] Osler traced twelve items before 1480 dealing with syphilis, in which he included Rolandus Capellutus Chrysopolitanus, *De curatione pestiferorum apostematum*, Rome, which he dated [*c*.1475], but which should more accurately be dated [*c*.1485]. Simone de Cordo's *Synonyma medicinae seu clavis sanationis*, the first printed medical dictionary, was first printed at Ferrara [1471–72?], of which edition a fragment of 21 leaves in the Bodleian Library appears to be the only recorded copy (see Osler, 11). It was also printed at Milan in 1473, and of this edition the British Library has a copy (catalogued under Simon Genuensis).

An exhaustive study of the incunable editions of the *Liber medicinalis Quinti Sereni* has recently been published by Joanne H. Phillips.[11] The work is a poem in 64 chapters, 1107 verses, which Miss Phillips says 'was probably intended as a formulary of practical medical instruction for the layman; it is devoid of theoretical discourse or directives'. It was written in the third century AD.

According to Leslie Cowlishaw,[12] the first medical book printed in

England is *A litil boke the which traytied and rehersed many gode thinges necessaries for the ... pestilence ... made by the ... Bisshop of Arusiens ...*, published in London by William of Machlinia in 1485.[13] This is usually attributed to Canutus, or Benedictus Kanuti, Bishop of Arusiens (Västers in Sweden), and occasionally bears alternative titles, such as *Regimen pestilentiae*, or *Treatise on the pestilence*. Duff lists three editions (nos 72–4), all printed by Machlinia, apparently all between 1486 and 1490. The STC gives these three editions (4589–91) with the respective dates [*c*.1486], [*c*.1488] and [*c*.1490], the last being noted as the first English book with a title-page. The same source also lists editions from Wynkyn de Worde, [*c*.1510] (4592), and one as [Amsterdam, *c*.1520] (4593). A more widely known book is the *Governayle of helthe*, printed by William Caxton in 1489.[14]

The earliest printed herbal, also probably the oldest existing illustrated herbal, is the translation of the Latin *Herbarium* of Apuleius Barbarus, Apuleius Platonicus or Pseudo-Apuleius. This compilation of medical recipes is mainly derived from fourth-century Greek material, and was the most influential early Latin herbal. First printed at Rome, probably in 1481, it has been issued in a modern edition by R. T. Gunther, Oxford, 1925. The *Herbarium* contains 132 chapters, each of which is devoted to a herb, and four early manuscripts of it survive.[15] Charles Singer wrote an authoritative paper on Greek herbals, stating that the earliest herbal was that of Diokles of Karystos, written about 350 BC, there being no Greek herbals before the fourth century BC. Diokles was followed by Theophrastus of Eresos (380–286 BC), whose *De historia et causis plantarum Latine, Theodoro Gaza interprete*, was first printed at Treviso in 1483.[16] Pedacius Dioscorides, a Greek army surgeon of the first century, was the author of *De materia medica*, which, with the Latin gloss of Petrus Paduanensis (Petrus de Abano) was printed at Colle di Valdelsa (near Siena) in 1478. The Greek text was first printed in 1499, and an English translation, edited by R. T. Gunther, was first published in 1934.[17]

After the Norman Conquest our herbals practically disappeared until the early days of printing, but about the middle of the thirteenth century Bartholomaeus Anglicus wrote *De proprietatibus rerum*, the seventeenth book of which is devoted to herbs. The work was translated into English in 1398 by John of Trevisa, and printed at Westminster by Wynkyn de Worde about 1495.[18] The first Latin edition was printed anonymously by Berthold Ruppel at Basle about 1470, at least 14 editions appearing before 1501.

The term 'incunabula' was first employed by Cornelius à Beughem in his *Incunabula typographiae*, 1688, which is the earliest printed catalogue of fifteenth-century publications.[19]

Certain other general lists of incunabula important from the medical viewpoint are noticed here before the strictly medical bibliographies of this material. The first prominent cataloguer of incunabula was Michel Maittaire (1668–1747), a Frenchman resident in England, who was a profound scholar, and who collected a large library that was sold in London in 1748. His *Annales typographici*, 1719–41, covers printed literature up to 1664, beginning with the block-book *Ars moriendi*, and proceeding in chronological order. Maittaire is not exhaustive as regards medical items, and his methods of entry are inconsistent. This list was supplemented by Michael Denis in 1789.

Georg Wolfgang Panzer (1729–1805) published his *Annalen der älteren deutschen Literatur* between 1788 and 1805, covering literature in the German language to 1526. Panzer also compiled *Annales typographici ad annum 1536*, eleven volumes, Nuremberg, 1793–1803, in which the entries are arranged in alphabetical order, with chronological and topographical indexes.

The most important bibliography up to that time, however, is Ludwig F. T. Hain's *Repertorium bibliographicum ad annum 1500*, four volumes, Stuttgart and Paris, 1826–38. Hain (1781–1836) based his catalogue upon the collection in the Munich Hofbibliothek, and the result is an alphabetical author list of 16 299 incunabula. The entries are very full and most reliable when they bear an asterisk (which means that Hain had seen the book), but are often suspect and incomplete when they do not.

Walter Arthur Copinger (1847–1910) published a supplement to Hain in three volumes, 1895–1902, correcting 7000 items and describing 6619 incunabula not seen or described by Hain. This list also is alphabetical, the final volume containing as an appendix Konrad Burger's *Printers and publishers of the 15th century, with lists of their works*. This was enlarged and issued separately in 1908. Dietrich Reichling published another supplement to Hain–Copinger in fascicules at Munich 1905–14, listing a further 1921 incunabula, in addition to numerous corrections. Reichling is very unreliable indeed on all typographical attributions and dating of undated works. He had a very poor eye for types.

Robert G. C. Proctor (1868–1903) was responsible for *An index to the early printed books in the British Museum ... to 1500, with notes of those in the Bodleian Library*, five volumes, 1898–1903. Arranged typographically by countries, towns, presses and dates, this has proved an invaluable bibliographical tool, and the arrangement has become known as 'Proctor order', which to this day is still the method of arrangement of the incunabula, which now number over eleven thousand, in the British Library. Full descriptions appear in the *Catalogue of books printed in the XVth century now in the British Museum*, the first volume of which was published in 1908. Three volumes covered the German incunabula, followed by four for Italy, then one large volume for France in 1949, one volume for the Low Countries in 1967, one for Spain and Portugal in 1971, and one slim supplementary volume for Italy in 1985. England still remains to be published. Hebrew incunabula in the British Library will be dealt with separately.

The Incunabula Short-title Catalogue (ISTC) is a computerized file compiled at the British Library which, currently recording over 22 000 editions (out of an estimated 30 000) forms the most comprehensive available listing of fifteenth-century items printed from movable type. It can be consulted via the British Library's on-line retrieval system BLAISE-LINE, which permits searching by words from titles, and by bibliographical references such as Arnold C. Klebs, *Incunabula scientifica et medica* and Sir William Osler, *Incunabula medica*, as well as the names of authors, editors, commentators, translators, printers, publishers and places of publication.

Among his numerous typographical studies Konrad Haebler of the Royal Berlin Library published *Typenrepertorium der Wiegendrucke*, six volumes, Halle and Leipzig, 1905–24, in which he analyses and classifies types, to form an invaluable source of reference for students of typography. Proctor in Britain and Haebler in Germany were the first real experts in typographical analysis of the fifteenth century. By contrast, Proctor was going blind when he lost his life in the Alps at the age of thirty-five, while Haebler lived to be over ninety.

Numerous catalogues covering special countries, private, public and university libraries have by now been published.[20] One of the most important of these is the catalogue of Mlle Marie Pellechet (1840–1900), *Catalogue général des incunables des bibliothèques de France*, Paris, 1897–1909, which was continued after her death by Marie Louis Polain. This list only reached the letter G. The manuscript part has been issued in facsimile by Kraus, but is maddeningly illegible, and many entries are incomplete. Most recently, the Bibliothèque Nationale has published its own catalogue of incunabula from G (where Polain left off) right down to Z, but, unlike Pellechet–Polain, this does not cover the rest of France. Regional catalogues of the French departments are, however, now appearing in a regular series, and are of high quality. Polain produced a national catalogue for Belgium in four volumes (Brussels, 1932), to which a supplementary volume was added in 1978. There are now up-to-date national catalogues of incunabula for Italy (six volumes, 1943–81), for Hungary (two volumes, 1970), for Poland (two volumes, 1970) and for Holland (two volumes, 1983).

The most authoritative list, however, which will, if ever completed, surpass all previous bibliographies of incunabula, is the *Gesamtkatalog der Wiegendrucke* (GW), which began publication in Leipzig in 1925, and in 1938 with Band 7 reached the heading 'Eigenschaften'. This is accurate to a minute degree, providing complete details of all items, references to other catalogues, and with a list of the important libraries possessing each item. After an interval of 34 years due to the Second World War, the publication of the GW was at last resumed in 1972, and had by 1985 reached the heading 'Gazius, Antonius'; but its progress is still lamentably slow.

These general catalogues of incunabula are followed by the strictly medical bibliographies, which begin with Ludwig Choulant's *Graphische Incunabeln für Naturgeschichte und Medizin* ..., 1858, which was reprinted in 1924.[21] This list of illustrated incunabula is not exhaustive, but gives full details of the books and plates, followed by particulars of the various editions, including place of publication, date, size (i.e. folio, etc.), name of printer, month and annotation. Bartholomaeus Anglicus, the Herbarius Moguntinus, Hortus sanitatis, Hieronymus Brunschwig, Hans von Gerssdorff, Albucasis, Eucharius Rösslin and others are included, followed by a section on anatomical illustration.

The first serious attempt at a complete list of medical incunabula was the *Incunabula medica* [*prodromus bibliographicus*], Trenton, 1889, compiled by John Stockton-Hough, and privately printed. This has been described by Garrison as 'eccentric in get-up, with a title-page in Latin, and a "sommaire de la table" in French, but otherwise not bad'. It lists 1626 items, of which 133 are later than 1500. A more scholarly bibliography, but limited to German incunabula, is Karl Sudhoff's *Deutsche medizinische Incunabeln* ..., Leipzig, 1908. This is a critical list, analysing each of the 460 items.

Giovanni Carbonelli's *Bibliographia medica typographica pedemontana saeculorum XV. et XVI.* ..., Rome, 1914 [1919], provides complete bibliographical details of 389 numbered entries, and contains numerous facsimiles of title-pages in a well-produced volume.

The *Incunabula medica. A study of the earliest printed medical books, 1467–1480*, Oxford, 1923, is generally known under the name of Sir William Osler, but actually the Presidential Address only, delivered to the Bibliographical Society in January 1914, is by him, the list being the work of other hands. It was begun by W. R. B. Prideaux (1880–1932), and later taken over by Osler's secretary, Miss J. P. Willcocks. Dr Victor Scholderer (1880–1971) is the editor of the list in printed form, which contains a preface by A. W. P.[ollard], Osler's Address, and an appendix entitled Synonyma, dictionaries, pandects, and antidotaria. Then comes Victor Scholderer's editorial note, the bibliographical list of 217 items, an index of authors and books, and an index of places and printers arranged geographically, then by printers, followed by chronological arrangement. A total of 16 facsimiles are provided at the end, while the frontispiece consists of a charming portrait of Osler.

Arnold Klebs (1870–1943) has provided a more recent list of medical incunabula in his *Incunabula scientifica et medica*, Bruges, 1938, which records over 850 editions of medical books published in the fifteenth century.[22] The compiler has endeavoured to present a complete list of incunabula devoted to medicine and science, showing the evolution of these subjects during the early days of printing. He lists over 3000 editions, and this is probably the most important study of incunabula in its class. Arrangement is alphabetical by authors, references to standard bibliographies are provided, and as all editions appear in chronological order under authors, one can note the popularity of the items, as evidenced by the number of times they appeared in print.

Two excellent guides to the subject of incunabula are provided by F. H. Garrison and by R. A. Peddie.[23] The latter's *Fifteenth-century books* contains lists of printed matter of initials, printers' marks or devices, colophons, title-pages, signatures and watermarks, together with a list of catalogues arranged by localities, etc., and is a most useful guide to the subject. Information on the cataloguing of incunabula is provided by A. C. Klebs and by Henry Guppy,[24] while much useful matter on the advanced treatment of bibliographical material is given by J. D. Cowley in his *Bibliographical description and cataloguing*, 1939.[25]

Medical incunabula are located in numerous national, university and other general collections, and the items housed by medical libraries also cover several branches of science.[26] Separate printed catalogues of incunabula contained in some of the larger medical libraries have been published, and a joint catalogue listing medical items in every collection and giving the location of copies still seems to be a major desideratum.

The monumental library collected by Erik Waller (1875–1955) and bequeathed to the University of Uppsala contains 150 incunabula, which are described in the first volume of the catalogue of the collection compiled by Hans Sallander.[27]

One of the largest collections housed in a British medical library is that of the Wellcome Historical Medical Library, London, a catalogue of which has been compiled by F. N. L. Poynter.[28] This contains 632 items, 117 of which were not in the British Museum at the time of publication (1954). Many of the items are devoted to science rather than to medicine, and 126 were printed before 1481. The catalogue contains indexes of names; subjects; signatures, inscriptions and other marks of ownership; printers; countries and towns; and a chronological list. Among the books listed are Avicenna's *Canon*, translated into Latin by Gerard of Cremona, Padua, 1479, Venice, 1486, 1489, 1490, with a translation into Hebrew from Arabic by Josef Lorki and Natan ha-Me'ati in three volumes, Naples, 1491, representing the first printing of a medical work in Hebrew. There are: Bartholomaeus Anglicus, *De proprietatibus rerum*, Strasbourg, 1485, and a Dutch translation, Haarlem, 1485; Celsus, *De medicina*, Florence, 1478, Venice, 1493 and 1497; John of Gaddesden, *Rosa anglica practica medicinae*, Pavia, 1492, being the first edition of the first medical book by an Englishman to be printed. John of Gaddesden (near Berk-hamsted, Herts) lived from *c*.1280 to 1361, and wrote the *Rosa* between

1305 and 1307. Both the Royal College of Physicians and the Royal College of Surgeons also own copies of this Pavia edition of 1492, that in the Physicians' Library being especially interesting because it belonged to Dr John Chambre, one of the founders of the College in 1518. The Wellcome also has: Galen, *Opera*, in Latin, Venice, 1490, and his *Therapeutica*, in Greek, Venice, 1500; Guy de Chauliac, *Chirurgia*, translated into Italian by Paulus de Vareschis, Venice, 1493, and his *Chirurgia parva*, Venice, 1500 [1501]; Hippocrates, *De natura hominis* [Rome, 1480 and c.1490]; Johannes de Ketham, *Fasciculus medicinae*, in Spanish with the title *Epilogo en medicina*, Pamplona, 1495, and a Latin edition, Venice, 1495; Moses Maimonides, *Aphorismi secundum doctrinam Galeni*, Bologna, 1489; several editions of the *Regimen sanitatis* [Louvain, 1480]; Louvain, [1480]; [Lyons, 1486]; Strasbourg, 1481; Cologne, 1494; Venice, [c.1500]; and a German translation, Ulm, 1482; Rhazes, *Cibaldone ovvero opera utilissima a conservarsi sano* [Venice, c.1475], and [Brescia, 1493]. There is also his *Liber nonus ad Almansorem*, Venice, 1490, 1493 and 1497 (two issues). These are also briefly recorded in *A catalogue of printed books in the Wellcome Historical Medical Library. I. Books printed before 1641*, London, 1962.

Other medical libraries in Great Britain containing incunabula, not all of which are devoted to medical subjects, are: Hunterian Library, Glasgow (534); Royal College of Physicians, London (107), of which a typescript catalogue exists; Royal College of Surgeons of England (58), a list of which was prepared by W. R. LeFanu and A. C. Klebs;[29] Royal Society of Medicine (15); Medico-Chirurgical Society of Aberdeen (15); and Royal Faculty of Physicians and Surgeons of Glasgow (7). In 1976 the Royal Medical Society of Edinburgh published *A catalogue of medical incunabula in Edinburgh libraries*, compiled by G. D. Hargreaves. The plate used as frontispiece shows a German almanac for 1492, listing days astrologically favourable for phlebotomy. This is GW 1473, recording this copy only, which is the property of Edinburgh Royal Observatory. It is ascribed with a query to the printer Georg Reyser at Würzburg. The catalogue describes one hundred books, of which, however, at least seven, and possibly as many as ten, were printed after 1500, and so are not incunabula. At least ten of the items are very rare books indeed.

Of the 107 incunabula at the Royal College of Physicians in London at least twenty, such as three Bibles, the first edition of Homer in Greek, Florence, 1488, a Juvenal of Venice, 1492, and Plutarch's *Lives*, Venice, 1478 are not medical books. Of the medical books in this library, mention must be made of the very rare tract of six leaves by Benedictus Kanuti, *Regimen contra epidemiam sive pestem*, with no imprint, but attributable to the press of Gerard Leeu at Antwerp about 1489. The British Library has the title-leaf only. Then there is one of the five or so different editions, all *sine nota* and very difficult to distinguish one from another, of Macer

Floridus, *De viribus herbarum*. These are nowadays usually ascribed to Louis Cruse at Geneva, but whether this one (Goff M 5, another copy in the Linnean Society) is before or after 1500 cannot be stated with certainty. There is also an edition of the *Regimen sanitatis*, which seems to vary from all other recorded editions. It is signed by the printer Bernardinus Venetus de Vitalibus at Venice, but is undated and may be after 1500. It collates A-T⁴V⁶. The rest of the incunabula at the RCP are all recorded in other copies by Goff, GW or the British Library catalogue.

Of the 58 incunabula in the Library of the Royal College of Surgeons, London, most are also in Goff, but a particularly rare one is Jacobus de Forlivio, *Expositio super libros Tegni cum questionibus eiusdem* ['Tegni' referring to the work of Galen], Venice, Bonetus Locatellus for Octavianus Scotus, 1 March 1495; and there is an apparently unrecorded tract of four leaves, a French translation of Aristotle's *Secreta secretorum* which seems to have been printed at Lyons in 1490.

The library of Thomas Linacre (*c.*1460–1524) has recently been studied.[30] Not more than 20 manuscripts and printed books have been traced, and, considering that he was one of the founders of the Royal College of Physicians, it is surprising that not one of these is a medical incunable. One, however, is a manuscript of Erotian's *Lexicon medicum*, another is Galen's *Anatomica* in manuscript, and a third is Galen, *De simplicium medicamentorum temperamentis ac facultatibus*. These three manuscripts are all now in libraries in the Low Countries.

In the United States of America there are several rich collections of medical incunabula, and the National Library of Medicine at Bethesda, Maryland, has increased its number of this material from the 232 items held in 1916 to the 493 listed in the catalogue compiled in 1950 by Dorothy M. Schullian and Francis E. Sommer.[31]

The College of Physicians of Philadelphia contained 409 incunabula in 1938, and a supplementary list published in 1960 records a further 14 items.[32] James F. Ballard prepared a catalogue of the 654 incunabula contained in the Boston Medical Library, and also listed the 52 manuscripts then held.[33]

The Huntington Library contained 532 items in 1931, when these were recorded in a list prepared by H. R. Mead.[34] A list of the incunabula in the New York Academy of Medicine prepared by Lesta Ford in 1930 contains 117 items.[35] Yale University (202), excluding the Klebs collection; the University of Michigan (*c.*78); the University of California; and numerous other universities and medical libraries' house collections of this material.

Writing in 1944, Curt F. Bühler provided figures for the holdings of scientific incunabula in a number of American libraries.[36]

Margaret Bingham Stillwell's census of incunabula in American libraries, published by the Bibliographical Society of America in 1940, listed 35 232 copies of 11 132 titles, of which 28 491 were housed in institutions and 6741 were then contained in private collections.[37] Of course, this national census of early books includes texts of every kind, not only medical. Miss Stillwell's work was superseded by her pupil Frederick R. Goff of the Library of Congress, who in 1964 published the third census of incunabula in North American libraries.[38] Figures now read: 12 599 titles in 47 188 copies. Unfortunately, Goff deliberately included in his enumeration at least 200 books which he knew to be printed in the sixteenth century, simply because they had been erroneously included in many previous and often unreliable sources. But why perpetuate errors? This seems an illogical procedure.

In France, the Faculté de Médecine de Paris owns about 100 incunabula, 90 of them being medical. In Italy, a complete survey of the country's holdings of medical incunabula could only be drawn up by a thorough reading of all six volumes of the *Indice Generale* referred to above.

Notes

1. Haebler, Konrad, *Hundert Kalendar-Inkunabeln* (Strasbourg, 1905).
2. *Pestblätter des XV. Jahrhunderts* (Strasbourg, 1901).
3. Viets, Henry R., and James F. Ballard, 'Notes on the plague tracts in the Boston Medical Library', *Bull. Hist. Med.*, 8 (1940) pp.370–80.
4. Singer, Dorothea Waley, 'Some plague tractates (fourteenth and fifteenth centuries)', *Proc. Roy. Soc. Med.*, 9 (1916) Section of History of Medicine, pp.159–212.
5. Correia, Fernanda da Silva, 'Regimento proveytoso contra ha pestenença – Lisboa, Valentim Fernandes, 1496(?)', *Boletim Clinico dos Hospitais Civis de Lisboa*, 24 (1960) pp.339–63.
6. Garrison, Fielding Hudson, *The principles of anatomic illustration before Vesalius: an inquiry into the rationale of artistic anatomy* (New York, 1926).
7. Jessup, Everett Colgate, 'Rabanus Maurus: "De sermonum proprietate, seu de universo", *Ann. Med. Hist.*, N.S.6 (1934) pp.35–41. This provides a translation of the portion on medicine.
8. Full bibliographical details provided in Sir William Osler's *Incunabula medica* (Oxford, 1923).
9. See Rhodes, Dennis E, 'A volume from the monastery library of Hayles', *Trans. Cambridge Bibl. Soc.*, 8 (1985) pp.598–603.
10. English translation of this by Casey A. Wood, 1929.
11. Phillips, Joanne H., 'The incunable editions of the *Liber medicinalis Quinti Sereni*. Estratto da "I testi di medicina Latini antichi: problemi storici e filologici" ', Atti del I. Convegno Internazionale (Macerata-S. Severino Marche, 26–28 aprile 1984). (Università di Macerata. Pubblicazioni della Facoltà di Lettere e Filosofia. 28), [Rome] (1985) pp.[215]–235.
12. 'Some early printed books: their authors and printers', *Med. J. Australia* (1926) II, pp.77–81.
13. This was produced in facsimile, Manchester, 1910.
14. A facsimile edition of this was published in 1858 but, as only 55 copies were printed, this reprint is rare (Cowlishaw, op. cit. in note 12 above, p.78). See Duff 165; STC 12138. There were also two other editions from the press of Wynkyn de Worde, STC 12139 (possibly 1506) and STC 12139.5 (*c*.1530). Much interesting material on fifteenth-century medical books is contained in Thomas E. Keys, 'The earliest medical books printed with movable type: a review', *Lib. Quart.*, 10 (1940) pp.220–30.
15. See Cockayne, Oswald, *Leechdoms, wort-cunning and starcraft of early England, being a collection of documents, for the most part never before printed, illustrating the history of science in this country before the Norman Conquest*, 3 vols (1864–6) reprinted 1961; see

also J. H. G. Gratton and Charles Singer, *Anglo-Saxon magic and medicine: illustrated specially from the semi-pagan text 'Lacnunga'* ... (London) 1952.

16. Singer, Charles, 'The herbal in antiquity', *J. Hellenic Studies*, 47 (1927) p.52 (contains ten coloured plates, illustrations and references); see also Stannard, Jerry, 'Medieval herbals and their development', *Clio Med.*, 9 (1974) pp.23–33.

17. *The Greek herbal of Dioscorides, illustrated by a Byzantine A.D. 512, Englished by John Goodyer, A.D. 1655, edited and first printed A.D. 1933 by Robert T. Gunther* (Oxford, 1934). This contains 396 illustrations.

18. Duff 40; STC 1536. See also Bartholomaeus Anglicus, 'De proprietatibus rerum. (Book seventh – On Medicine)', translated and annotated with an introductory essay by James J. Walsh, *Medical Life*, 40 (1933) pp.449–602.

19. Beughem, Cornelius à, *Incunabula typographiae, sive catalogus librorum scriptorumque proximis ab inventione typographiae annis, usque ad annum Christi M.D. inclusive, in quavis lingua editorum* (Amsterdam, 1688). This is arranged alphabetically by authors. Second edition, 1733.

20. For a more complete list, see Garrison, F. H., 'Progress in the cataloguing of medical incunabula ...', *Bull. N.Y. Acad. Med.*, 2nd ser., 6 (1930) pp.386–9; also Cowley, J.D., *Bibliographical description and cataloguing* (1939) pp.214–48.

21. Choulant, Ludwig, *Graphische Incunabeln für Naturgeschichte und Medizin. Enthaltend Geschichte und Bibliographie der ersten naturhistorischen und medizinischen Drucke des XV. und XVI. Jahrhunderts, welche mit illustrierenden Abbildungen versehen sind. Nebst Nachträgen zu des Verfassers Geschichte und Bibliographie der anatomischen Abbildung* ... [Leipzig, 1858] (Munich, 1924).

22. *Osiris*, 4, i (1938); reprinted Hildesheim, 1963.

23. Garrison, Fielding H., op. cit. in note 20 above, pp.365–435 (contains a chronological tabulation of printers in German cities, lists of leading printers, and other useful matter); Peddie, R. A., *Fifteenth-century books: a guide to their identification. With a list of the Latin names of towns, and an extensive bibliography of the subject* (1913).

24. Klebs, Arnold C., 'Desiderata in the cataloguing of incunabula; with a guide for catalogue entries', *Papers of the Bibl. Soc. of America*, 10 (1916) pp.143–63; Guppy, Henry, *Rules for the cataloguing of incunabula*, 2nd edn rev. (1932).

25. See also Bühler, Curt F., James G. McManaway and Lawrence C. Wroth, *Standards of bibliographical description* (Philadelphia, 1949) in which Bühler deals exhaustively with the correct rules for cataloguing incunabula.

26. See also chapter on scientific incunabula in Thornton–Tully.

27. *Bibliotheca Walleriana, The books illustrating the history of medicine and science collected by Dr. Erik Waller and bequeathed to the Library of the Royal University of Uppsala. A catalogue compiled by Hans Sallander*, 2 vols (Stockholm, 1955).

28. Poynter, F. N. L., *A catalogue of incunabula in the Wellcome Historical Medical Library* (London, 1954).

29. LeFanu, W. R., and A. C. Klebs, 'Incunabula in the Library of the Royal College of Surgeons of England', *Ann. Med. Hist.*, N.S.3 (1931) pp.674–6.

30. Barber, Giles, 'Thomas Linacre: a bibliographical survey of his works', *Linacre Studies* (1977) pp.290–336. Books from Linacre's library are listed on pp.331–6.

31. Schullian, Dorothy M., and Francis E. Sommer, *A catalogue of incunabula and manuscripts in the Army Medical Library* [now the National Library at Bethesda, Maryland] New York [1950].

32. McDaniel, W. B., 'Census of incunabula in the Library of the College of Physicians of Philadelphia, 1938', *Trans. Stud. Coll. Phys. Philad.*, 4th ser., 6 (1938) pp.159–93; and Supplement 1, 1960, ibid., 4th ser., 28 (1960–1) pp.191–2.

33. Ballard, James F., *A catalogue of the medieval and Renaissance manuscripts and incunabula in the Boston Medical Library* (Boston, 1944), privately printed. By the same author, see also 'Medical incunabula in the William Norton Bullard Collection', *Boston Med. Surg. J.*, 196 (1927) pp.865–75. Readers of this article should beware of the illustration on p.872, which purports to show 'John of Gaddesden, "Rosa Anglica", Pavia, 1492. Title page of first edition.' The title is certainly of that edition, but the ornamental border surrounding it is of the seventeenth, if not the eighteenth, century.

34. Mead, Herman Ralph, 'Incunabula medica in the Huntington Library', *Huntington Lib. Bull.*, No. 1 (1931) pp. 107–51.
35. Ford, Lesta, 'Incunabula in the New York Academy of Medicine', *Ann. Med. Hist.*, N.S.2 (1930) pp.340–5.
36. Bühler, Curt F., 'Scientific and medical incunabula in American libraries', *Isis*, 35 (1944) pp.173–5; see also Bühler, C.F., *The Fifteenth-century book. The scribes, the printers, the decorators* (Philadelphia, 1960).
37. *Incunabula in American libraries: second census of fifteenth-century books owned in the United States, Mexico and Canada*, ed. by Margaret Bingham Stillwell (New York, 1940).
38. Goff, Frederick R. (ed.), *Incunabula in American libraries: third census* (New York, 1964) reprinted by Kraus Reprint Co., Millwood, N.Y., 1973; Supplement, New York, 1972.

3 Medical books of the sixteenth century

Yvonne Hibbott

> The middle of the sixteenth century witnessed a revolution in the treatment of
> the sick poor of London, and produced a number of books written by men who
> had the interest of surgery at heart, and who strove to raise their calling from a
> trade to a profession. Vicary, Gale, Clowes, Banester, Read, and Maister Lowe
> wrote books which are still a joy to read. Their language is charming, their
> invective is fierce, their poetry is vile, but they give so lively a picture of the
> times in which they lived that many a profitable hour may still be spent in their
> company.
>
> (Sir D'Arcy Power)

With the Renaissance and the revival of learning medicine began to pass
from medieval to modern conditions. The prime causes of this dramatic
evolution were the invention of printing, the development of humanism,
and the advancement of scientific and artistic anatomy.

The rapid development of printing in the second half of the fifteenth
century had ensured the widespread dissemination of the classics. The new
communications network created by the printing press made possible the
recovery of classical scientific knowledge and, by fixing it in print, sub-
jected it to critical appraisal. Thus typography 'set the stage' for the
scientific revolution by initiating a process of information retrieval.[1] This
scientific revolution was aided by the creation of new universities and
centres of learning; philosophy was separated from science, and the latter
began to develop into specialist disciplines.

The Renaissance was a period of incessant intellectual ferment and
activity. The Byzantine Greek scholars, who sought refuge in Italy after
the destruction of Constantinople in 1453, brought to Europe a knowledge of the Greek language and a dissemination of the literature. The
humanist scholars made critical studies of the original classical sources
which were crucial to the development of medicine.

The revival of learning led to a new interest in anatomy and, therefore,
dissection. The natural prejudice against the examination of the dead had
prevented the art of medicine from developing beyond the stage reached
by the Greeks. With the scientific revival, however, the human mind
became more open to reason so that a knowledge of structure and function, and also of the changes caused by disease and accident, was obtained
by autopsy and dissection. Both artists and anatomists dissected and
recorded their observations, and this determination to investigate the
human body was the foundation of outstanding advances in medicine and
surgery.

Bibliographically the sixteenth century is no longer the 'neglected' century that it was, and several outstanding catalogues and bibliographies have been produced – in particular the *Catalogue of sixteenth century books in the National Library of Medicine* compiled by Richard J. Durling, and *A Catalogue of sixteenth-century medical books in Edinburgh libraries*, compiled by D. T. Bird.[2] Other valuable sixteenth-century catalogues and bibliographies include the work of E. M. Parkinson, J. Linet and P. Hillard, P. Limacher, H. J. H. Drummond, H. M. Adams, M. B. Stillwell and K. F. Russell.[3] The medical and scientific Renaissance has been the study of several excellent works by A. G. Debus, C. D. O'Malley, J. W. Shirley and F. D. Hoeniger, A. Wear *et al.*, C. Webster and W. P. D. Wightman.[4]

The history of herbals in the sixteenth century reflects the transition from an era of folk medicine, magic and superstition to an era of science. F. J. Anderson[5] defines a herbal as

> ... a book that is descriptive of plants. It is, however, a great deal more than that. For one thing, herbals generally concern themselves most with plants that have medicinal properties, and they usually include some information as to how to identify them, extract their useful properties, and then apply them to cure certain disorders, wounds, and diseases. But it would be erroneous to give the impression that herbals are only about plants, for they draw their medicaments from other sources as well.

Excellent studies of herbals have been made by Eleanour S. Rohde, Agnes Arber, Wilfrid Blunt and F. J. Anderson.[6] A scholarly history and bibliography of English botanical books has been written by B. Henrey.[7]

The sixteenth-century German authors of herbals exercized a strong influence on the advancement of science in that they encouraged accurate observation of natural phenomena, and this influence spread far beyond botany and medicine. Two of the most beautiful of these early herbals were the *Herbarum vivae eicones*, Strasbourg, 1530, by Otto Brunfels and *De historia stirpium*, Basle, 1542, by Leonhart Fuchs, both of which were illustrated with exceptional woodcuts. Fuchs closely supervized the illustrations for his book as he was concerned at errors made by readers through improper identification of plants. An outstanding publication from an Italian botanist was the commentaries on Dioscorides of Pietro Andrea Mattioli, first published in Venice in 1544. Mattioli's commentaries provided the focus which the botanical movement needed.[8]

The first printed English herbal, devoted entirely to herbs, is that published by Richard Banckes at London in 1525. The author is unknown, but the book was generally known as *Banckes' Herbal*, and was very popular, going into many editions. It was also issued by other publishers under various titles, among editions recorded being those dated 1525, 1526, 1530, 1532–1537, 1541, 1546, 1548, 1550 and 1552.[9] Probably the most famous of all herbals was the *Grete herball* printed by Peter

Treveris in 1526 (STC 13176–13179), which is actually a translation of *Le grand herbier*. It is arranged alphabetically, but is poorly illustrated, and editions have been recorded for 1516,[10] 1525,[11], 1526, 1529, 1539, 1550 and 1561.[12] The complications of the authorship and printers of *Banckes' Herbal* and Treveris' *Grete herball* have been investigated by H. M. Barlow.[13]

English botany can truly be said to begin with the herbals of William Turner (1510–68) who was the first to study the subject in a scientific manner. Turner was twice exiled to the continent for his religious beliefs during the reign of Henry VIII and Mary Tudor, but he used this time wisely to gather material for his herbals, and to study with European scientists such as Gonrad Gesner and Luca Ghini. Turner's first botanical work was *Libellus de re herbarium novus*, printed by John Byddell at London in 1538 (STC 24358). In 1548 appeared another short work entitled *The names of herbes in Greke, Latin, Englishe, Duche, and Frenche wyth the commone names that herbaries and apotecaries use, gathered by William Turner* (STC 24359). This was followed by his most notable contribution to the subject, *A new herball*, the first part of which was printed by Steven Mierdman at London in 1551 (STC 24365), the second and third parts by Arnold Birckman at Cologne in 1561 (STC 24366). The latter also printed the 1568 edition containing all three parts (STC 24367). This herbal is particularly noteworthy for the numerous beautiful woodcuts with which it is illustrated. His other books are noted in STC 24351–24368.[14]

One of the most beautiful, and certainly one of the most popular of the sixteenth-century herbals was written by John Gerarde (1545–1612). Gerarde had a house in Holborn where he grew a thousand herbs of which he published a catalogue in 1596,[15] and a second edition three years later. His larger work, *The herball, or generall historie of plantes*, was printed by John Norton of London in 1597 (STC 11750). The second edition of this was even more successful, being greatly enlarged and amended by Thomas Johnson, and published in 1633 (STC 11751).[16] Thomas Johnson was born in Selby, Yorkshire, about 1597. He made many botanizing expeditions of which he published details, and also translated the works of Ambroise Paré (1634).[17] A facsimile of Johnson's 1633 edition of Gerarde's *Herball* was published in 1975.[18] A study of the title-page has been made by M. Corbett.[19]

The woodcuts used in the early herbals were often crude, and the same illustration would be used for different plants, often being copied from author to author. The skill of woodcutting in Gerarde's *Herball* reached a new level, and when this was combined with hand colouring, a very fine volume resulted.

The sources of vegetable drugs were thus increased by the advances in botany, and the extension of geographical knowledge particularly the exploration of America and the Indies, brought new drugs onto the market. Plants of the East Indies were described by Garcia da Orta (*c*.1500–*c*.1568) in his book *Coloquios dos simples e drogas*, published at Goa in 1563.

The humanist scholars of the Renaissance examined the extensive Greek texts which now became available. The writings of Aristotle were printed for the first time in Greek by Aldus Manutius (1450–1515). Aldus also published the first Greek text of *De materia medica* by Dioscorides in 1499. The first Greek editions of Galen and Hippocrates were published after Aldus's death (1525 and 1526) by his successors, Girolamo Rossi and Francesco Torresano.[20] Almost alone, the Aldine Press supplied the demand for classical medical texts. It was left to rival firms, like the Giuntas (established in Florence, but with connections in Lyons and Venice) to fill such gaps that might remain. The Giunta Press, for instance, supplied a demand for Latin editions of medieval Arabic writers, notably Avicenna and Mesue.

This return to Greek learning in medicine, particularly the Galenic sources,[21] was considered a progressive step. It was looked upon as a return to the wisdom of the classical physicians, which was only known previously through the filterings of medieval writers. However the oppressive authority of Galen was not lifted until the work of Andreas Vesalius.

The sixteenth-century advances in scientific anatomy and artistic anatomy were closely interwoven. The great artists of the Renaissance – Pollaiolo, Michelangelo, Leonardo da Vinci, Raphael and Dürer – began to make detailed studies of the human form. They soon found that to represent it accurately some knowledge of anatomy, especially of the bones and muscles, was needed. The artists therefore began to dissect.[22]

Leonardo da Vinci (1452–1519) was the most versatile scientist of any century, although his fame as an artist tends to overshadow his contributions to science. Leonardo had carried out anatomical dissection for many years, and he later worked on the preparation of a textbook of anatomy and physiology in collaboration with a medical teacher at Padua, Marcantonio della Torre (1473–1506). Owing to the death of della Torre this work was never finished (thus leaving Vesalius to become the founder of scientific anatomy), but many of Leonardo's beautifully illustrated notebooks have survived. He was one of the first to question the views of Galen, and believed that a scientific knowledge of artistic anatomy could be gained only at the dissecting table. This unrelenting search for representational accuracy was the leading characteristic of Renaissance art.

Leonardo executed some 750 separate anatomical drawings, which he bequeathed to Francesco Melzi, from whom they were obtained by Pompeo Leoni the sculptor. They were purchased from the latter in 1623 by Prince Charles, and were deposited, with drawings by Hans Holbein, in a secret cupboard in the Royal Library at Windsor. Richard Dalton, librarian to George III, found them and showed them to William Hunter, who pronounced that Leonardo 'was the best anatomist at that time in the world'.[23] Leonardo contributed in no uncertain measure to anatomy, embryology, physiology, and to many other branches of science.[24] He wrote a treatise on painting, the *Trattato della pittura*, while other volumes containing his work (published posthumously) include *Tabula anatomica ...*, Lüneburg, 1830; *I manoscritti di Leonardo da Vinci della reale biblioteca di Windsor ...*, two volumes, Paris, Turin, 1898–1901; *Notes et desseins*, twelve volumes, Paris, 1901; and *Quaderni d'anatomia. I–VI Fogli della Royal Library di Windsor ...*, six volumes, Oslo, 1911–16. In addition to the drawings at Windsor there is a small collection in Paris, but the majority are located in the Ambrosian Library in Milan. Leonardo's drawings would undoubtedly have been extremely important had they been published during or shortly after his lifetime. He was one of the first and most successful experimental scientists, and it is one of the tragedies of his career that his vast accumulation of new knowledge was not available to his contemporaries and successors. Leonardo's notes and drawings have been the subject of excellent studies by K. D. Keele, K. Clark, C. D. O'Malley and J. B. de C. M. Saunders, E. MacCurdy, E. Belt, M. Kemp, and others.[25]

A Renaissance artist whose writings were also of anatomical interest was Albrecht Dürer (1471–1528), painter and engraver, who was born in Nuremberg. He wrote books on botany, chemistry, mathematics and perspective, but lived to see only two of these works printed. Dürer concentrated on the outline and proportion of the human body rather than the structure and mechanism which had occupied Leonardo. His treatise on human proportion, *Vier Bücher von menschlicher Proportion* was published at Nuremberg in 1528, a Latin translation appearing six years later. This work was the first application of anthropometry to aesthetics.[26] Dürer also wrote a work on symmetry, published in Nuremberg in 1532, *De symmetria patrium in rectis formis humanorum corporum ...*, an Italian translation being printed in Venice in 1591. Many translations and editions of these two books were produced, again reflecting the enquiring spirit of the Renaissance artists.

Medicine in the early sixteenth century was still dominated by the writings of Galen, and the revival of Greek scholarship tended to consolidate this position. Although scientific anatomy is generally dated from the period of Vesalius, several of his predecessors paved the way for his modernistic approach to the subject by challenging the Galenic view of anatomy. In particular the writings of Alessandro Achillini, Niccolo Massa, Charles Estienne and Berengario da Carpi are outstanding examples of pre-Vesalian anatomy.[27] Although Vesalius may have been influenced by these works, it does not detract from his achievement in establishing anatomy as a scientific foundation of medicine.

Alessandro Achillini (1463–1512) of Bologna was the author of *De humani corporis anatomia*, Venice, 1516. Niccolo Massa (1499–1569) a medical graduate of Padua and successful practitioner in Venice, published *Liber introductorius anatomiae* ..., Venice, 1536 – the best brief anatomical textbook prior to Realdo Colombo's *De re anatomica* (1559) and containing good independent observations on the heart.[28] Massa emphasized the necessity of dissection. Charles Estienne (Stephanus) (1504–64) completed his *De dissectione partium corporis humani* in 1539, although it was not printed until 1545 in Paris, followed by a French translation from the same press in 1546. Legal proceedings had delayed publication, as Estienne wished to omit the name of his co-author, Estienne de la Rivière. In the meantime, however, Vesalius had stolen the show. The woodcut illustrations of *De dissectione* are mannered in style and its influence upon the development of medical illustration was transient.[29]

Probably the most outstanding of these forerunners was Jacopo Berengario da Carpi (*c*.1460–1530) a noted anatomist and physician, whose true name was Barigazzi, a fact only revealed in his last will. He qualified at Bologna in 1489 and became lecturer in surgery there in 1502. Berengario was the first to describe the vermiform appendix, the thymus and the valves of the heart. His first book bore the title *Anothomia Mundini noivter* [sic] *impressa ac per Carpum castigata*, Bologna, 1514, and was also printed in Venice in 1529, 1530 and 1538. This was followed by his *Tractatus de fractura calve sive cranei*, Bologna, 1518, with a second edition from Venice in 1535. It was reprinted at Leyden in 1629, 1651, 1715 and 1728. The best known work by Berengario da Carpi, however, is undoubtedly his short introduction to anatomy, bearing the title *Isagogae breves* ... This was printed in Bologna, 1522; Venice, 1523, 1533 and 1535; Cologne, 1529; and Strasbourg, 1530 and 1533. An English translation by Henry Jackson was published as Μικροκομογραφια [*Mikrokosmographia*] *or a description of the little world or body of man* ..., London, 1660, and a 'second edition', apparently a reissue with slightly different title was printed in 1664. The 1660 edition is very rare, and at least one copy of the 1664 printing has the name of the translator on the title-page as Jackeson.[30] An English version by L. R. Lind was published in 1957.[31] Berengario da Carpi was also the author of *Commentaria cum amplissimis additionibus super anatomia Mundini...*, Bologna, 1521, and *Galeni Pergameni Libri anatomici ...*, Bologna, 1529.

The earliest work published in England devoted entirely to anatomy was the *Introduction to anatomy* published in 1532 by David Edwardes (Edguardus) (1502–*c*.1542) (STC 7483). Edwardes was educated at Oxford and practised around Cambridge. His book contained two treatises, *De indiciis et praecognitionibus* and *In anatomicen introductio loculenta et brevis*, with a common title-page, but with separate dedications. The anatomical part consists of fifteen pages only, and the sole remaining copy is preserved in the British Library. It has been reproduced in facsimile, with an introductory essay by C. D. O'Malley and K. F. Russell.[32]

Jacques Dubois, more generally known as Jacobus Sylvius (1478–1555), was a native of Picardy, and had Vesalius, Charles Estienne and Servetus among his pupils, but remained a staunch Galenist, and later became an opponent of Vesalius. Sylvius influenced the development of anatomical terminology,[33] and his advice for poor medical students has been translated by C. D. O'Malley.[34] This was first printed anonymously as *Victus ratio, scholasticis pauperibus partu facilis & salubris*, Paris, 1542, of which possibly a unique copy is preserved at Yale, and was reprinted in *Thesaurus sanitatis paratu facilis electus ex variis authoribus, per Joannem Liebaultium*, Paris, 1577. His *Opera medica* was printed in Geneva in 1634.[35]

The central place in the unfolding drama of the sixteenth century was occupied by Andreas Vesalius of Brussels (1514–64), whose work *De humani corporis fabrica libri septem* has been called 'the greatest medical work ever printed' (William Osler). The first edition was printed by Oporinus in Basle in 1543, and marked the foundation of medicine as a science.

Vesalius was born at Brussels in 1514, and studied first at the University of Louvain, and later at Paris where he was a pupil of Sylvius. He was appointed Professor of Anatomy and Surgery at Padua in 1547, when only twenty-four years of age, and established a scientific tradition at Padua which that University still retains. After the publication of *De fabrica* Vesalius entered imperial service as court physician to Emperor Charles V. He died on the island of Zante in 1564.

The greatness of Vesalius has been well served by two outstanding works – Harvey Cushing, *A bio-bibliography of Andreas Vesalius*, and C. D. O'Malley, *Andreas Vesalius of Brussels 1514–1564*.[36] O'Malley's full-scale biography contains an exhaustive study of Vesalius, his life and writings, with translations from *De fabrica*.

Two of the earliest literary efforts of Vesalius were his commentary on the Almansor of Rhazes, *Paraphrasis in nonum librum Rhazae* ..., Louvain, 1527, with a second, revised edition from Basle [1537], and later printings from Basle [1544]; Lyons, 1551; and Wittenberg, 1586 and 1592; and a revision of Johann Günther's *Institutionum anatomicarum secundum Galeni sententiam* ..., Venice, 1538, which went into several editions.

In 1538 Vesalius published a set of six anatomical plates, the *Tabulae anatomicae*, Venice, of which edition only two copies are known. The plates were intended as an aid to his students in their anatomical and physiological studies. Although the work reflects the teaching of Galen and Aristotle, Vesalius now began to question their views, and his scepticism led him to put the statements of his predecessors to the test of experiment. In 1874 the plates of the *Tabulae anatomicae* were reprinted in facsimile by Sir William Stirling Maxwell, but only 30 copies were printed. Another facsimile edition appeared from Leipzig, 1920, and was issued by Moriz Holl and Karl Sudhoff. This was followed by a further facsimile edition, New York and Munich, 1934, and by a scholarly study with reproductions of the plates by Charles Singer and C. Rabin entitled *A prelude to modern science*.[37] A facsimile of the Cologne and Augsburg editions appeared in 1965.[38] Vesalius was also the author of a venesection epistle, *Epistola, docens venam axillarem dextri cubiti in dolore laterali secandam & melancholicum succum ... pertinentibus, purgari*, Basle, 1539, [Venice] 1544, and Amsterdam, 1930. This was edited and translated into English by John B. de C. M. Saunders and C. D. O'Malley in 1949.[39]

In 1543 appeared the book which was to revolutionize anatomical knowledge – *De humani corporis fabrica libri septem*, published by Joannes Oporinus at Basle in 1543. This contains 663 folio pages and over 300 illustrations (a facsimile edition was published in Brussels in 1964). An unillustrated pocket edition was published in Lyons, 1552. In 1555 Vesalius was persuaded to publish a second edition of *De fabrica*. This contains certain changes in point of view that are important for the subsequent development of anatomy and physiology. Vesalius now no longer merely suggests his doubts as to the character of Galen's physiology; he openly asserts that he had been unable to verify its fundamental bases.[40]

At the time of writing *De fabrica* Vesalius was professor of Anatomy at Padua University where his revolutionary scientific approach to anatomy was a sharp contrast to the previous following of Aristotle and Galen. Vesalius insisted that students study the cadaver at first hand as he believed that careful dissection and observation should be the basis of anatomical research. At that time it was unheard of for the professor to perform the dissection himself – this was performed by the *demonstrator* (a barber or surgeon), with an *ostensor* pointing out the structures. The new Vesalian method of investigation was carefully followed in the most successful of the seven books of the *Fabrica* – books I and II, which are devoted to the bones and muscles. An excellent study of the accuracy of *De fabrica* has been made by C. D. O'Malley.[41]

The art of woodcut illustration reached its highest peak in the publication of *De fabrica* which contains over 300 illustrations, the work of Venetian block cutters. Apart from their scientific content, the woodcuts of *De fabrica* are among the great landmarks in the history of the woodcut and of book illustration (see Plate 4). Vesalius carefully supervised the drawings made from his dissections. The magnificent illustrations are believed to have come from Titian's studio, and to be the work of Johann Stephan van Calcar and other pupils.[42] The identity of the artist or artists is not, however, conclusive, and the van Calcar attribution is doubted by

O'Malley.[43] Vesalius himself gave no indication of the identity of the artist either in *De fabrica* or in any later publication or correspondence. This was in marked contrast to the praise given to van Calcar for his work on three skeletal figures in Vesalius's earlier *Tabulae anatomicae sex*, 1538 – but all later references to artists were hostile and derogatory.[44]

The evidence suggesting that van Calcar was the artist is based on Vasari's attribution,[45] van Calcar's earlier contributions to the *Tabulae anatomicae sex*, and Vesalius's reference to him in the *Epistola docens*.[46] The illustrations are undoubtedly the work of a fine artist and keen observer. The figures of muscles and of skeletons are not diagrammatically displayed front, back and side, but posed as in the living body. They are given tone and movement, and provided with a landscape background.[47]

The blocks for the illustrations of *De fabrica* had a colourful history and have been the subject of several studies.[48] After the death of Vesalius they were taken over by his heirs and later purchased by Andreas Maschenbaur for Ludwig König, and some were published as being the work of Titian. After being lost, the blocks were recovered in 1777, and eventually found their way to Munich, where they were found in an attic of Munich University Library in 1893. Samuel W. Lambert was responsible for tracing the remainder in 1932, and the New York Academy of Medicine sponsored their publication in 1935, although the title-page bears the date 1934, as *Icones anatomicae of Andreas Vesalius*. The blocks were unfortunately destroyed in Munich during the Second World War. The illustrations were reproduced with annotations and translations by J. B. de C. M. Saunders and C. D. O'Malley.[49] Several interesting studies have been made of the woodcut initial letters.[50]

The title-page of *De fabrica* shows Vesalius carrying out a dissection at Padua surrounded by students, doctors, attendants and members of the lay public. The spectators are divided into two main groups – professional men and students surround Vesalius, and the lay public stand beyond the furthermost barrier, forming a gallery. An articulated skeleton presides over the scene to emphasize the importance of osteology. Two assistants, who would previously have carried out the dissection, are seen in front of the dissection table. This crowded scene of the title-page is not exaggerated, as an eyewitness account exists of Vesalius's public demonstrations at Bologna in 1540. This account (a manuscript in the Royal Library, Stockholm) was written by Baldasar Heseler, a student of Vesalius. Heseler's detailed notes have been edited and translated into English by R. Eriksson.[51] Despite the opposition to Vesalius's new theories, Heseler realized the great significance of the demonstrations he witnessed: 'Vesalius corrected many false opinions very carefully by means of the dissection ... and showed the doctors and us students many things neither heard of nor seen before.'

During the same month of publication as *De fabrica*, but probably after the main work, appeared the Epitome, *Suorum de humani corporis fabrica librorum epitome*, Basle (1543). This was an abridgement of the larger *Fabrica*. The plates of the *Epitome* were issued unbound, like the *Tabulae* – they were ephemeral, and hence perfect copies are excessively rare. A German edition appeared in the same year, Basle [1543], and a reissue of the Latin edition was also published there in 1555, the only known copy being in the Waller Library. The book was published without illustrations in Paris, 1560, Wittenberg, 1582 and 1603, and a Dutch translation was printed in Bruges in 1569. A pirated edition containing the full Latin text of the *Epitome*, with 40 engraved plates copied from the 1545 Geminus was printed and published in Cologne with the date 1600 on the title-page and 1601 in the colophon.[52] A translation into Dutch was printed in Brussels, 1947, and an English translation by L. R. Lind was published in New York in 1949.

Among other books by Vesalius were *Radicis chynae usus*, Basle, 1546, which went into several editions. This was Vesalius's answer to his former teacher, Jacobus Sylvius, who accused him of having damaged the authority of Galen. Vesalius's defence is based on his belief that the errors of Galen occurred because he did not use dissections. Vesalius's last publication was *Gabrielis Fallopii Observationum examen*, Venice, 1564, and Hanau, 1609. Five years after the death of Vesalius one of his students, Prospero Borgarucci, published *Chirurgia magna ...*, Venice, 1569, which is not considered to be the work of Vesalius.[53] The *Opera omnia anatomica & chirurgica*, edited by Herman Boerhaave and B. S. Albinus, was printed in Leyden in 1725.

Contemporaries attacked Vesalius for his revolutionary work, but its true value was immediately apparent to many, and the Vesalian influence spread throughout Europe.[54] Vesalius has attracted the attention of many medical historians, and various aspects of his work have been studied.[55] Recent research includes the work of R. J. Wolfe and H. R. Tyler who discovered variant copies of the 1543 *Fabrica* with preliminary leaves that differ typographically from those of the regular first edition. This research was continued by M. Horowitz and J. Collins.[56]

Plagiarism of text and illustrations was rife in the sixteenth and seventeenth centuries. However, these plagiarisms did contribute greatly to the dissemination of the Vesalian ideas and methods. Illustrations were copied exactly, or in a modified form from author to author across Europe. Thomas Geminus copied illustrations completely from Vesalius's *Epitome* and *De fabrica*, and Valverde de Hamusco copied from *De fabrica*, modifying certain illustrations for his *Historia de la composicion del cuerpo humano*, Rome, 1556.[57] Authors acquired blocks or plates, and used them with their own texts, or had new blocks or cuts made with slight modifications from the originals. Intensive investigation is necessary to disentangle the intricacies of plagiarism upon plagiarism. Some of the most unscrupulous plagiarisms of Vesalius, and other authors, were carried out by the printers of the broadsides, or so called 'fugitive sheets' (fliegende Blätter).[58] These were single sheets, printed and sold separately, of anatomical figures reproduced from woodcuts. Superimposed flaps were often used to show the anatomical relationships in depth. Fugitive sheets were widely reproduced in the middle years of the sixteenth century and continued in use well into the seventeenth century.

A plagiarism which, unusually, holds an important place in the history of medical books is Thomas Geminus, *Compendiosa totius anatomie delineatio*, 1545 (STC 11714). Geminus (born Thomas Lambrit) came from Flanders, and was both a printer and engraver. He engraved the copperplate illustrations in the *Compendiosa* which make the book such an important landmark in the transition from woodcut to copperplate illustration (see Plate 5).[59] This atlas was the first medical work in England, together with Thomas Raynalde's *The byrth of mankynde*, to have illustrations printed from copperplates.

Henry VIII had commissioned Thomas Geminus to produce a version of Vesalius's atlas. The *Compendiosa* was printed for Geminus by Nicholas Hyll and published by John Herford in London, 1545. The first English edition, translated by Nicholas Udall, was published in 1553, and the text bears more resemblance to the *Anatomie* of Thomas Vicary than to Vesalius. This edition has been reproduced in facsimile, with interesting introductory matter by C. D. O'Malley.[60] The 1559 edition is substantially a reissue, but was dedicated to Queen Elizabeth. Editions in Latin and French were published in Paris in 1564 and 1565.

The work of Geminus represented a great advance in English anatomical illustration, although Vesalius complained that the woodcuts had been inaccurately copied. It is evident, however, that the copper engraving gave finer detail than was possible with woodcuts. The engraved title-page is clearly cut, in little but outline, and is of interest as one of the earliest examples of the mixture of strap-work and grotesque which became so popular all over Europe, especially in the Netherlands in the latter half of the century.[61] The 1559 edition has added interest in the portrait of Elizabeth I which replaced the royal arms on the title-page, and is the earliest printed portrayal of the Queen.

The Geminus plates were used in several Latin and English issues of the *Compendiosa* before being sold to a Parisian printer, André Wechel, who also brought out a Latin version as late as 1564. Crummer[62] has suggested that Geminus engraved two of the plates in the second edition of Thomas Raynalde's *The byrth of mankynde*, 1545, using duplicate plates for his own book. He also refers to the interesting evidence of repair in the plates.

The value and success of the *Compendiosa* resulted in the publication of plagiarisms in England and on the continent, particularly those of Jacques

Grévin and Jacob Bauman, and the influence of Geminus continued to be felt for at least a century after the publication of his book – 'Few plagiarisms have been flattered by so much imitation'.[63]

Gabriele Falloppio (Fallopius) (1523–62) of Modena was a pupil and successor of Vesalius at Padua. He wrote works on anatomy, medicine and pharmacy, including *Observationes anatomicae*, Venice, 1561, which includes his description of the oviduct (Fallopian tubes); *De morbo Gallico*, Padua, 1563; and *De parte medicinae, quae chyrurgia nuncupatur ...* of which the second edition was printed at Venice in 1571. Falloppio also described the cochlea and labyrinth of the ear and the chorda tympani. His work on the cranial nerves in the *Observationes* is important and has been studied by O'Malley.[64] An edition of the letters of Falloppio has been published by Di Pietro.[65]

Bartholomeo Eustachi (Eustachius) (1500/10–74) of San Severino was a contemporary of Vesalius and Falloppio, and spent most of his professional life in Rome. Later he became physician to the Duke of Urbino, and in 1547 to the Duke's brother, Cardinal Giulio della Rovere, whom he followed to Rome in 1549. There he joined the medical faculty of the Sapienza as teacher of anatomy. Eustachi strongly defended Galenic anatomy, but this did not prevent him from making original and accurate observations on the anatomy of the ear, kidney and venous system. Eustachi's hostility to Vesalius may have been caused by his frustration at the international acclaim of *De fabrica* in comparison to the lack of recognition for his own work in Rome.

Eustachi is remembered especially for his remarkable description of the auditory or Eustachian tube and his important contributions to medical illustration. He drew many of the figures for his *Opuscula anatomica*, printed in Venice in 1564, with a second edition, Leyden, 1707. Together with Pier Matteo Pini, Eustachi made the drawings and supervised the copperplates (engraved by Guilio de' Musi of Rome) for a work which was never to be published. The 38 copperplates, completed in 1552, were left to Pini on Eustachi's death. The plates were later rediscovered by Giovanni Maria Lancisi, physician to Pope Clement XI, and published at Rome in 1714 as *Tabulae anatomicae*, with Lancisi adding his own descriptions to the plates which did not have a commentary by Eustachi. The subjects are depicted in elegant, classically formal poses, and although they may be less artistic than the *Fabrica* illustrations, some show greater accuracy. A ruled graduated border, surrounding each figure on three sides, was used to give reference numbers to each anatomical structure, in the same way that references to latitude and longitude can be used to locate a place on a map. This method of grid referencing allowed Eustachi to present his figures without superimposed lettering or numbering.[66]

The delay of 150 years in the publication of Eustachi's work deprived him of the recognition he deserved. In particular his contribution to the knowledge of the ear was a notable scientific achievement; this appeared on pages 148–64 of his *Opuscula anatomica*, which was the first separate treatise on the ear. The work has been translated by C. D. O'Malley.[67]

The first printed textbook for midwives went through at least 40 editions and was first printed in 1513 as *Der swangern frauwen und hebammen roszgarten*, by Eucharius Rösslin (Röslin or Rhodion) (died 1526), a physician at Worms and later at Frankfort-on-Main. Mainly compiled from Soranus of Ephesus, it was illustrated with quaint woodcuts, being first printed at Strasbourg in 1513. It was reissued twice in that year, once probably at Strasbourg, and once from Hagenau, after which reprints and translations followed rapidly. It was reprinted at Strasbourg in 1522, 1524 and 1528, at Augsburg in 1524, 1528, 1544 and 1551, at Erfurt in 1529, and at Frankfort in 1561 and 1568. There appeared translations into Dutch (1516), Czech (1519), French (1536), and into Latin as *De partu hominis*, Frankfort, 1532. This was reprinted at Paris in 1536 and at Venice in 1537, while an English translation of it was printed in 1540 as *The byrth of mankynd newly translated out of laten into Englysshe*. Two issues of this, which are identical except for the title-page, appeared in 1540 (STC 21153). The four illustrations in the 1540 edition are believed to be the first copperplate engravings to be printed in a medical book. The engravings contain an illustration of a birth-stool and 17 figures of positions of the foetus *in utero*. The engraving is crude in style and inaccurate, even though the copperplates show a finer detail than the woodcuts of previous editions. In 1545 a new edition appeared of *The byrth of mankynde*... (STC 21154). This contains an extensive prologue by Thomas Raynalde or Raynolde (also the name of the printer), who edited and enlarged the work. The new edition published in 1552 (STC 21155), and subsequent editions, all bore the name of Thomas Raynalde. The book was later taken over by the printers Richard Jugge and John Cawood who, together with their descendants, issued the editions of 1560, several undated issues between 1560 and 1565, two editions dated 1565 (STC 21156–21159) and one of 1588 (printed by Richard Watkins, who had married Jugge's daughter) (STC 21160). The editions of 1604 and 1613 were both printed 'for Thomas Adams' (STC 21161–21162), and those of 1626 and 1634 were both printed 'for A. H.' (STC 21163–21164). The last edition, dated 1654, was printed 'for J[ohn] L[egat], Henry Hood, Abel Roper, and Richard Tomlins'. On the title-page this is called the fourth edition. Rösslin's *Roszgarten* and *The byrth of mankynde* profoundly influenced the practice and art of midwifery for more than three centuries. The popularity and numerous editions of the work have caused it to become of great bibliographical interest, and Sir D'Arcy Power made an exhaustive study of the editions of the book, recording details of the printers and publishers, while J. W. Ballantyne, LeRoy Crummer and E. Ingerslev have written interesting papers on the subject.[68]

Rösslin's *Roszgarten* was used by Jacob Rueff in the preparation of his *De conceptu et generatione hominis*, Zurich, 1554. Rueff (1500–58), a surgeon in Zurich, was responsible for the training of midwives. An edition of his book in German also appeared in 1554: *Trostbüchle von den Empfengknussen und Geburten der Menschen und jren vilfaltigen Zuofälen und Verhindernussen* ..., or 'a comforting booklet of encouragement concerning the conception and birth of man, and its frequent accidents and hindrances ...'. Further editions were printed in 1580 and 1587 at Frankfort. A study has been made by Koelbing of the differences in the Latin and German texts.[69] Rueff's use of Rösslin's *Roszgarten* has been examined by H. L. Houtzager.[70] In many texts, the opinion is adopted that Rueff's *Manual for Midwives* is nothing more than a 'revised edition' of Rösslin's *Der swangern frauwen und hebammen Roszgarten*. The contents of both books, however, overlap only in part. It is of great significance that Rueff for the first time placed emphasis on anatomical knowledge in obstetrics. He therefore writes not only for midwives, but also for surgeons, in whose hands the responsibility for gynaecology was being placed. This was primarily instruction in midwifery, but Rueff's text also regards participation in the birth process itself. The interesting woodcuts in the books of Rösslin and Rueff have been studied by K. B. Roberts.[71] A facsimile of the 1587 edition of Rueff was printed in 1971.[72]

Another important book devoted to obstetrics was that written by Geronimo Scipione Mercurio (1550–1616), a native of Rome, who studied medicine at Bologna and Padua, where he later practised medicine, before proceeding to Milan, and finally to Venice. Mercurio introduced into Italy the operation of Caesarean section on living women, and his *La comare o riccoglitrice* was printed in Venice in 1596, the first two books being dated 1595. There were editions in 1601 and 1606, both printed in Venice, and a total of about 20 editions was published. It was the first Italian book devoted to obstetrics.[73]

In 1541 there died at Salzburg one of the most enigmatic characters in the history of medicine. Described by Garrison as the 'most original thinker of the sixteenth century', by Osler as 'the Luther of medicine', and by Singer as 'alchemist, quack, rebel, prophet, and genius', Paracelsus was, indeed, a most curious combination of vices and virtues. Philippus Aureolus Theophrastus Bombastus von Hohenheim was born at Einsiedeln, near Zurich, in 1493 or, according to Walter Pagel, more probably 1494. He later adopted the name Paracelsus. He took a doctor's degree at Ferrara in 1515 under Leonicenus, and then travelled extensively in Europe and possibly the East, mixing with barbers, gipsies, midwives and quacks, from whom he acquired an extensive knowledge of folk-medicine. Paracelsus became town physician and professor of medicine at Basle in 1527, but his career there was of short duration, firstly because he lectured in German, and secondly because he publicly burned the works of Galen and other classic authors. He continued his travels, always affected by *Wanderlust*. Paracelsus was a successful physician and surgeon, a pioneer of experimental chemistry and chemical medicine.[74] He taught physicians to substitute chemical therapeutics for alchemy, and introduced into the pharmacopœia laudanum (tincture of opium), antimony, lead, copper sulphate, and zinc (which he discovered). Although attacking quackery, his writings are interspersed with astrology and the occult sciences, and this led to the neglect of his work until Karl Sudhoff studied the subject. The latter's writings on Paracelsus enable us to appreciate his true position in the history of medicine, and Sudhoff's bibliography was the first scientific analysis of his editions and manuscripts, being the standard source.[75] Paracelsus had prejudiced his contemporaries by his bombastic bearing, but his work on miners' disease, open wounds, and the use of mercury in syphilis entitle him to recognition as an original thinker.

Paracelsus was a prolific writer, but the dates of issue of the early editions of his works are obscure. Many of his books were not published until after his death, and numerous writings have been falsely attributed to him. Among his works are *Von der frantzösischen Kranckheit*, Nuremberg, 1530; *Der grossen Wundartzney*, Augsburg and also Ulm, 1536; *De Gradibus ...*, 1562; *Das Buch Paramirum*, 1562; and *Chirurgia Magna*, 1572. The first collected edition of the writings of Paracelsus was edited by John Huser and published in ten volumes at Basle, 1589–90, with reprints in 1603–5. Karl Sudhoff edited the *Sämtliche Werke* in fourteen volumes, 1922–3, and a reprint of this commenced publication in 1954. Walter Pagel has contributed a thoroughly documented study of Paracelsus, which also provides a guide to his writings and to biographical studies of him.[76] A more recent study by Pagel places the scientific and medical discoveries of Paracelsus in their philosophical and religious setting.[77]

The sixteenth century saw the development of humanism, with a renewed interest in the achievements of classical antiquity combined with a new insight into human understanding. The Renaissance humanists included Erasmus, John Colet, Sir Thomas More and the scholar–physician Thomas Linacre (1460–1524).[78] Born at Canterbury, Linacre was educated at Padua and Oxford where he graduated MD. He later became tutor to Prince Arthur, eldest son of Henry VII, and, subsequently, Physician to Henry VIII.

While he was in Italy Linacre met Aldus the printer, for whom he later translated Proclus's *De sphera* from the Greek, published in 1499. He is remembered especially for his works on grammar and his part in the foundation of the Royal College of Physicians of London in 1518.

Linacre translated several of Galen's works from Greek into Latin, the following being particularly noteworthy: *De sanitate tuenda*, Paris, 1517, and *Methodus medendi*, Paris, 1519, both of which were dedicated to Henry VIII, and went through several editions; also *De temperamentis*,

Cambridge, 1521,[79] printed by Siberch, and dedicated to Leo X. Linacre also compiled a popular Latin grammar, *De emendata structura Latini sermonis*, printed by Pynson in 1524 after Linacre's death (STC 15634). He deeply influenced current thought and has been called by Osler 'one of the most distinguished of the medical humanists'.[80] An excellent collection of essays on the life and work of Linacre was published in 1977, edited by Francis Maddison, Margaret Pelling and Charles Webster (this includes a detailed bibliographical survey of Linacre's works).[81]

One of the earliest of the French humanists was Symphorien Champier (1472–1539) of Lyons, a medical graduate of Pavia, and physician to Charles VIII and Louis XII. He was a prolific writer, 99 editions of his 55 works having been recorded by James F. Ballard and Michel Pijoan,[82] and many other works have been falsely attributed to him. The following are among his more important contributions to medicine: *Hortus Gallicus*, Lyons, 1533; *De medicinae claris scriptoribus* ..., Lyons, 1506, which is the earliest and best history of medicine of his period; *Vocabulorum medicinalium et terminorum difficilium explanatio*, Lyons, 1508, the first medical dictionary since that of Simone de Cordo; *Rosa Gallica*, Nancy, 1512, Paris, 1514 and 1518; and *Practica nova in medicina*, Lyons, 1517. Champier also wrote biographies of Arnold of Villanova and Mesue, entitled *Arnald de Villanova vita*, Lyons, 1520, Basle, 1525[?], Venice, 1527, and Lyons, 1535; and *Joanis Mesüe Nazareni vita* in *Oeuvres de Mesüe*, Lyons, 1523.[83]

The first significant theory on infection was the contribution of the Renaissance scholar Girolamo Fracastoro (Hieronymus Fracastorius) whose work *De contagione* anticipated the modern germ theory of disease. Fracastoro (1478?–1553) was born in Verona, and was eminent as a poet, physician, astronomer and mathematician.[84] He is best known for the poem which gave the name to syphilis, a disease which had reached epidemic proportions in the sixteenth century. The poem *Syphilis, sive morbus gallicus*, first printed at Verona in 1530, became an outstanding success, of which one hundred editions have been traced.[85] The first two books were probably written between 1510 and 1512, and the third probably added just before the work was printed. It came from the press of Stefano Nicolini da Sabbio, while the second edition, printed by Antonio Blado d'Asola at Rome in 1531 was supervised by Fracastoro, and is the more important edition, containing two lines previously omitted. A complete Italian translation appeared from Naples in 1731, although fragments had previously been published. The poem has been translated into six languages, and there are 15 Italian versions, and seven English. There are 29 Italian editions, 13 English, nine French, six German, one Spanish and one Portuguese, while there are 45 Latin editions (11 in *Opera omnia*), and 22 bilingual editions.[86] The first translation into English was by Nahum Tate, the poet laureate, printed at London in 1686; the first

French translation was published at Paris in 1753, and the first German translation came from Vienna in 1827. This was incomplete, and a full German version did not appear until 1881, being printed at Leipzig. The poem remained popular for centuries, and was translated again into English by W. Van Wyck in 1934.[87] A recent translation was made by G. Eatough in 1984.[88]

Fracastoro's work on infectious diseases was published in Venice in 1546. *De sympathia et antipathia rerum liber unus* and *De contagione et contagiosis morbis et curatione libri iii* show an understanding of the role of living micro-organisms in communicable disease. Fracastoro believed infection to be caused by the passage of minute bodies from the infector to the person infected.[89] *De contagione* also contains an early account of typhus fever. The work was translated by W. Cave Wright.[90] Fracastoro's collected works appeared as *Opera omnia ...*, Venice, 1555, and numerous editions were published.

The development of Renaissance physiology was stimulated by the work of Jean Fernel (1497–1558) who has been called 'the greatest physician of the Renaissance'. A remarkable study of him was made by Sir Charles Sherrington, whose reconstruction of the life and achievements of Jean Fernel includes a bibliography of his writings, and stresses the value of the scholarly contributions of the man who gave the name 'physiology' to the subject.[91] Jean Fernel was born in 1497, and in 1516 entered the Collège de Ste Barbe of the University of Paris. Here he obtained the MA degree, and in 1526 was lecturing on philosophy. He was also keenly interested in mathematics, his first book describing a kind of astrolobe he had devised. This was *Monalosphaerium ..*, Paris, 1527,[92] which was accompanied by an album of plates, but of which no copy is known (Sherrington, p.15). The following year appeared his *Cosmotheoria ...*, Paris, 1527,[93] which dealt with the size and shape of the earth, and the same year Fernel published *De proportionibus ...*, also accompanied by a volume of plates. After obtaining the degree of MD in 1530, Fernel settled in Paris, but he appears still to have studied astronomy, and designed several instruments for the purpose. He later devoted himself entirely to medicine, and in 1536 began teaching that subject in the Collège de Cornouailles.

Fernel was a precise, orderly thinker and writer, who preferred to observe for himself and to draw conclusions from his own observations. This is reflected in his work on physiology, which was to become the standard book on the subject for over a century. It was entitled *De naturali parte medicinae ...*, Paris, 1542, of which it is believed only two copies exist outside France (one is in the Hunterian Library, Glasgow). Other editions were printed at Venice, 1547, and Lyons, 1551, while it was reissued in 1554 as part of his *Medicina*. In this work Fernel rejected all magic and superstition as irrelevant to the study of bodily functions, and clearly stated that anatomy shows only the location and not the nature of these processes. Among Fernel's other printed works are *De vacuandi ratione* ..., Paris, 1545; Lyons, 1548; Venice, 1548 and 1549; and Lyons, 1549; *De abditis rerum causis* ..., Paris, 1548, which Fernel had referred to in his previous writings as the 'Dialogues', and which had circulated in manuscript for many years. This was also printed in Venice, 1550; Paris, 1551 and 1560, and was later included in his other works. Fernel's *Medicina* was first printed in Paris, 1554, editions following from Venice, 1555 and 1566–67 (in two volumes); Lyons, 1564; Leyden, 1728; and Paris, 1879. He died on 26 April 1558, and posthumous publications include his *Opera medicinalia*, Venice, 1565 and 1566, and his *Universa medicina* ..., Paris, 1567, of which many other editions appeared. There are several other books by Fernel, or attributed to him, some of which are very rare. Jean Fernel's writings on physiology, pathology and therapeutics indicate a distinct advancement as the result of his labours,[94] while his mathematical and astronomical researches are of significant value in the history of those subjects.

Important precursors of Harvey's great work on the circulation appeared in the sixteenth century, with Michael Servetus and Realdo Colombo who both described the lesser circulation through the lungs. Realdo Colombo described the pulmonary circulation in *De re anatomica* (published posthumously at Venice in 1559) and Harvey's notes, in 1616, acknowledge his contribution. Book XV of *De re anatomica* was translated by R. J. Moes and C. D. O'Malley.[95] A Latin translation of the work of an Arabian writer, Ibn an-Nafis (1210–88), was published in 1547, and this includes the earliest known description of the lesser circulation.[96] Singer and Underwood have written of the rival claims:

> Colombo was possibly teaching these views [on pulmonary circulation] as early as 1546. His work is superior to that of Servetus, which may have been an inspired guess. Both may have had the same idea; or either may have been influenced by the ideas of the other; or either or both may have heard of the views of Ibn an-Nafis. For over twenty years it has been known that Colombo may have had indirect contact with a translation of the works of Ibn an-Nafis.[97]

Michael Servetus (1511–53), a Spanish theologian and physician, was born at Vilanova de Xixena, now Villanueva de Sigena, but when going under the name of Michael Villanovanus he stated that he had been born in Tudela, Navarra.[98] He graduated at Paris (having studied with Fernel and Sylvius), becoming a lecturer there, and first came into conflict with the theologians on the publication of *De Trinitatis erroribus* [Hagenau], 1531. A spurious edition was issued [Regensburg, 1721?]; a Dutch translation appeared [Amsterdam], 1620; and an English translation by Earl Morse Wilbur was published in *The two treatises of Servetus on the Trinity*, Cambridge, Mass., 1932,[99] the other treatise being *Dialogorum de*

Trinitate libri duo, first printed in [Hagenau], 1532, with later printings and translations as for *De Trinitatis erroribus*.

Servetus's account of the blood in the pulmonary circulation passing into the heart, after having been mixed with air in the lungs, is recorded in his *Christianismi restitutio*[100] on pages 168–73. For the heretical doctrines expressed in the book Calvin had Servetus burned at the stake in Geneva a few months later. *Christianismi restitutio* was first printed secretly at Vienna in 1553, but had been circulated in manuscript in 1546.[101] One thousand copies were printed, but most were burnt, only three copies surviving. One, formerly belonging to Richard Mead, is in the Bibliothè-que Nationale, Paris; a second is in the Imperial Library, Vienna (formerly in the possession of a Hungarian, Markos Szent Ivanyi, who was living in London in 1665); and the third is in the University Library, Edinburgh (this copy has the title-page and first sixteen pages missing, and is said to be the copy sent to Calvin).

Fragments of *Christianismi restitutio* were printed in 1569 [London, 1723] and a Polish fragment [Pińczów, 1568?]. A German translation in three volumes was published in Wiesbaden, 1892–6, with a second edition of volume one in 1895. It has been asserted that Richard Mead was responsible for a reprint undertaken in London in 1723, but this was actually for a Dutchman, Gysbert Dummer. After 250 pages had been printed the sheets were confiscated, but Mead was not directly implicated. This imperfect London reprint is very rare, there being two copies in the British Library, one in the Medical Society of London, a set of proofs in the Bodleian, and a copy in the Bibliothèque Nationale, which originally came from Mead's library, and has a transcript of the rest of the book appended.[102] A Nuremberg reprint made in 1790 for C. G. von Murr is sometimes wrongly given the date 1791, but the year 1790 is printed in very small type at the end of the book, which might otherwise be mistaken for the original issue, it being a page-for-page facsimile reprint. On page 170 is found a description of the pulmonary circulation (see also p.13). Servetus was the author or editor of the following items, of which a bibliography has been compiled by Madeline E. Stanton:[103] *In Leonardum Fuchsium apologia* [Lyons], 1536, with a facsimile edition from Oxford, 1909, and an English translation by C. D. O'Malley with certain other of his writings;[104] a revision of Ptolemy's *Geography*, Lyons, 1535 and 1541, with a Spanish translation, Madrid, 1932; *Syruporum universa ratio* …, Paris, 1537, Venice, 1545, Lyons, 1546, Lyons 1547, Lyons, 1548, and possibly another edition from Venice, 1548. A Spanish translation was published in Madrid in 1943, and an English translation by C. D. O'Mal-ley in 1953 in his collection which also includes *Disceptatio pro astrologia*. This was first printed in [Paris, 1538], and reprinted in Berlin, 1880. Servetus also edited *Biblia sacra* …, Lyons, 1542, in both folio and octavo editions, with a seven-volume edition from Lyons in 1545. The execution of Michael Servetus is a tragic instance of man's inhumanity to man. Undoubtedly this remarkable Spaniard was a bold, original thinker and his untimely death destroyed a potentially brilliant career.[105]

The new anatomical knowledge acquired by Renaissance artists and anatomists was applied to surgery by Ambroise Paré, a French military surgeon, who served in the civil and religious wars of the period. Paré (1510–90) was born in Laval, France, and became a dresser at the Hôtel Dieu in Paris. He began his service career in 1536 and followed the French armies in France, Flanders, Italy and Germany during the greater part of the next 40 years. He was successively surgeon to Henry II, Francis II, Charles IX and Henry III.

Paré's contributions to surgery included the introduction of artificial limbs, the reintroduction of the ligature, the abandonment of cauterization with boiling oil as treatment for gunshot wounds, and the invention of many surgical instruments. Paré was looked upon with some disfavour by the 'qualified' surgeons because of his ignorance of Latin. However this did not prevent him from questioning the causes of illness and carefully observing the results of his treatments.

It was during his first campaign, in 1536, that Paré discovered that cauterization with boiling oil was not a necessary treatment for gunshot wounds. Surgeons believed that the wounds were poisoned burns which needed to be counteracted by dressing with boiling oil.[106] After the French troops had captured the castle of Villaine, Paré treated the wounded in the usual manner, but he did not have sufficient oil to treat all the injuries:

> Now because there were some few left to be dressed, I was forced ... to apply a digestive made of the yolk of an egg, oil of roses, and turpentine. I could not sleep all that night ... Therefore I rose early in the morning. I visited my patients, and beyond expectation, I found such as I had dressed with a digestive only, free from vehemence of pain, to have had good rest, and that their wounds were not inflamed, nor tumified; but on the contrary the others that were burnt with the scalding oil were feverish, tormented with much pain, and the parts about their wounds were swollen.[107] (*Apologie et Treatise*).

The first book written by Ambroise Paré dealt with the treatment of gunshot wounds, being *La méthode de traicter les playes faictes par hacquebutes et aultres bastons à feu* ..., Paris, 1545, of which a second enlarged edition appeared dated 1551 and 1552, with the title *La manière de traicter les playes* ..., Paris. The 1545 edition was translated into Dutch in 1547, one copy only of which survives, in the University of Ghent, and the 1551 edition was similarly translated in 1556. The English translation by Walter Hamond entitled *The method of curing wounds made by gun-shot* ..., London, 1617 (STC 19191) is also very rare, the only known copy being in the Bodleian Library.[108] Paré's *Briefve collection de l'administration anatomique* ... was published in Paris in 1549 and reissued in 1550. It was enlarged and rewritten as *Anatomie universelle du corps humain* ...,

Paris, 1561. The same year appeared his work on the head, *La méthode curative des playes, et fractures de la teste humaine. Avec les pourtraits des instruments nécessaires pour la curation d'icelles*, Paris. In 1564 this was followed by *Dix livres de la chirurgie avec le magasin des instrumens nécessaires à icelle*, Paris, which also contained Paré's treatise on gunshot wounds. A translation by R. W. Linker and N. Womack appeared in 1969.[109] An interesting variant in one of the woodcuts appears in *Dix livres de la chirurgie*.[110]

One of Paré's best works was *Traicté de la peste, de la petite verolle et de rougeolle: avec une brefve description de la lepre*, Paris, 1568, which was reissued with a new title-page in 1580, and translated into English as *A treatise of the plague ...*, London, 1630, the translation probably being the work of Thomas Johnson (STC 19192). An Italian translation was published at Bologna in 1720. Paré's *Cinq livres de chirurgerie ...*, Paris, 1571 and 1572, is his most important book. No copy of the 1571 edition is known. His *Deux livres de chirurgerie ...*, Paris, 1573, was written for students. In 1575 appeared his *Oeuvres ...*, Paris, in a splendid folio. A second edition was published in 1579, but there was no third French edition; a Latin translation appeared in 1582, which is considered the finest of all. The fourth edition of 1583, which was reprinted in facsimile in 1962 (Lyons), is the best French edition, and Paré revised the fifth, which was published in 1598 (after his death). Editions followed in 1607, 1614 and the eighth in 1628, the last of the Paris editions. Then followed those with Lyons imprints, all of which were badly printed, becoming worse with each edition, these being dated 1633, 1641, 1652, 1664 and the thirteenth edition, 1685. The next was J. F. Malgaigne's edition of Paré's *Oeuvres complètes*, in three volumes, 1840–1. Thomas Johnson published an English translation from the Latin edition in 1634 (STC 19189), there being four other English printings, in 1649, 1665, 1678 and 1691 respectively. A German translation appeared from Frankfort-on-Main in 1601, and a Dutch translation from Amsterdam in 1636. It was also published in Japanese. Paré issued several other works, including numerous replies to his critics, and many extracts from his works have been printed.[111] He wrote a book on mummies and unicorn's horn, entitled *Discours ... à scavoir de la mumie, de la licorne, des venins, et de la peste ...*, Paris, 1582, and a book on monsters and marvels, *Des monstres et prodiges*, which has been translated by J. L. Pallister.[112] Geoffrey Keynes has written of Paré's contributions to surgery:

> He was, by virtue of his personality and his independent mind, the emancipator of surgery ... There was no comparable practitioner, during his time, in England or any other country, and his influence was felt in every part of Europe. He left in his collected works a monument to his own skill and humanity which is unsurpassed in the history of surgery.[113]

For Ambroise Paré the foundation of the healing art was love of his fellow men. His kindness and compassion is revealed to us in the famous aphorism which appears many times in his writings: 'Je le pansais, Dieu le guérit.' (I dressed him, and God healed him.)[114]

The curious conflict which existed during the Renaissance between progressiveness and the cult of antiquity is reflected in the literature. The humanists continued to edit the Greek texts of ancient medical authorities, and the students and practitioners who did not read Greek provided a ready market for new Latin translations. Works in the vernacular were also well established by the middle of the century, with the publication of books for surgeons, midwives and laymen. The publishers particularly aimed their books at surgeons and midwives, who, because they had no knowledge of Latin, had previously had to learn simply by following tradition and example.[115] In a study made by P. Slack[116] it has been possible to identify 153 medical titles published in the vernacular in England before 1605. Sir Thomas Elyot defended his use of the vernacular in his manual of domestic medicine *The Castel of Helth ...*, London, 1541: 'If phisitions be angry that I haue wryten phisike in englyshe, let theym remembre that the grekes wrate in greke, the Romanes in latyne, Auicena and the other in Arabike, whiche were their owne propre and maternal tonges'.[117]

The first English anatomy printed in the vernacular was *The Englisheman's Treasure* by Thomas Vicary, a work which has aroused controversy concerning its origins. Thomas Vicary (*c*.1490–1561/2) was in practice in Maidstone when he was called to treat Henry VIII who was on a Royal Progress through Kent. The King was troubled with his 'sorre leg', which Vicary successfully treated. In gratitude, the King appointed Vicary his surgeon and in 1536 he became Sergeant Surgeon to the King, an office which he also held under King Edward VI, Queen Mary and Queen Elizabeth. Vicary undoubtedly influenced the King to organize the profession of surgery by combining the Company of Barbers with the Guild of Surgeons. The presentation of the Charter to Vicary by Henry VIII is depicted in Holbein's famous painting. In 1541 Vicary was elected Master of the Company, an office he held on three further occasions.

It has been suggested that Vicary published a first edition of *A treasure for Englishmen containing the anatomie of man's body* in London, 1548, but no copy of this has survived. The evidence for its existence is based upon a comment of John Halle (1529?–68) in his *Anatomy or dissection of the body of man*, published in 1565. Vicary's work was not original in any respect, being derived from Henri de Mondeville and Lanfranc, and was not an accurate reflection of contemporary anatomy. The surgeons of Vicary's hospital, St Bartholomew's, published (after his death) *A profitable treatise of the anatomie of man's body*, London, 1577, only two copies of this work now being extant, in the British Library and the University Library,

Cambridge. The book appeared with numerous alterations and additions from various publishers, and with several changes of title. It was printed in London with the title *The English-man's treasure; with the true anatomy of mans bodie*, in 1586 (STC 24707), 1587 (STC 24708), 1596 (STC 24709), 1599 (STC 24709.5) (only recorded copy in the National Library of Medicine, Bethesda), 1613 (STC 24710), 1626 (STC 24711), 1633 (STC 24712), 1641 and 1651. This 1651 edition bears the title *The surgions directorie for young practitioners*, but is not a separate work. The Early English Text Society published the text in 1888, edited by F. J. and Percy Furnivall, and it was reprinted in 1930. D. P. Thomas has contributed an unpublished invaluable study of Vicary's life and times, with particular emphasis on the bibliographical aspects of his book.[118] Although much controversy still surrounds Vicary's works, there can be no doubt about his devotion to the 'sick pore' and the value of his contribution to the craft of surgery.

Thomas Gale (1507–87) was a military surgeon who later practised in London. His works are remarkable for their sound practical teaching and marked a turning-point in English surgery which was now basing itself on first-hand experience. His printed works include *Certaine workes of chirurgerie ...*, London, 1563 (STC 11529), which contains *An excellent treatise of wounds made with gunneshot*, 1563, *An institution of a chirurgean* and *An enchiridion of chirurgerie ...*, all bound together, but they were also issued separately.[119] This was followed by a second edition in 1586 (STC 11529a) but a second volume of the first edition had been printed in 1567, the only copy traced being in the National Library of Medicine, Bethesda. The title-page is mutilated, but it probably read *The [second part of the] institucion of chyrurgerie: newly published by Thomas Gale, master in surgerie* (STC 11530.5).[120] Gale also wrote *An antidotarie conteyning hidde and secrete medicines, simple and compounde, as also all suche as are required in chirurgerie*, London, 1563, but the history of his treatises and collected works is complicated and requires careful investigation, as the known copies vary considerably.

Gale was succeeded by William Clowes (1544–1604), 'the greatest Elizabethan surgeon'. Clowes possessed wide practical knowledge of military and naval surgery. He was appointed surgeon to Queen Elizabeth in 1596, and served in the fleet which defeated the Spanish Armada. With years of experience in the Navy he was expert in treating the injuries and wounds of men on active service.

Clowes was also a specialist in syphilis and in 1576 he published a book on the subject, but no copies of this edition have survived. A new edition published in 1579 had the title *A short and profitable treatise touching the cure of the disease called (morbus gallicus) by unctions*, London. The book was again printed in 1585 with the title *A briefe and necessarie treatise touching the cure of the disease called morbus gallicus, or lues venerea ...*

(STC 5447–8) It was later published as pages 145–229 of his *A profitable and necessarie booke of observations*, but with a separate title-page, in 1596 (STC 5445.5), and was once more reprinted in a 'third edition' in 1637 (STC 5445.7) as *A profitable and necessarie booke of observations, for all those that are burned with the flame of gun-powder* ... A facsimile of the 1596 edition was published in 1945 by de Witt T. Starnes and C. D. Leake.[121] The chief value of this work on syphilis was the detailed description of mercurial treatment, which remained the only useful remedy against the disease until this century.

Clowes' *Profitable and necessarie booke* was also a useful book on wounds, of which the first edition was issued in 1588 (STC 5444)[122] under the title *A prooved practice for all young chirurgians concerning burnings with gun-powder and wounds made with gunshot, sword, halbard, pike, launce, or such other* ... This was reissued in London, 1591 (STC 5445). The 1596 edition mentioned above includes the first description in the English language of the ligation of arteries (Chapter VIII). Clowes acknowledges the work of Jacques Guillemeau, and gives his own description of the procedure.

Clowes also wrote a book on struma (scrofula) or the King's evil, entitled *A right frutefull and approoved treatise, for the artificial cure of that malady called in Latin struma, and in English the evill cured by kinges and queenes of England. Very necessary for all young practizers of chyrurgery*, London, 1602 (STC 5446). This book discusses the disease, for the first time, from a medical standpoint.[123] Copies of Clowes' books are rare, but a selection from his writings was edited by F. N. L. Poynter in 1948.[124]

Peter Lowe (1552–1612), a Scottish army surgeon, wrote the first student surgical textbook in English. Lowe practised in France and Flanders for 22 years before returning to Scotland, where he founded the Faculty of Physicians and Surgeons of Glasgow in 1599 – a considerable achievement after centuries of separation of physicians and surgeons. Lowe made the first English translation of Hippocrates in 1597, but his *Whole course of chirurgerie*, which went through four editions, was his most popular work, being a students' textbook, written partly in the form of a catechism. The book differs from those of Gale and Clowes because it is written for the use of students who were to be examined in surgery, while Lowe's predecessors had written for surgeons already in practice. The first edition of 1597 (STC 16869.5) is not illustrated but the later editions contain woodcuts, and are much enlarged. The second edition is entitled *A discours of the whole art of chyrurgerie* ..., London, [1612] (STC 16870), the third edition appeared in 1634 (STC 16871), and the fourth in 1654.[125]

William Bullein (c.1515–76) was born on the Isle of Ely, but little is known of his life except that it was an adventurous one, as judged from his writings. These are fascinating popular works, entertainingly written, containing many personal anecdotes, and representing fine examples of

Elizabethan prose. Among his books must be noted *A newe booke, entitled the governement of healthe, wherein is uttered manye notable rules for mannes preservacion* ..., London, 1558 (STC 4039), of which a corrected edition entitled *A new booke of physick* was published in the same year (STC 4040), with others in 1559 (STC 4041) and 1595 (STC 4042). *Bulleins bulwarke of defence againste all sicknes, sornes, and woundes* ..., 1562 (STC 4033) and 1579 (STC 4034), consists of four separate treatises, separately foliated and bearing different dates.[126] The *Bulwarke* was written while Bullein was in prison, and was inspired by Sir Thomas Elyot's *Castle of Health* (1539). Another popular work of his was *A comfortable regiment and a very wholesome order against the most perilous pleurisi* ..., 1562.

Bullein's most successful work was written after an outbreak of plague in 1563: *A dialogue bothe pleasaunte and pietifull, wherin is a goodly regiment against the fever pestilence* ..., 1564 (STC 4036), with later editions in 1569, 1573 (STC 4037) and 1579 (STC 4038). This *Dialogue*, edited by Mark W. Bullen and A. H. Bullen, was also published in 1888 by the Early English Text Society. Another work doubtfully attributed to Bullein was *A brief discourse of vertue and operations of balsome and diet for healthe*, 1585.[127] In 1946 a bookseller advertised a copy of Bullein's *Bulwarke of defence*, 1562, containing marginal notes believed to be in the handwriting of the author,[128] and a copy of the same book, bound for the author, is now in the Houghton Library, Harvard University.[129] Bullein's works are noteworthy as popular handbooks of medical advice for laymen but his primary importance undoubtedly lay in his early awareness of continental medical innovation, especially in iatrochemistry.[130]

John Caius (1510–73), born John Key or Kaye in Norwich in 1510, was a man of many talents: humanist and man of culture, writer of books of wide interests, President of the Royal College of Physicians and physician to Henry VIII, Edward VI, Mary Tudor and Elizabeth I. He also found time to lecture on anatomy for 20 years.[131] Caius was taught by Joannes Baptista Montanus and Paulus Crassus, among others, and had shared a house with Vesalius at Padua.[132] Caius was, however, a staunch Galenist, despite his personal acquaintanceship with Vesalius, and he edited certain of Galen's writings for publication. An interesting study has been made by V. Nutton of Caius's notes and annotations in the Eton Galen.[133]

Caius returned to England in 1544 and became physician to Henry VIII. He introduced the study of practical anatomy into England, and lectured and demonstrated to surgeons. In 1564, just after Caius's second period as President, and probably at his instance, the College obtained from Queen Elizabeth a charter which allowed the public dissection of four bodies annually.

Caius wrote *De medendi methodo libri duo* ..., Basle, 1544, and *A boke or counseill against the disease commonly called the sweate or sweatying sicknesse*, London, 1552 (STC 4343), the first book to be published in this country describing a single disease in detail.[134] The sweating sickness remains a mystery but was clearly a well-defined epidemic disease which struck Britain on five occasions between 1485 and 1551. A facsimile edition of the *Sweatyng sicknesse*, edited by Archibald Malloch, was published in 1937. Also written by Caius was a work on dogs, *De canibus Britannicis*, London, 1570. This was based on notes sent by Caius to Gesner for his *Historiae animalium* but Gesner died before using the material, and Caius published it himself. In 1556 appeared an alleged translation by Abraham Fleming as *Of Englishe dogges* (STC 4347), but it was actually based on Caius's work, and was chiefly the material of Fleming.[135] An authentic translation is contained in a book by E. C. Ash.[136] Caius's works were reprinted in 1912, with a memoir of his life by John Venn. Caius is today best remembered for his endowment of Gonville Hall, later known as Gonville and Caius College.[137]

A neglected figure in Tudor medicine is Andrew Boorde (Borde or Boarde) (*c*.1490–1549) who wrote two popular works on family medicine. Born about 1490 at Boorde's Hill, near Cuckfield, in Sussex, h᾿ became a priest, physician and traveller. Boorde first entered a Carthusian monastery but left the religious life to study medicine at Montpellier. He returned to England and later went on a pilgrimage to Spain. It was during a fourth tour of the Continent, while again at Montpellier, that he wrote his *Fyrst boke or the introduction of knowledge*, which is believed to be the first guide-book to the Continent written in English and printed in England. It was printed in [1548] (STC 3383); 1555 (STC 3384), and [1562?] (STC 3385). His handbook of domestic medicine, the first medical book by a medical man to be originally written and printed in English, was entitled *Breviary of healthe*, 1547 (STC 3373.5) and further editions were published in 1552 (STC 3374), 1557 (STC 3374.5), 1575 (STC 3376), 1587 (STC 3377) and 1598 (STC 3378). It is arranged alphabetically (from Abstinence to Zirbus), consisting of 384 short chapters, with an appendix called 'The second booke', of 73 chapters. Among other writings Boorde published his *Compendyous regyment, or a dyetary of helth made in Montpyllor*, [1542?] (STC 3378.5); 1564 (STC 3378.7); 1567 [1547] (STC 3380); 1562 (STC 3381); and 1576 (STC 3382). This work contains much sound advice on diet for the healthy and the sick.

The *Breviary* and *Dyetary* are pioneer works in family medicine and convincing evidence that Boorde was not the 'buffoon' of reputation but a shrewd and sensible physician who held views far in advance of his time. He was a happy and good-natured man who appears to have taken as his motto his oft-quoted remark that 'Myrth is one of the chiefest thynges in physicke.'[138]

Felix Platter (Plater, Platerus) (1536–1614) was a member of a famous Swiss medical family, and went to Montpellier in 1552, keeping a diary of his travels. He persuaded his father, Thomas, to write his autobiography, which was completed in 1572 when he was seventy-three, and also caused the younger Thomas to keep a journal when he went to Montpellier in 1595. Thomas the elder had remarried at the age of seventy-three and had six more children, the eldest of these being Thomas the younger (born 1574), who was brought up by Felix, his half-brother. English versions of the journals of Felix and of Thomas have been published, and contain further information and references on the family.[139] Felix Platter was the author of *De corporis humani structura et usa*, Basle, 1583; *Praxeos, seu de cognoscendis, praedicendis, praecavendis curandisque affectibus homini incommodanibus. Tractatus tres*, Basle, 1602–8, which was translated into English as *A golden practice of physick ... By Felix Plater, R. W., Abdiah Cole, Nich. Culpeper*, London, 1662; and *Observationum in hominis affectibus plerisque ... libri tres*, Basle, 1614, which is said to contain the first account of meningioma,[140] and was translated as *Platerus. Histories and observations upon diseases offending the body and mind; hurt of functions, pain or troubles and infirmities: in three books ... By Felix Plater, Nich. Culpeper, Abdiah Cole*, London, 1664. Both these English translations are rare.[141] A German translation of Book I by Günther Goldschmidt has been edited by H. Buess.[142]

Without attempting to name every prominent person connected with sixteenth-century medicine it is impossible to omit certain others who contributed through their writings to the history of their craft. François Rabelais (1494–1553) is better remembered for his literary work, and it is not generally known that he was professor of pathology at Montpellier, and later attached to the Lyons Hospital. Rabelais translated Hippocrates's *Aphorisms* into Latin, and was also prominent in the advancement of medical education.[143]

The medical references in Shakespeare's plays are the fascinating subject of a book by R. R. Simpson. Shakespeare's knowledge of Elizabethan medicine is examined, together with the possible role of his son-in-law, the physician John Hall, in providing medical material for the plays.[144]

The scientific revolution of the Renaissance saw the subdivision of medicine into specialized subjects – infectious diseases with the work of Girolamo Fracastoro (see pp. 58–9 above), plastic surgery with Gaspare Tagliacozzi, dermatology with Girolamo Mercuriale, paediatrics with Thomas Phaire, and psychiatry with Timothy Bright.

An outstanding pioneer of plastic surgery was Gaspare Tagliacozzi (1545–99) of Bologna, who revived the operation of rhinoplasty and introduced his own methods. His surgery involved skin grafts for the remodelling and repair of the nose, ears and lips, but this work was strongly opposed by the Church, and denounced by other surgeons. Tagliacozzi wrote the first book devoted to reconstructive surgery, *De curtorum chirurgia per insitionem* ... Much of this was in manuscript form as early as 1586, and was printed by Gasparo Bindoni in Venice in 1597. A pirated edition was issued by Roberto Meietti in the same year, but is on cheaper paper, with smaller type, and is generally much inferior. Editions were printed in Frankfort, 1598, and Berlin, 1831, and a complete reprint appeared in J. J. Manget's *Bibliotheca chirurgica*, volume one, pages 333–485. No complete translation into English has been published, but a summary of Book II appeared in Alexander Read's *Chirurgorum comes* ..., London, 1687, and is reproduced in Martha T. Gnudi and Jerome P. Webster's well-documented biographical study of Tagliacozzi.[145]

Diseases of the skin became a specialist discipline,[146] and the first treatise on the subject was written by Girolamo Mercuriale (1530–1606): *De morbis cutaneis*, Venice, 1572. Mercuriale also produced a treatise on medical gymnastics, *Artis gymnasticae* ..., Venice, 1569, which went to six editions. Effective woodcut illustrations were introduced in the second edition, 1573. It was the first book dealing with the relationship between medicine, sport and the role of exercise.[147]

The first book written in English on paediatrics was by Thomas Phaire (Phaer, Faer, Phyre, Phayer, etc.) (*c*.1510–60). It examines forty diseases and their 'remedyes', which are mainly herbal. Phaire was probably born at Norwich, and was educated at Oxford, before studying law. After practising medicine for twenty years, he took the BM and then MD Oxford. Phaire's work, *The boke of children*, was first published in 1545 as an addition to *The regiment of life*, which he had translated from a French version of *Regimen sanitatis Salerni*, and went into later editions in 1550, 1553, 1560, 1565, 1567, 1570 and 1596 (STC 11967–11976). The 1553 edition was published in London as *The regiment of life, whereunto is added a treatise of the pestilence, with the Boke of children, newly corrected and enlarged by Thomas Phaire*,[148] and the section devoted to paediatrics was reprinted in 1955.[149]

The first book on psychiatry in English, *A Treatise of Melancholie*, was written by Timothy Bright (1550–1615), who studied medicine at Cambridge, and later practised there. He wrote *A treatise: wherein is declared the sufficiencie of English medicines, for cure of all diseases, cured with medicine*, London, 1580 (two issues) (STC 3750–3751) which was reprinted in 1615 with the addition of *A collection of medicines, growing (for the most part) within our English climat* ... Only the initials 'T. B.' appear in this book. In 1582 Bright wrote *Hygieina, id est de sanitate tuenda* ..., London, 1582 (STC 3744) with a second part *Medicinae therapeuticae pars prima* ..., London, 1583 (STC 3746). These were also printed in Frankfort, 1589 and 1598, and in Mainz, 1647. His *In physicam Gulielmi Adolphi Scribonii* ..., Cambridge, 1584 (STC 3745) is very rare, and was reprinted in Frankfort in 1593 (and possibly in 1587). Bright became physician to St Bartholomew's Hospital, London in 1585, and while there produced his famous *Treatise of melancholie* ..., 1586 (STC 3747), of which there were two printings, one by Thomas Vautrollier and the other by John Windet. A third edition was published in 1613, all of these being rare. A facsimile of the first edition was printed for the Facsimile Text Society in New York. Bright explained in his *Treatise of melancholie* the causes and reasons of the strange effects that melancholy works in minds and bodies, and promised 'physick cure, and spiritual consolation' for those in need of treatment. This book was read and quoted by Robert Burton, author of *Anatomy of melancholy*, 1621, and was also probably used by Shakespeare, in particular for the melancholy of Hamlet.[150]

Bright's method of shorthand was published as *Characterie. An arte of shorte, swifte, and secrete writing by character*, London, 1888 (STC 3743), few copies of which survive. A type-facsimile reprint issued in 1888 was limited to one hundred copies. Bright was twice warned for neglecting his patients at St Bartholomew's Hospital, and finally was dismissed. He took up the living at Methley, in Yorkshire, and also published *An abridgement of the booke of acts and monumentes of the Church ...* (STC 11229) by John Fox, London, 1589. A manuscript of 28 leaves, bound in vellum and written by Bright, was found in the Bodleian Library. Entitled 'De clandestino scripto methodica tractation ...', and dated 1587, it is a summary of the second and third books of Giovanni Battista della Porta's *De furtivis literarum notis, vulgo de ziferis*, Naples, 1563, dealing with secret writing.[151] Sir Geoffrey Keynes produced a study of the life of Bright, with a bibliography of his writings, from which the above is derived.[152]

On the continent Wilhelm Fabry of Hilden (Guilhelmus Fabricius Hildanus) (1560–1634) continued Paré's work and introduced the method of amputation above the gangrenous area in a limb. His principal surgical writings are arranged in the form of case records. Fabricius went to school at Cologne, but had no university education, and was apprenticed to a surgeon in 1576. He travelled widely in France, Germany and Switzerland, and died at Berne on 15 February 1634. He was the author of *De gangraena et sphacelo ...*, Cologne, 1593, which was published in later editions and translations in Geneva, 1598 (Latin) and 1669 (French); Lyons, 1598, 1658 and 1696; Basle, 1598, 1600, 1603 and 1615; and Oppenheim, 1617. His *Observationum et curationum chirurgicarum XXV*, Oppenheim, 1598, contained his first 25 observations, which were then included in a volume containing 100 observations printed in Basle, 1606. A second hundred observations were published in Geneva and Basle, 1611; a third from Oppenheim and Basle, 1614; a fourth, Basle, 1619; a fifth, Frankfort, 1627; and a sixth printed in Lyons, 1641, and Flensburg, 1780–3. These were published together as *Observationum et curationum nunc simul in unum opus congestae ...*, two volumes, Lyons, 1641, which was translated into Dutch, Rotterdam, 1656; into French, Geneva, 1669; and into German, Leipzig, 1914. After his death appeared *Opera observationum et curationum medico-chirurgicarum quae extant omnia* from Frankfort, 1646, with a German translation by Friedrich Greiffen with the title *Wundartzney*, Frankfort, 1652, and a further Latin edition, also from Frankfort, 1682.

Fabricius wrote *Traité de la dysenterie*, Payerne, 1602, which was translated into Latin, Oppenheim, 1610, and into German, 1616. His *Epistolarum ad amicos ... centuria prima* was published at Oppenheim in 1619. This was followed by his classic treatise on stone, *Lithotomia vesicae*, published in Basle, 1626 (German) and 1628 (Latin), with an English translation from London in 1640. His *Von geschossenen Wunden*, Basle, 1615, was followed by his description of a medical field chest, *Cista militaris*, Geneva, 1633; Basle, 1634; a Dutch translation, Amsterdam, 1664; and an English translation from London in 1674 and 1686. *Anatomia praestantia et utilitas*, Berne, 1624, was written in German, and a second edition in that language was prepared by Fabricius, but he died before it was published. It was eventually issued as *Von der Furtrefflichkeit und Nutz der Anatomy*, Berlin, 1936, edited by F. de Quervain and Hans Bloesch. Fabricius also wrote on burns, *De combustionibus*, Basle, 1607, and Oppenheim 1614; with a Dutch translation from Amsterdam, 1634; and an English translation by John Steer from London in 1643. Also on mineral baths, *De conservanda valetudine*, Frankfort, 1629 and 1655. His collected writings appeared as *Opera omnia ...*, Frankfort-on-Main, 1682.[153]

Although printing was invented in the middle of the fifteenth century, it did not become established in the New World until the sixteenth century. The first American medical printed book was Francisco Bravo's *Opera medicinalia*, printed in Mexico in 1570. It is in four books, being written in Latin, and is very rare, three copies only being known. Other important medical works of the same century published in America include *Summa y recopilacion de cirugia* by Alphonso Lopez de Hinozoso, published in 1578 (second edition, 1595), and the *Tracto breve de medicina* of Fray Agustin Farfán, 1592, both printed in the city of Mexico. Farfán's *Tractado brebe de anothomia y chirurgia*, the first text on anatomy in America, was published in 1579.[154]

Works of a more general nature that are of particular use in studying sixteenth-century medical literature are Conrad Gesner's monumental *Bibliotheca universalis ...*, Zurich, 1545–9; A. Hahn and P. Dumaître, *Histoire de la médecine et du livre médical*, Paris, 1962; William Osler, *Bibliotheca Osleriana*, Montreal and London, 1969; and two catalogues of the Wellcome Institute for the History of Medicine: *A catalogue of printed books, Vol. I, Books printed before 1641*, edited by F. N. L. Poynter, London, 1962; and the *Subject catalogue of the history of medicine and related sciences*, London, New York, 1980, 18 vols.

The sixteenth century was marked by a revival of learning and a Renaissance of art. This period was distinguished by intellectual perception, freedom of thought and artistic gifts – an ideal foundation for the growth of medical science and its literature and illustration.

Acknowledgements I am grateful to John Thornton, David Bird and Richard Palmer for their expert advice.

Notes

1. Eisenstein, E., *The printing press as an agent of change*, 2 vols, (Cambridge, 1979); Eamon, W., 'Arcana disclosed: the advent of printing, the books of secrets tradition and the development of experimental science in the sixteenth century', *Hist. Sci.*, 22 (1984) pp.111–50.
2. Durling, R.J. (comp.), *A catalogue of sixteenth century books in the National Library of Medicine* (Bethesda, 1967); Supplement, compiled by P. Krivatsky: *A catalogue of incunabula and sixteenth century printed books in the National Library of Medicine*, Bethesda, 1971; Bird, D. T. (comp.), *A catalogue of sixteenth-century medical books in Edinburgh Libraries* (Edinburgh, 1982).
3. Parkinson, E. M., *Catalogue of medical books in Manchester University Library, 1480–1700* (Manchester, 1972); Linet, J. and P. Hillard, *Catalogue des ouvrages imprimés au XVIe siècle. Sciences, techniques, médecine* (Paris, 1980); Limacher, P., *Inventaire des livres du XVIe siècle de la Bibliothèque de la Sorbonne. Vol. 1, Sciences, science politique, médecine* (Paris, 1964); Drummond, H. J. H. (comp.), *A short-title catalogue of books printed on the continent of Europe, 1501–1600 in Aberdeen University Library* (Oxford, 1979); Adams, H. M. (comp.), *Catalogue of books printed on the continent of Europe, 1501–1600 in Cambridge Libraries*, 2 vols (Cambridge, 1967); Stillwell, M. B., *The awakening interest in science during the first century of printing 1450–1550: an annotated checklist of first editions viewed from the angle of their subject content* (New York, 1970); Russell, K. F., *British anatomy 1525–1800*, revised and enlarged (Winchester, 1986).
4. Debus, A. G. (ed.), *Science, medicine and society in the Renaissance: essays to honour Walter Pagel*, 2 vols, (New York, 1972); O'Malley, C. D., 'Tudor medicine and biology', *Huntington Lib. Quart.*, 32 (1968) pp.1–27; Shirley, J. W. and Hoeniger, F. D. (eds), *Science and the arts in the Renaissance* (Cranbury, NJ, 1985); Wear, A., R. K. French and M. Lonie, *The medical Renaissance of the sixteenth century* (Cambridge, 1985); Webster, C. (ed.), *Health, medicine and mortality in the sixteenth century* (Cambridge, 1979); Wightman, W.P.D., *Science in a Renaissance society* (London, 1972).
5. Anderson, F. J., *An illustrated history of the herbals* (New York, 1977) pp.1–2.
6. Rohde, Eleanour Sinclair, *The old English herbals* ... (New York, 1922); (contains bibliographies of manuscript herbals, of printed English herbals, and of certain foreign herbals); Arber, Agnes, *Herbals, their origin and evolution in the history of botany, 1470–1670. A new edition* ... (Cambridge, 1938); Arber, Agnes, 'From medieval herbalism to the birth of modern botany', in *Science, medicine and history*, Vol.1 (1953) pp.317–36; Blunt, Wilfrid, *The art of botanical illustration* ..., (London, 1950); Anderson, F. J., *An illustrated history of the herbals* (New York, 1977).
7. Henrey, B., *British botanical and horticultural literature before 1800: comprising a history and bibliography of botanical and horticultural books printed in England, Scotland and Ireland from the earliest times until 1800*, Vol. 1, The sixteenth and seventeenth centuries history and bibliography (London, 1975).
8. Palmer, R., 'Medical botany in northern Italy in the Renaissance', *J. Roy. Soc. Med.*, 78 (1985) p.152.
9. See Rohde, Eleanour Sinclair, op. cit. in no.6 above, pp.204–6, for complete list.
10. No record except mention by Ames.
11. No record except mention by Hazlitt.
12. Rohde, Eleanour Sinclair, op. cit. in no.6 above, pp.207–8.
13. Barlow, H. M., 'Old English Herbals 1525–1640', *Proc. Roy. Soc. Med.*, 6 (1913) pp.108–49.

14. See also Thornton–Tully, pp.76–7.
15. The only known copy of this work is in the British Library. It was privately reprinted in 1876.
16. A second edition of this appeared in 1636, and this has been partly reproduced as *Gerard's Herball; the essence thereof distilled by Marcus Woodward from the edition of Th. Johnson, 1636* (Edinburgh, London, 1927).
17. See Kew, H. W. and H. E. Powell, *Thomas Johnson, botanist and royalist ...* (1932) which contains a list of his works, editions, etc.; and Power, Sir D'Arcy, 'Thomas Johnson (1597–1644), botanist and barber surgeon', *Glasgow Med. J.*, 133 (1940) pp.201–5, who corrects the dates and facts in Kew–Powell.
18. Gerarde, J., *The Herbal or general history of plants. The complete 1633 edition as revised and enlarged by Thomas Johnson* (New York, 1975).
19. Corbett, M., 'The engraved title-page to John Gerarde's "Herball or Generall Historie of Plantes", 1597', *J. Soc. Bibliog. Nat. Hist.*, 8 (1977) pp.223–30.
20. Bird, D. T. (comp.), *A Catalogue of sixteenth-century medical books in Edinburgh libraries* (Edinburgh, 1982) pp.xii, xvii.
21. Durling, R. J., 'A chronological census of Renaissance editions and translations of Galen', *J. Warburg & Courtauld Inst.*, 24 (1961) pp.230–305; Wear, A., 'Galen in the Renaissance', in V. Nutton (ed.), *Galen: problems and prospects* (London, 1981); Temkin, O., *Galenism* (New York, 1973).
22. Singer, C. and E. A. Underwood, *A short history of medicine*, 2nd edn (Oxford, 1962) pp.88–90.
23. See Finch, Sir Ernest, 'The forerunner (Leonardo da Vinci). Thomas Vicary Lecture delivered at the Royal College of Surgeons of England on 29th October, 1953', *Ann. Roy. Coll. Surg. Engl.*, 14 (1954) pp.71–91.
24. See also Thornton–Tully, pp. 57–8.
25. See Keele, Kenneth D., 'Leonardo da Vinci's influence on renaissance anatomy', *Med. Hist.*, 8 (1964) pp.360–70; Keele, K. D., *Leonardo da Vinci on movement of the heart and blood ...* (London, 1952); Keele, K. D., 'Leonardo da Vinci on vision', *Proc. Roy. Soc. Med.*, 48 (1955) pp. 384–90; Keele, K. D., 'Leonardo da Vinci's "Anatomia naturale" ' (Inaugural John F. Fulton Lecture), *Yale J. Biol. Med.*, 52 (1979) pp. 369–409; Keele, K. D. and C. Pedretti, *Leonardo da Vinci, corpus of the anatomical studies in the collection of Her Majesty the Queen at Windsor Castle*, 3 vols (London and New York, 1978–80); Keele, K. D., *Leonardo da Vinci's elements of the science of man* (London, 1983); Clark, K., *The drawings of Leonardo da Vinci in the collections of Her Majesty the Queen at Windsor Castle*, 2nd edn, revised with the assistance of Carlo Pedretti (London, 1968); O'Malley, C. D. and J. B. de C. M. Saunders, *Leonardo da Vinci on the human body*, (New York, 1952); Saunders, J. B. de C. M., 'Leonardo da Vinci as anatomist and physiologist: a critical evaluation', *Texas Rep. Biol. Med.*, 13 (1955) pp.1010–26; MacCurdy, E., *The notebooks of Leonardo da Vinci*, 2nd edn, 2 vols (London, 1956); Belt, Elmer, *Leonardo the anatomist* (Logan Clendening Lectures on the History and Philosophy of Medicine, 4th series) (Lawrence, Kansas, 1955); Belt, Elmer, 'Leonardo da Vinci, medical illustrator', *Postgrad. Med.*, 16 (1954) pp.150–7; Kemp, M., *Leonardo da Vinci: the marvellous works of nature and man* (London, 1981); and 'Dissection and divinity in Leonardo's late anatomies', *J. Warburg & Courtauld Inst.* (1972) 35, pp.200–25; Smith, Marshall, 'Leonardo da Vinci and Andreas Vesalius: a comparison', *Trans. Stud. Coll. Phycns Philad.*, 25 (1958) pp.167–77; Murphy, Leonard, 'Leonardo da Vinci and the anatomy of the genito-urinary system', *Med. J. Australia*, 2 (1964) pp.556–60; Pegus, L., 'Leonardo da Vinci – anatomical drawings', *Med. Biol. Illus.*, 1 (1978) pp.63–9; Eastwood, B., 'Alhazen, Leonardo and late medieval speculation on the inversion of images in the eye', *Ann. Sci.*, 43 (1986) pp.413–46; Bottger, Herbert, 'Die Embryologie Leonardos da Vinci', *Centaurus*, 3 (1953–4) pp.222–35; Heydenreich, Ludwig H., *Leonardo da Vinci*, 2 vols (1954).
26. Gysel, C., 'La typologie d'Albrecht Dürer', *Janus*, 57 (1970) pp.104–11.
27. See Rath, Gernot, 'Pre-Vesalian anatomy in the light of modern research', *Bull. Hist. Med.*, 35 (1961) pp.142–8; Premuda, L., 'L'Anatomia nelle Università dell'Italia settentrionale prima di Vesalio', *Arch. Ital. Anat. Embryol.*, 79 (1965) pp.115–40;

Coleman, Ruth B., 'Illustration of human anatomy before Vesalius', *Surg. Gynec. Obstet.*, 90 (1950) pp.500–7; Herrlinger, R., *History of medical illustration from antiquity to A.D. 1600* (London, 1970); Garrison, Fielding Hudson, *The principles of anatomic illustration before Vesalius: an inquiry into the rationale of artistic anatomy* (1926); Lind, L.R., *Studies in pre-Vesalian Anatomy* (Philadelphia, 1975).

28. O'Malley, C.D., 'Niccolo Massa', *Physis*, 11 (1969) pp.458–68; Palmer, R., 'Nicolo Massa, his family and his fortune', *Med. Hist.*, 25 (1981) pp.385–410.

29. See Kellett, C. E., 'Two anatomies', *Med. Hist.*, 8 (1964) pp.342–53; Kellett, C. E., 'Perino del Vaga et les illustrations pour l'anatomie d'Estienne', *Aesculape*, 37 (1955) pp.74–89; Kellett, C. E., 'A note on Rosso and the illustrations to Charles Estienne's *De dissectione*', *J. Hist. Med.*, 12 (1957) pp.325–36; Rath, Gernot, 'Charles Estienne: contemporary of Vesalius', *Med. Hist.*, 8 (1964) pp.354–9; Herrlinger, R., 'Carolus Stephanus and Stephanus Riverius (1530–1545)', *Clio Med.*, 2 (1967) pp.275–87.

30. See Russell, K. F., 'Jacopo Berengario da Carpi', *Australian N.Z.J. Surg.*, 23 (1953) pp.70–2; Larkey, Sanford V. and Linda Tum Suden, 'Jackson's English translation of Berengarius of Carpi's "Isagogue Breves", 1660 and 1664', *Isis*, 21 (1934) pp.57–70; Govons, S. R. and W. M. Seaman, 'Berengario on "Signa cerebri commoti" ', *Bull. Hist. Med.*, 43 (1969) pp.473–6.

31. *Jacopo Berengario da Carpi. A short introduction to anatomy (Isagogae breves). Translated with an introduction and historical notes by L. R. Lind, and with anatomical notes by Paul G. Roofe* (Chicago, 1957).

32. Edwardes, David, *Introduction to anatomy, 1532. A facsimile reproduction with English translation and an introductory essay on anatomical studies in Tudor England by C. D. O'Malley and K. F. Russell*, 1961.

33. See Elze, Curt, 'Jacobus Sylvius, der Lehrer Vesals, als Begründer der anatomische Nomenklatur', *Zeits. Anat. Entwicklungsgesch.*, 114 (1949) pp.242–50.

34. 'Jacobus Sylvius' Advice for poor medical students', translated by C. D. O'Malley, *J. Hist. Med.*, 17 (1962) pp.141–51.

35. See also Kellett, C. E., 'Sylvius and the reform of anatomy', *Med. Hist.*, 5 (1961) pp.101–16.

36. Cushing, Harvey, *A bio-bibliography of Andreas Vesalius … Second edition*, (Hamden, Conn., London, 1962); (consists of a facsimile of the first edition of 1943, with the addition of corrigenda and addenda, and a list of Vesaliana published since that edition); O'Malley, C. D., *Andreas Vesalius of Brussels 1514–1564* (Berkeley, Los Angeles, 1964).

37. Singer, Charles and C. Rabin, *A prelude to modern science: a discussion of the history, sources and circumstances of the 'Tabulae anatomicae sex' of Vesalius* (Cambridge, 1946).

38. *Tabulae anatomicae. Facsimilé des sept planches de l'édition de Cologne et des six planches de l'édition d'Augsburg* (Brussels, 1965).

39. Saunders, John B. de C. M. and Charles Donald O'Malley (eds), *Andreas Vesalius Bruxellensis: The bloodletting letter of 1539. An annotated translation and study of the evolution of Vesalius's scientific development* (1949).

40. Singer, Charles and E. Ashworth Underwood, *A short history of medicine*, 2nd edn (Oxford, 1962) p.93; Schiller, J., 'La place de Vésale dans l'histoire de la physiologie', *Hist. et Biol.*, Fasc. 1 (1968) pp.25–43.

41. O'Malley, C. D., *Andreas Vesalius of Brussels 1514–1564* (Berkeley, Los Angeles, 1964) pp.139–86.

42. Roth-Woelfle, L., 'Jan Stephan von Kalkar als Illustrator der Anatomie des Andreas Vesal', *Imprimatur*, 11 (1980) pp.86–100; Goodrich, J. T., 'John Stephen of Calcar: the identification of the anatomical illustrators of the "De Humani Corporis Fabrica" (1543)', *J. Biocommun.*, 5 (1978) pp.26–32.

43. O'Malley, C. D., *Andreas Vesalius of Brussels 1514–1564* (Berkeley, Los Angeles, 1964) p. 124.

44. Petrucelli, R. J., 'Giorgio Vasari's attribution of the Vesalian illustrations to Jan Stephan of Calcar: a further examination', *Bull. Hist. Med.*, 45 (1971) pp.29–37.

45. Vasari, G., *Le vite de'piv eccellenti pittori, scultori, e architettori*, 2nd edn, Vol. 3, pt 1 (Florence, 1568) p.309 (incorrectly numbered 319).

46. Vesalius, A., *Epistola, docens venam axillarem dextri in dolore laterali secandam*, (Basle, 1539) p.66.

47. Kemp, M., 'A drawing for the Fabrica: some thoughts upon the Vesalius muscle-men', *Med. Hist.*, 14 (1970) p.281; Lambert, S. W., W. Wiegand and W. M. Ivins, *Three Vesalian essays to accompany the Icones Anatomicae of 1934* (New York, 1952) pp.40–1; Cavanagh, G.S.T., 'A new view of the Vesalian landscape', *Med. Hist.*, 27 (1983) pp.77–9.

48. Lambert, S. W., W. Wiegand and W. M. Ivins, *Three Vesalian essays to accompany the Icones anatomicae of 1934* (New York, 1952) (pp.1–24 deal with the initial letters, and pp.25–42 are devoted to the wanderings and discovery of the blocks).

49. *The illustrations from the works of Andreas Vesalius of Brussels*, with annotations and translations by J. B. de C. M. Saunders and Charles D. O'Malley (New York, 1950).

50. The woodcut initial letters for different editions varied in size. See Ollerenshaw, Robert, 'The decorated woodcut initials of Vesalius' "Fabrica" ', *Med. Biol. Ill.*, 2 (1952) pp.160–6; Wells, L. H., 'Notes on a historiated initial letter in the Fabrica of Vesalius', *Med. Hist.*, 6 (1962) pp.287–8; Anson, Barry J, 'Anatomical tabulae and initial letters in Vesalius' Fabrica and in imitative works', *Surg. Gynec. Obstet.*, 89 (1949) pp.97–120; Herrlinger, R., 'Die Initialen in der "Fabrica" des Andreas Vesalius', *Acta Med. Hist. Patav.*, 10 (1963–4) pp.97–117.

51. Heseler, Baldasar, *Andreas Vesalius' first public anatomy at Bologna, 1540, an eyewitness report by Baldasar Heseler together with his notes on Matthaeus Curtius' lectures on Anatomia Mundini. Edited, with an introduction, translated into English and notes by R. Eriksson* (Uppsala, Stockholm, 1959); (Lychnosbibliothek, 18); see also Eriksson, R., 'Notes on medical manuscripts of the Royal Library, Stockholm, especially MS. Hol X.93, B. Heseler's account of Vesalius' public anatomy at Bologna, 1540', *Libri*, 11 (1961) pp.355–63.

52. Keynes, G., 'The Epitome of Vesalius: another notable acquisition for the Library', *Ann. Roy. Coll. Surg. Engl.*, 29 (1961) pp.385–8; see also Spencer, W. G., 'The "Epitome" of Vesalius on vellum in the British Museum Library', in *Essays on the history of medicine presented to Karl Sudhoff ... Edited by Charles Singer and Henry E. Sigerist* (London, Zurich, 1924) pp.237–44.

53. Cushing, H., *A bio-bibliography of Andreas Vesalius*, 2nd edn (Hamden, Conn., London, 1962) pp.216–17.

54. O'Malley, C. D., 'The Vesalian influence in England', *Acta Med. Hist. Patav.*, 10 (1963–4) pp.11–20; Pinero, J. M. L., 'The Vesalian movement in sixteenth-century Spain', *J. Hist. Biol.*, 12 (1979) pp.45–81.

55. See, for example, Fontana, Velarde Perez, *Andreas Vesalius Bruxellensis y su epoca* (Montevideo, 1963); O'Malley, Charles D., 'Andreas Vesalius 1515–1564: in memoriam', *Med. Hist.*, 8 (1964) pp.299–308; O'Malley, C. D., 'A review of Vesalian literature', *Hist. Sci.*, 4 (1965) pp.1–14; Pagel, Walter, 'Vesalius and the pulmonary transit of venous blood', *J. Hist. Med.*, 19 (1964) pp.327–41; Singer, C., (ed.), *Vesalius on the human brain* (London, 1952); Schulte, B.P.M., 'Vesalius on the anatomy of the brain', *Janus*, 53 (1966) pp.40–9; Saunders, John B. de C. M., 'Andreas Vesalius, 1564–1964 – his work and inspiration', *J. Amer. Med. Assn*, 192 (1965) pp.127–30.

56. Horowitz, M. and J. Collins, 'A census of copies of the first edition of Andreas Vesalius' "De humani corporis fabrica" (1543), with a note on the recently discovered variant issue', *J. Hist. Med.*, 39 (1984) pp.198–221.

57. Wells, L. H., 'A note on the Valverde muscle-man', *Med. Hist.*, 3 (1959) pp.212–14; 12 (1979) pp.45–81; and his further note, 'The "M.F." engraving and the Valverde muscle-man; a correction', *Med. Hist.*, 5 (1961) p.197. Also O'Malley, Charles D., 'The anatomical sketches of Vitus Tritonius Athesinus and their relationship to Vesalius' *Tabulae anatomicae*', *J. Hist. Med.*, 13 (1958) pp.395–7.

58. Lindberg, Sten G., 'Chrestien Wechel and Vesalius: twelve unique medical broadsides from the sixteenth century', *Lychnos* (1953) pp.50–74; Wells, L. H., 'A remarkable pair of anatomical fugitive sheets in the Medical Center Library, University of Michigan', *Bull. Hist. Med.*, 38 (1964) pp.470–6; Choulant, L., *History and bibliography of anatomic illustration* (New York, 1945) pp.156–67.

59. Hind, A. M., *Engraving in England in the sixteenth and seventeenth centuries* (Cambridge, 1952) Part 1: The Tudor Period, pp.39–52.
60. Thomas Geminus, *Compendiosa totius anatomie delineatio. A facsimile of the first English edition of 1553 in the version of Nicholas Udall. With an introduction by C. D. O'Malley* (London, 1959). See also Larkey, Sanford V., 'The Vesalian compendium of Geminus, and Nicholas Udall's translation: their relation to Vesalius, Caius, Vicary, and de Mondeville', *Lib. Trans. Bib. Soc.*, 4th ser., 13 (1933) pp.367–94; and Keynes, Sir Geoffrey, 'The Anatomy of Thomas Geminus: a notable acquisition for the Library', *Ann. Roy. Coll. Surg. Engl.*, 25 (1959) pp.171–5.
61. Hind, A. M., *A history of engraving and etching*, 3rd rev. edn (New York, 1923), pp.134–5.
62. Crummer, L., 'The copper plates in Raynalde and Geminus', *Proc. Roy. Soc. Med.*, 20 (1926) pp.53–6.
63. Payne, L., 'A plagiarist plagiarised', *J. Roy. Coll. Phycns Lond.*, 19 (1985) pp.44–7.
64. O'Malley, C. D., 'Gabriele Falloppia's account of the cranial nerves', *Sudhoffs Archiv* (1966) issue 7, pp.132–7.
65. Di Pietro, P., *Epistolario di Gabriele Falloppia* (Ferrara, 1970).
66. Roberts, K. B., 'Eustachius and his anatomical plates', *Canad. Soc. Hist. Med. Newsletter* (April 1979) pp.9–13.
67. O'Malley, C. D., 'Bartolomeo Eustachi: an epistle on the organs of hearing. An annotated translation', *Clio Med.*, 6 (1971) pp.49–62.
68. Power, Sir D'Arcy, *'The birth of mankind, or the woman's book*; a bibliographical study', *Trans. Bib. Soc.*, 4th ser., 8 (1927–8) pp.1–37 (the reprint of this contains a table of comparison of the ornamental initial letters, not incorporated in the original paper); Ballantyne, J. W., 'The "Byrth of mankynde" ', *J. Obstet. Gynaec.*, 10 (1906) pp.297–325; 12 (1907) pp.175–94, 255–74 (many plates, and list of editions); Crummer, LeRoy, 'The copper plates in Raynalde and Geminus', *Proc. Roy. Soc. Med.*, 20, i–ii (1927) pp.53–6; Ingerslev, E., 'Rösslin's "Rosegarten": its relation to the past (the Muscio Manuscripts and Soranos), particularly with regard to podalic version', *J. Obstet. Gynaec.*, 15 (1909) pp.1–25, 73–92.
69. Koelbing, H. M., ' "De conceptu et generatione hominis" – die lateinische Fassung von Jakob Rueffs "Trostbüchle", Zürich, 1554,' *Gesnerus*, 38 (1981) pp.51–8.
70. Houtzager, H. L., 'Jacob Rueff', *Europ. J. Obstet. Gynaec. Reprod. Biol.*, 13 (1982) pp.105–7.
71. Roberts, K. B., 'Illustrations in a sixteenth-century book on obstetrics', *Can. Bull. Med. Hist.*, 1 (1984) pp.80–95.
72. Rueff, J. *Ein schön lustig Trostbüchle von den Empfengknussen und Gerburten der Menschen* ... (Editions Medica Rara, Zurich, 1981).
73. See Spencer, Herbert R., 'Lloyd Roberts Lecture: the renaissance of midwifery', *Trans. Med. Soc. Lond.*, 48 (1925) pp.71–105; also issued separately.
74. For his scientific contributions, see Thornton–Tully, pp.72–3; see also Webster, C., *From Paracelsus to Newton: magic and the making of modern science* (Cambridge, 1982); Debus, A. G., 'The Paracelsians and the Chemists: The chemical dilemma in Renaissance medicine', *Clio Med.*, 7 (1972) pp.185–99; and Debus, A. G., 'The chemical philosophers: chemical medicine from Paracelsus to Van Helmont', *Hist. Sci.*, 12 (1974) pp.235–59.
75. Sudhoff, Karl, *Versuch einer Kritik der Echtheit der paracelsischen Schriften*, 2 vols (Berlin, 1894–9); see also *Registerband zu Sudhoffs Paracelsus Gesamtausgabe bearbeitet von Martin Müller. Nova Acta Paracelsica Supplementum* (Basle, 1960).
76. Pagel, Walter, *Paracelsus: an introduction to philosophical medicine in the era of the Renaissance* (Basle, New York, 1958); see also the companion volume by Walter Pagel, dealing mainly with the chemical achievements of Paracelsus, *Das medizinische Weltbild des Paracelsus: seine Zusammenhänge mit Neuplatonismus und Gnosis* (Wiesbaden, 1962); see also Pagel, Walter, 'Paracelsus', *DSB*, 10 (1974) pp.304–13; *Paracelsus. Selected writings, edited with an introduction by Jolande Jacobi. Translated by Norbert Guterman* (1951); (published in German as *Theophrastus Paracelsus: Lebendiges Erbe* (Zurich, 1942); Stoddart, Anna M., *The life of Paracelsus Theophrastus von Hohenheim, 1493–1541* ... (1911); Debus, A. G., *The English Paracelsians*

78   Thornton's medical books, libraries and collectors

(London, 1965); Braun, L., *Paracelse* (Paris, 1980); and 'Paracelsus, Kreatur und Kosmos, internationale Beiträge zur Paracelsusforschung (Prof. Dr. phil. Kürt Goldammer … zum 65. Geburtstag)', *Medizinhist. J.*, 16 (1981) issues 1/2, pp.1–198.
77. Pagel, W., *Paracelsus: an introduction to philosophical medicine in the era of the Renaissance*, 2nd edn (Basle, 1982).
78. See O'Malley, C. D., *Logan Clendening Lectures on the History and Philosophy of Medicine, 12th series. English medical humanists; Thomas Linacre and John Caius* (Lawrence, Kansas, 1965); and Gemmill, Chalmers L., 'Thomas Linacre and John Caius', *Virginia Med. Monthly*, 89 (1962) pp.15–18.
79. This was reproduced in facsimile, with an introduction by Joseph Frank Payne, Cambridge, 1881.
80. Osler, Sir William, *Thomas Linacre. (Linacre Lecture, 1908, St John's College, Cambridge)* (Cambridge, 1908); (contains portraits, and facsimiles of title-pages); see also Johnson, John Noble, *The Life of Thomas Linacre … Edited by Robert Graves* (1835); Thornton, John L., 'Andrew Boorde, Thomas Linacre and the "Dyetary of helth" ', *Bull. Med. Lib. Assn*, 36 (1948) pp.204–9; Thornton, John L., 'Andrew Boorde's *Dyetary of helth* and its attribution to Thomas Linacre', *Lib. Trans. Bib. Soc.*, 5th ser. (1947) pp.172–3; Cameron, Sir Roy, 'Thomas Linacre at the portal to scientific medicine', *Br. Med. J.* (1964) , pp.589–94; Newman, Charles, 'Thomas Linacre, founder of the Royal College of Physicians', *Lond. Hosp. Gaz.*, 64 (1961) pp.20–4; and Sharpe, William D., 'Thomas Linacre, 1460–1524: an English physician scholar of the Renaissance', *Bull. Hist. Med.*, 34 (1960) pp.233–56.
81. Maddison, F., M. Pelling and C. Webster (eds), *Essays on the life and work of Thomas Linacre, c.1460–1524* (Oxford, 1977); (includes Barber, G., 'Thomas Linacre: A bibliographical survey of his works', pp.290–336).
82. Ballard, James F. and Michel Pijoan, 'A preliminary check-list of the writings of Symphorien Champier, 1472–1539', *Bull. Med. Lib. Assn*, 28 (1940) pp.182–7.
83. Copenhaver, B. P., *Symphorien Champier and the reception of the occultist tradition in Renaissance France* (Hague, Paris, 1978).
84. Chakravorty, K. C., 'Girolamo Fracastoro: a man of the Renaissance', *Hist. Med.*, 6 (1975) pp.65–7.
85. Baumgartner, Leona and John F. Fulton, *A bibliography of the poem Syphilis sive morbus gallicus, by Girolamo Fracastoro of Verona* (New Haven, London, 1935).
86. Ibid.
87. *The sinister shepherd: a translation of Girolamo Fracastoro's Syphilidis sive de morbo gallico libri tres by William Van Wyck* (Los Angeles, 1934).
88. *Fracastoro's 'Syphilis'. Introduction, text, translation and notes, with a computer-generated word index by G. Eatough* (Liverpool, 1984); See also Abraham, J. Johnston, 'The early history of syphilis', *Br. J. Surg.*, 32 (1944–5) pp.225–37; and Sudhoff, Karl, *The earliest printed literature on syphilis; being ten tractates from the years 1495–1498. In complete facsimile, with an introduction and other accessory material by Karl Sudhoff, adapted by Charles Singer* (Florence, 1925); (Monumenta Medica, III).
89. Fracastoro, G., 'Da Gerolamo Fracastoro ad Athanasius Kircher ed Antony van Leeuwenhoek', *Fracastoro*, 64 (1971) pp.196–228; Howard-Jones, N., 'Fracastoro and Henle: a re-appraisal of their contribution to the concept of communicable diseases', *Med. Hist.*, 21 (1977) pp.61–8.
90. *De contagione*, translated into English by Wilmer Cave Wright (New York, 1930).
91. Sherrington, Sir Charles, *The endeavour of Jean Fernel; with a list of the editions of his writings* (Cambridge, 1946); (bibliography of Fernel's writings, pp.187–207).
92. Two variants of the title-page, one giving 1526, and the other 1527.
93. Two variants of the title-page, one giving 1527, and the other 1528.
94. See Brown, Alfred, 'Old masterpieces in surgery. The universal medicine of Jean Fernel', *Surg. Gynec. Obstet.*, 51 (1930) p.876; Long, Esmond R., 'Jean Fernel's conception of tuberculosis', *Science, medicine and history*, 1 (1953) pp.401–7.
95. Moes, Robert J. and C. D. O'Malley, 'Realdo Colombo: "On those things rarely found in anatomy". An annotated translation from the *De re anatomica* (1559)', *Bull. Hist. Med.*, 34 (1960) pp.508–28.

96. See O'Malley, Charles Donald, 'A Latin translation of Ibn Nafis (1547) related to the problem of the circulation of the blood', *J. Hist. Med.*, 12 (1957) pp.248–53.

97. Singer, C. and E. A. Underwood, *A short history of medicine*, 2nd edn (Oxford, 1962) p.119; see also Ghalioungui, P., 'Was Ibn al-Nafis unknown to the scholars of the European Renaissance?', *Clio Med.*, 18 (1983) pp.37–42.

98. See Trueta, Josep, 'Michael Servetus and the discovery of the lesser circulation', *Yale J. Biol.*, 21 (1948) pp.1–15; Trueta, J., 'The contribution of Michael Servetus to the scientific development of the Renaissance', *Br. Med. J.* (1954) , pp.507–10; and Ongaro, G., 'La scoperta della circolazione polmonar e la diffusione della "Christianismi restitutio" di Michele Serveto nel XVI secolo in Italia e nel Veneto', *Episteme*, 5 (1971) pp.3–44.

99. *Harvard Theological Studies*, vol. 16.

100. See also Bainton, Roland H., 'The Fielding H. Garrison Lecture. Michael Servetus and the pulmonary transit of the blood', *Bull. Hist. Med.*, 25 (1951) pp.1–7; Wilson, L. G., 'The problem of the pulmonary circulation', *J. Hist. Med.,* 17 (1962) pp.229–44.

101. Mackall, Leonard L., 'A manuscript of the "Christianismi restitutio" of Servetus, placing the discovery of the pulmonary circulation anterior to 1546', *Proc. Roy. Soc. Med.*, 17 (1924) section of Hist. of Med., pp.35–8.

102. See McDaniel, W. B., 'The unfinished London reprint of Servetus' "Restoration of Christianity" ', *Ann. Med. Hist.*, N.S.8 (1936) pp.270–1; see also Osler, Sir William, *Michael Servetus* (1909). Unfortunately Osler gives the date of the Vienna reprint as 1791 (p.32) and also involves Mead too closely in the attempted London reprint of 1723 (p.33).

103. See Fulton, John F., *Michael Servetus humanist and martyr ... With a bibliography of his works and census of known copies. By Madeline E. Stanton* (New York, 1953).

104. O'Malley, Charles Donald, *Michael Servetus. A translation of his geographical, medical and astrological writings with introductions and notes* (Philadelphia, 1953).

105. See Bainton, Roland H., *Hunted heretic: the life and death of Michael Servetus, 1511–1553* (Boston, 1953); (contains a bibliography of works by Servetus, pp.220–3, and a selected list of writings about him, pp.223–41); Willis, R., *Servetus and Calvin: a study of an important epoch in the history of the Reformation* (1877); Friedman, J., *Michael Servetus: a case study in total heresy* (Geneva, 1978); Bayon, H. P., 'William Harvey, physician and biologist: his precursors, opponents and successors. Part IV', *Ann. Sci.*, 4 (1939) pp.65–106; and Bloch, H., 'Michael Servetus 1511 to 1553: heresies in theology and medicine', *NY State J. Med.*, 78 (1978) pp.2114–16.

106. Wangensteen, O. H., S. D. Wangensteen and C. F. Klinger, 'Wound management of Ambroise Paré and Dominique Larrey, great French military surgeons of the 16th and 19th centuries', *Bull. Hist. Med.*, 46, (1972) pp.207–34.

107. *The Workes of that famous chirurgion Ambrose Parey translated out of Latine and compared with the French by Thomas Johnson* (London, 1634) p.409.

108. See Doe, Janet, *A bibliography of the works of Ambroise Paré, premier chirurgien and conseiller du roy* (Chicago, 1937) p.63 (reprinted 1976). This bibliography contains portraits, facsimiles of title-pages, complete bibliographical details, annotations and location of copies; an extensive list of authors consulted, and a chronological table of Paré's books. See also Addenda to Miss Doe's Bibliography of Ambroise Paré, *Ann. Med. Hist.*, 3rd ser, 2 (1940) pp.443–4.

109. *Ten books of surgery with the magazine of the instruments necessary for it*, translated by R. W. Linker and N. Womack (Athens, 1969).

110. Lindskog, G. E., 'A note concerning Ambroise Paré's *Dix livres de la chirurgie*', *Surgery*, 70 (1971) pp.452–4.

111. For example, *Selections from the works of Ambroise Paré; with short biography, and explanatory and bibliographical notes by Dorothea Waley Singer ...,* 1924; *The Apologie and Treatise of Ambroise Paré, containing the voyages made into divers places, with many of his writings upon surgery. Edited, and with an introduction by Geoffrey Keynes* (1951); a German translation by Erwin Ackerknecht of the *Apologie*, in 2 volumes (Bern, 1963); and *The case reports and autopsy records of Ambroise Paré. Compiled and edited by Wallace B. Hamby. Translated from J. P. [i.e. F.] Malgaigne's "Oeuvres*

complètes d'Ambroise Paré", Paris, 1840 (Springfield, Ill., 1960); contains 'Professional chronology of Ambroise Paré', pp.xv–xx.

112. *On monsters and marvels*, translated with an introduction and notes by J. L. Pallister (Chicago, 1982).

113. *The Apologie and Treatise of Ambroise Paré, containing the voyages made into divers places, with many of his writings upon surgery. Edited, and with an introduction by Geoffrey Keynes* (1951) pp.xx–xxi.

114. See Packard, Francis R., *Life and times of Ambroise Paré [1510–1590]; with a translation of his Apology and an account of his journeys in divers places ... Second edition* (New York, 1926); Paget, Stephen, *Ambroise Paré and his times, 1510–1590* (New York, London, 1897); Dumaître, P., *Ambroise Paré, chirurgien de quatre rois de France* (Paris, 1986); Malgaigne, J. F., *Surgery and Ambroise Paré*, translated from the French and edited by W. B. Hamby (Oklahoma, 1965); Hill, Boyd Howard, 'Ambroise Paré: sawbones or scientist?', *J. Hist. Med.*, 15 (1960) pp.45–58; Chauvelot, R., 'Les sources d'Ambroise Paré. Introduction à la chirurgie', *Presse Méd.*, 63 (1955) pp.1717–19; Anson, B. J., 'XXV Wherry Memorial Lecture. The ear and the eye in the collected works of Ambroise Paré, Renaissance surgeon to four kings of France', *Trans. Amer. Acad. Ophthal. Otolaryng.*, 74 (1970) pp.249–77; and Peltier, L. F., 'Compound fracture of the leg, Paré's personal care', *Clin. Orthop.* (1983) no.178, pp.3–6.

115. Eccles, A., 'The reading public, the medical profession and the use of English for medical books in the 16th and 17th centuries', *New-philol. Mitt.*, 75 (1974) pp.143–56.

116. Slack, P., 'Mirrors of health and treasures of poor men: the uses of the vernacular medical literature of Tudor England', in Webster, C. (ed.), *Health, medicine and mortality in the sixteenth century* (Cambridge, 1979), ch.7, pp.237–73.

117. Elyot, T., *The Castel of Helth* (Scholars Facs, New York, 1937).

118. Thomas, Duncan Porter, 'The life and works of Thomas Vicary. The Wix Prize Essay', St Bartholomew's Hospital Medical College (London, 1953) (typescript). See also Thomas, Duncan Porter, 'Thomas Vicary ... (Being a summary of part of the Wix Prize Essay, 1953)', *St Bart's Hosp. J.*, 57 (1953) pp.255–9; Thomas, Sir Clement Price, 'Vicary amongst his contemporaries. Thomas Vicary Lecture delivered at the Royal College of Surgeons of England on 26th October, 1961', *Ann. Roy. Coll. Surg. Engl.*, 30 (1962) pp.137–54; MacDonald, G. G., 'General medical practice in the time of Thomas Vicary', *Ann. Roy. Coll. Surg. Engl.*, 40 (1967) pp.1–20; Power, Sir D'Arcy, 'Notes on the bibliography of three sixteenth-century books connected with London Hospitals. ii. Vicary's Anatomy of man', in his *Selected writings, 1877–1930* (1931) pp.111–19; see also his 'The beginnings of the literary renaissance of surgery in England', *Proc. Roy. Soc. Med.*, 22 (1929) pp.77–82.

119. Power, Sir D'Arcy, 'Epoch-making books in British surgery. II. Certain works of chirurgerie by Thomas Gale, Maister in Chirurgerie', *Br. J. Surg.*, 15 (1927–8) pp.177–81.

120. See Wilson, William Jerome, 'Thomas Gale, educator of surgeons', *Bull. Cleveland Med. Libr.*, 1 (1954) pp.79–83.

121. See Clowes, William, *Profitable and necessarie booke of observations ... With introductions, general and medical, by De Witt T. Starnes and Chauncey D. Leake* (New York, 1945); (bibliographical note, pp.xxi–xxii).

122. Power, Sir D'Arcy, 'Epoch-making books in British surgery. III. A proved practice for all young chirurgians, by William Clowes, Maister in Chirurgery', *Brit. J. Surg.*, 15 (1927–8) pp.353–9.

123. Morgenstern, S., ' "A right fruitefull and approved treatise, for the artificiall cure of ... struma ..." by William Clowes – An outstanding gift of the friends', *Acad. Bkman*, 24 (1971) pp.2–15.

124. *Selected writings of William Clowes 1544–1604. Edited, with a introduction, and notes by F. N. L. Poynter* (1948); (contains bibliographical material and information on location of copies). See also Major, Ralph H., 'William Clowes and his "Profitable and necessarie booke of observations" ', *Ann. Med. Hist.*, N.S.4 (1932) pp.1–11.

125. See Finlayson, James, *Account of the life and works of Maister Peter Lowe, the founder of the Faculty of Physicians and Surgeons of Glasgow* (Glasgow, 1889); Guthrie,

Douglas, 'The achievement of Peter Lowe, and the unity of physician and surgeon', *Scottish Med. J.*, 10 (1965) pp.261–8; Edington, G. H., 'The "Discourse" of Master Peter Lowe: extracts and comments', *Glasgow Med. J.*, 108 (1922) pp.43–50; and Power, Sir D'Arcy, 'Epoch-making books in British surgery. IV. *The whole course of chirurgerie* compiled by Peter Lowe, Scotchman', *Br. J. Surg.*, 15 (1927–8) pp.533–7.

126. See Matthews, Leslie G., 'William Bullen and his "Bulwarke" ', *Pharmaceutical Journal*, 186 (1961) pp.69–73.

127. See Mitchell, William S. 'William Bullein, Elizabethan physician and author', *Med. Hist.*, 3 (1959) pp.188–200.

128. Catalogue of R.C. Pearson, Cambridge, Pt 1, [1946] item 54.

129. See Nixon, Howard M., 'English bookbindings, xxxvii. A binding for William Bullein by the initial binder, 1562', *Book Collector*, 10 (1961) p.184.

130. Mambretti, C. C., 'William Bullein and the "Lively fashions" in Tudor medical literature', *Clio Med.*, 9 (1974) pp.285–97.

131. Lister, I., 'John Caius: the versatile doctor', *Practitioner*, 183 (1959) pp.637–40.

132. O'Malley, D., 'The relations of John Caius with Andreas Vesalius and some incidental remarks on the Giunta Galen and on Thomas Geminus', *J. Hist. Med.*, 10 (1955) pp.147–72.

133. Nutton, V., 'John Caius and the Eton Galen: medical philology in the Renaissance', *Med. Historisch. J.*, 20 (1985) pp.227–52; Nutton, V., *John Caius and the manuscript of Galen* (Cambridge, 1987).

134. Cooke, A. M., 'Dr John Caius, 1510–1573', *J. Roy. Coll. Phycns Lond.*, 7 (1973) p.366.

135. See Barber-Lomax, J. W., 'De canibus Britannicus', *Journal of Small Animal Practice*, 1 (1960) pp.24–31; and Barber-Lomax, J. W., 'A further illustrated note on De canibus Britannicus – London, 1570', ibid., pp.109–12.

136. Ash, E. C., *Dogs and their history*, Vol. 1 (1927) pp.74–84.

137. See O'Malley, Charles Donald, 'The relations of John Caius with Andreas Vesalius and some incidental remarks on the Giunta Galen and on Thomas Geminus', *J. Hist. Med.*, 10 (1955) pp.147–72; O'Malley, C. D., 'Logan Clendening Lectures on the History and Philosophy of Medicine. Twelfth series', *English medical humanists: Thomas Linacre and John Caius* (Lawrence, Kansas, 1965); Gemmill, Chalmers L., 'Thomas Linacre and John Caius', *Virginia Med. Monthly*, 89 (1962) pp.15–18; Nutton, V., 'John Caius and the Linacre tradition', *Med. Hist.*, 23 (1979) pp.373–91; Langdon-Brown, Sir Walter, 'John Caius and the revival of learning', *Proc. Roy. Soc. Med.*, 35 (1941–2) pp.61–9 (also in his *Some chapters in Cambridge medical history*, Cambridge, 1946, Ch.1, pp.1–19).

138. Guthrie, Douglas, 'The "Breviary" and "Dyetary" of Andrew Boorde (1490–1549), physician, priest and traveller' [Synopsis] *Proc. Roy. Soc. Med.*, 37 (1944) pp.507–9.

139. Platter, Felix, *Beloved son Felix. The journal of Felix Platter, a medical student in Montpellier in the sixteenth century. Translated and introduced by Sean Jennett ...* (1961); Platter, Thomas, *Journal of a younger brother. The life of Thomas Platter as a medical student in Montpellier at the close of the sixteenth century. Translated and introduced by Sean Jennett ...* (1963).

140. See Netsky, Martin G. and Jean Lapresle. 'The first account of meningioma', *Bull. Hist. Med.*, 30 (1956) pp.465–8.

141. See Cranefield, Paul, 'Little known English versions of the "Praxis" and "Observationes" of Felix Platter', *J. Hist. Med.*, 17 (1962) pp.309–11.

142. *Observationes. Krankheitsbeobachtungen in drei Büchern. 1. Buch: Funktionelle Störungen des Sinnes und der Bewegung ...* (Bern, Stuttgart, 1963); (Hübers Klassiker der Medizin und der Naturwissenschaften, Band 1).

143. See Carter, H. S., 'Dr François Rabelais', *Glasgow Med. J.*, 36 (1955) pp.267; Antonioli, R., *Rabelais et la médecine* (Geneva, 1976); and Enselme, J., 'L'ambiance médicale au XVIe siècle à travers les œuvres de Rabelais et de Shakespeare', *Rev. Lyon. Méd.*, 17 (1968) pp.301–20.

144. Simpson, R. R., *Shakespeare and medicine* (Edinburgh and London, 1959).

145. Gnudi, Martha Teach and Jerome Pierce Webster, *The life and times of Gaspare Tagliacozzi, surgeon of Bologna, 1545–1599 ...* (New York, 1950); see also Dumaître,

Paule, 'Le traité de chirurgie plastique de Gaspard Tagliacozzi, chirurgien de Bologna en XVIe Siècle', *Aesculape* (1955) pp.343–55.

146.   Copeman, P. W. M. and W. S. C. Copeman, 'Dermatology in Tudor and early Stuart England', *Br. J. Derm.*, 82 (1970) pp.78–88, 182–91.

147.   For details of other writings by Mercuriale, see the following papers by Alfred Brown: 'Old masterpieces in surgery. Girolamo Mercuriale (Hieronymus Merculiaris)', *Surg. Gynec. Obstet.*, 44 (1927) p.420; 'Concerning diseases of women – Hieronymus Mercurialis', *Surg. Gynec. Obstet.*, 46 (1928) p.300; 'Concerning the gymnastic art, by Hieronymus Mercurialis', *Surg. Gynec. Obstet.*, 46 (1928) p.145; and Peltier, L. F., 'Geronimo Mercuriali (1530–1606) and the first illustrated book on sports medicine', *Clin. Orthop.*, No. 198 (1985) pp.21–4.

148.   Phaire, Thomas, *The boke of children* (Edinburgh, London, 1955).

149.   See also Still, Sir George Frederic, *The history of paediatrics: the progress of the study of diseases of children up to the end of the XVIIIth century* (1931) pp.108–27.

150.   See Riesenfeld, Kurt, 'Timothy Bright und Shakespeare', *Sudhoffs Archiv*, 41 (1957) pp.244–54.

151.   See Carlton, W. J., 'An unrecorded manuscript by Dr Timothy Bright', *Notes and Queries*, N.S.11 (1964) pp.463–5.

152.   Keynes, Sir Geoffrey Langdon, *Dr Timothie Bright 1550–1615. A survey of his life with a bibliography of his writings* (1962); (Publications of the Wellcome Historical Medical Library, N.S.1). See also Carlton, William J., *Timothie Bright, doctor of phisicke: a memoir of 'the father of modern shorthand ...'* (1911).

153.   See Jones, Ellis W. P., 'The life and works of Guilhelmus Fabricius Hildanus (1560–1634)', *Med. Hist.*, 4 (1960) pp.196–209; Hoffmann, Karl Frz., 'Wilhelm Fabry von Hilden, genannt Fabricius Hildanus (1560–1634), der Begründer der klinischen Chirurgie', *Medizinische Monatsschrift*, 14 (1960) pp.391–4; and Scharli, A. F., 'Kinder mit Mißbildungen in der Renaissance (nach den Aufzeichnungen von Fabricius Hildanus, 1560–1634)', *Z. Kinderchir.* (1984) 39, pp.296–301.

154.   See Malloch, Archibald, 'Certain old American works', *Bull. N.Y. Acad. Med.*, 2nd ser., 12 (1936) pp.545–65; Buño, W., 'El primer texto da anatomia publicado en America, Anothomia, por Fr. Agustin Farfán, Mexico, 1579', *Arch. Iberoamer. Hist. Med.*, 10 (1958) pp.105–9.

4   Seventeenth-century medical books

Christine R. English

Truth must be discovered by the light of nature, not recovered from the
darkness of the past.
                                                                    Francis Bacon

The seventeenth century can be seen as the cradle of modern science,
rocked as it was in parts of Europe by political unrest, particularly the
Civil War in England. It was certainly this century that saw the beginnings
of organized scientific research and experimentation and the setting aside
of structures of thought about the natural world which had limited its
understanding since late antiquity. Medicine benefited from the new spirit
of investigation. Knowledge of anatomy and physiology advanced at a
startling rate during this period, revolving around the discovery of the
circulation of the blood made by William Harvey in the early years of the
century, which overturned the accepted anatomical model; the development of a new instrument, the microscope, brought into focus the world of
micro-organisms and expanded the scope of anatomical observation
beyond the limits of the unassisted eye, enabling the existence of the
capillaries, which Harvey had posited, to be established; experimentation
in chemistry introduced new therapeutic agents into the pharmacopœia
and began to provide the explanation of physiological processes,
especially respiration.[1]

The background to this scientific renaissance has been much studied; its
literature is more elusive. A principal source will be the National Library
of Medicine's catalogue of printed books covering this period, companion
to the volumes already published on the sixteenth and eighteenth centuries. Publications in English and published in Great Britain are recorded by
Pollard and Redgrave's *Short-title catalogue of books … 1475–1640* and
by Wing's *Short-title catalogue of books … 1641–1700* commonly referred
to as STC and Wing. These are not descriptive bibliographies although
they do attempt to list different editions and issues; the revised STC is
particularly thorough. The division of the century at 1641 recognizes the
impact of the Civil War and although this date is only significant for
British publications it is used also to divide the catalogue of the printed
books of the Wellcome Institute for the History of Medicine, which is still
in progress. This catalogue is complemented by the published Subject
Catalogue, which is a valuable source for the secondary literature on the
history of medicine of all periods.[2]

Standards of book production varied according to the market. It was
common for a book to make its first appearance in a handsome folio or

quarto edition and for subsequent editions to decrease in size. Cheaper octavo and duodecimo editions enabled texts to reach a wider readership than was previously possible. A new phenomenon in this century was the increased cooperation between publishers in England and Holland, which led to books appearing simultaneously in both countries, often in a single edition with different title-pages. Engravings became more widely used to illustrate scientific works and some reached very high standards; copper-plates were still expensive to produce, however, and plagiarism or re-use of plates was very common.

Although most of the books described in this chapter were issued from the major centres of printing in Europe, it is worth mentioning the very few items with any medical association printed in America in this period, if only because of their rarity. The first American imprint of this kind was a reprint of a sermon by Thomas Vincent (1634–78) with the title *Gods terrible voice in the city of London*, describing the plague of 1665 and the Great Fire, which was printed in Cambridge, Massachusetts in 1668. Another sermon by John Oliver, *A present to be given to teeming women ... containing directions for women with child*, originally published in London, 1663, was reprinted in Boston, Mass. in 1694. The only indigenous medical item printed in this period was by Thomas Thacher (1620–78), *A brief rule to guide the common-people of New-England how to order themselves and theirs in the small pocks, or measels*, Boston, 1677 [i.e. 1673], survives in only one copy in the Massachusetts Historical Society, Boston. Two further American editions of this title are known and all were published in facsimile in 1937.[3]

The communication of ideas was aided by the increasing availability of printed books in the seventeenth century but as important were the organizations which provided a meeting place for ideas to be exchanged. The volume of correspondence which survives from this period, for example in the archives of the Royal Society or among the manuscripts of Sir Hans Sloane in the British Library, bears witness to the stimulus which these institutions gave to research of all kinds. The early scientific societies fostered the development of experimental science in all fields and medical men were usually among their members. The earliest of the early modern scientific societies were Italian; Giambattista della Porta organized in 1560 a group of friends who met at his home and were known as the Academia Secretorum Naturae or Accademia del Segreti. This short-lived society was followed by the Accademia dei Lincei founded at Rome in 1603 by Prince Federigo Cesi. Its members included Della Porta and Galileo. Like the earlier society, it was threatened by suspicion of sorcery but it was revived in 1609 and began recording the proceedings of its meetings in the earliest publication of its kind, the *Gesta Lynceorum*. Cesi died in 1630 and the society followed suit in 1657, though the name was revived in the Accademia Nazionale dei Lincei, founded in 1784 and still extant. In the year of the demise of the Lynxes, another society, the Accademia del Cimento (1657–67), was established at Florence. Nine scientists pursued their researches for the ten years of the academy's life and the results were published in *Saggi di Naturali esperienze fatte nell'Accademia del Cimento*, which first appeared in 1666 with a second edition in 1667. This was published in English, translated by Richard Waller, in 1684; a Latin translation by P. von Musschenbroek appeared in 1731 and a French version in 1755.

Joachim Jungius (1587–1657), a physician, naturalist and mathematician, founded in 1622 what was probably the earliest scientific academy, the Societas Ereunetica of Rostock. The society ceased to exist in 1625 and left no publication to record its activities. The Academia Naturae Curiosorum was founded in 1652 by Johann Lorenz Bausch (1605–55), a physician of Schweinfurt. The society, which still survives, aimed to publish monographs principally on medicine and pharmacy and from 1670 published a periodical modelled on the *Philosophical Transactions* of the Royal Society – the *Miscellanea curiosa medico-physica*. The society changed its name in 1677 to the Academia Caesarea Leopoldina.[4]

The Royal Society originated in informal meetings which began about 1645 in London and later in Oxford. The London meetings were held at Gresham College and the society was formally constituted in 1660. The first Fellows included fourteen medical men, among them Francis Glisson, George Ent, Thomas Willis, and Daniel Whistler. A Royal Charter was granted on 15 July 1662. The first periodical published by a learned society, the *Philosophical Transactions* began publication on 6 March 1665. The first number included three papers taken from the *Journal des Sçavans* which had begun publication two months earlier. The *Philosophical Transactions* has been published ever since with only minor breaks; although it did not appear between 1677 and 1683, Robert Hooke edited a replacement with the title *Philosophical Collections* for most of this time. The first secretary of the Royal Society, Henry Oldenburg (1615?–77), was instrumental in establishing both the *Philosophical Transactions* and the correspondence with foreign scientists; his role in the society's development has been explored by A. Rupert Hall and Marie Boas Hall, who have edited his voluminous correspondence. Thomas Sprat published *The history of the Royal Society of London, for the improving of natural knowledge*, 1667, and Nehemiah Grew (1641–1712) wrote an account of the society's collections in *Musaeum Regalis Societatis. Or a catalogue and description of ... rarieties belonging to the Royal Society*, 1681.[5]

The *Philosophical Transactions* were printed by John Martyn and James Allestry, printers to the Royal Society, who also printed a number of the monographs which appeared under the society's imprimatur. The first book to be published thus was John Evelyn's *Sylva, or a discourse of forest trees*, 1664, and Robert Hooke's *Micrographia*, 1665, and Malpighi's treatise on the silkworm were among the works which followed.[6]

Although both German and English societies were under royal patronage, of the Emperor Leopold and Charles II respectively, they remained independent of the court; the Académie des Sciences, however, founded in 1666, was more closely tied to the French court of Louis XIV and was more generously funded, with pensions to allow the members to concentrate on scientific research. The Académie used the *Journal des Sçavans* to publish in until after the reorganization of the Académie in 1699, when its own periodical appeared, the *Histoire de l'Académie des Sciences*, 1702–97. The researches of the Académie's early period were collected in the *Histoire de l'Académie des Sciences depuis son établissement en 1666 jusqu'à 1699*, issued in eleven volumes in 1733. Like the Royal Society, the Académie encouraged the publication of monographs, the first of which was Perrault's *Mémoires pour servir à l'histoire naturelle des animaux*, Paris, 1671–6. This was translated into English by Alexander Pitfield and published by the Royal Society in 1688.[7]

The subjects addressed by these societies were as diverse as the interests of the virtuosi but comparative anatomy, physiology and chemistry figured prominently among them. Institutions specifically devoted to medicine consisted of the professional bodies, such as colleges of physicians, which tended to devote themselves to upholding the traditional orthodoxy rather than encouraging experimentation and innovation. The College of Physicians of London, established in 1518, although supporting traditional medical teaching based on Galen and hostile towards chemical medicine, was nevertheless the scene for the demonstrations of William Harvey's revolutionary theory of the circulation of the blood, when Harvey was Lumleian lecturer there from 1616. The College occupied premises at Amen Corner for most of the century, and here a botanical garden was planned, an anatomical theatre built and a museum and library established. The building was destroyed in the Great Fire of 1666 and although Christopher Merrett, the Harveian Librarian, managed to save about 140 books, the rest were lost. New buildings designed by Robert Hooke were erected in Warwick Lane in 1670–5. Harvey was part of the committee which prepared the first official pharmacopœia which was published in 1618; the first version of the *Pharmacopœia Londinensis* appeared in May but was withdrawn and a revised and enlarged text was issued in December; facsimile reprints of both versions were published in 1944. A second pharmacopœia was issued in 1650 and a third, entitled *Pharmacopœia Collegii Regalis Londini*, was published in 1677. Although a number of medieval receipts continued to inhabit the pharmacopœias into the eighteenth century, each successive edition reflected some changes in medical thinking. The Royal College of Physicians of Edinburgh, founded in 1681, issued its first pharmacopœia in 1699.[8]

The London pharmacopœia was intended to be observed by both physicians and apothecaries who had their own governing body, the Society of Apothecaries of London, from 1617. The society was first incorporated by a charter from James I dated 9 April 1606, when the apothecaries were united with the grocers. Their independence was secured by a Charter of 6 December 1617. The society's Hall in Blackfriars Lane was procured in 1632 and although the original building was destroyed in the Great Fire of 1666, a new one was erected in 1668. Two men closely involved with the foundation of the society were Gideon Delaune (1565–1659), Apothecary to Anne of Denmark, and Sir Theodore Turquet de Mayerne (1573–1655), physician to James I and Charles I, who emigrated to England after his pamphlet on chemical medicines was condemned by the Faculty of Medicine of Paris in 1603. Mayerne published little in his lifetime but some volumes of his manuscript day-books are among the Sloane manuscripts in the British Library. Mayerne's clinical practice is preserved in the *Praxeos Mayernianae*, London, 1670, which was extracted from the day-books by his son-in-law, and his treatise on the gout, published posthumously in Geneva in 1674, was translated into English by Thomas Sherley, physician in ordinary to Charles II, in 1676. Some of Mayerne's remedies were incorporated in the London pharmacopœia.[9]

Medical education still revolved around a few centres of excellence and there is no doubt that universities had a significant role in furthering investigative research despite the traditional Galenic bias of the medical curriculum. At the beginning of the seventeenth century, Padua retained its prominence as a place of study for medicine.

One of the teachers based at Padua was Sanctorius Sanctorius (Santorio Santorio) (1561–1636), the founder of the physiology of metabolism. Sanctorius is particularly remembered for his experiments on the changes in weight of the human body, which he conducted on himself by means of a steelyard balance in which he took his meals and even slept. His published writings include *Methodi vitandorum errorum*, Venice, 1602, which went into several editions, and *Ars ... de statica medicina*, Venice, 1614, his most famous publication, which had a second revised edition in 1615 with the title *De medicina statica* and was reprinted many times and translated into English (1676) and other languages. Sanctorius also produced commentaries on Galen (Venice, 1612) and on Avicenna's *Canon* (Venice, 1625) and his last work was *Liber de remediorum inventione*, Venice, 1629. His collected works were issued in four volumes, *Opera omnia*, Venice, 1660.[10]

Hieronymus Fabricius ab Aquapendente (Girolamo Fabrizio) (1533–1619) studied under Fallopius at Padua and succeeded him as teacher of anatomy; Fabricius was appointed to lecture on anatomy and surgery in 1565. He was responsible for building the anatomy theatre which still exists. In 1574, while dissecting, he first noticed the valves of the veins, which he illustrated in his most famous work, *De venarum ostiolis*, Padua, 1603, issued separately although usually found bound with other of his works with a general title-page dated 1625. Fabricius was not the first to discover these valves, nor did he appreciate their function or significance; this was understood by his pupil, William Harvey. Fabricius's medical interests were wide and among his works are *Dissertatio de lue pestifera*, 1585 and *Pentateuchos cheirurgicum*, Frankfort, 1592, a collection of his surgical work edited by Johann Hartmann Beyer. Fabricius intended to publish a huge work surveying all of anatomy; this was not completed but he published parts of it in various treatises; *De visione, voce, auditu*, Venice, 1600, *De locutione et ejus instrumentis liber*, Venice, 1601, *De musculi artificio, ossium de articulationibus*, 1614, and works on respiration and the digestive system. Fabricius may have bequeathed his interest in embryology to his most illustrious pupil; it is the subject of the late works *De formato foetu*, Venice 1600 and *De formatione ovi et pulli*, Padua, 1621. The collected writings of Fabricius were printed as *Opera chirurgica*, Frankfort, 1620, translated into French, German and Italian; *Opera anatomica*, Padua, 1625 and *Opera omnia anatomica et physiologica*, Leipzig, 1687.[11]

William Harvey (1578–1657) exemplifies the spirit of empirical investigation which enabled medical science to make such advances in this century. Harvey was born at Folkestone on 1 April 1578; he graduated from Caius College, Cambridge, with a BA in 1597 and went to Padua, where he studied under Fabricius, becoming Doctor of Medicine in 1602. On his return to England he received the same degree from Cambridge. In 1604 Harvey settled in London, became a Fellow of the College of Physicians (1607), serving as Censor and from 1615, Lumleian Lecturer, a position he held until his retirement in 1656. He was physician to St Bartholomew's Hospital from 1609. During the Civil War Harvey followed the King to Oxford and was for a time Warden of Merton College. Much of his work was lost when a mob raided his London lodging in 1642 and after the reversal of the Royalist cause, in 1645, Harvey retired from public life; he died on 3 June 1657 at his brother Eliab's home in Roehampton. The definitive biography of Harvey is the work of Sir Geoffrey Keynes, who was also responsible for the bibliography of Harvey's writings, first published in 1928 to celebrate the tercentenary of the publication of Harvey's major work.

Like his teacher Fabricius, Harvey was slow to publish, accumulating evidence to construct an irrefutable argument. His concise and logical demonstration of the circulation of the blood was contained in the 72 pages of his first published work, *Exercitatio anatomica de motu cordis et sanguinis in animalibus* 1628. This work, commonly referred to by the shorter title *De motu cordis*, is probably the most famous medical book ever published, and its pre-eminence is reflected in the high prices which the first edition, despite its unimpressive appearance, can command. It was published in Frankfort by the Englishman, William Fitzer; the bulk of the edition was printed on poor quality paper which has been subject to foxing, though a few of the sixty-odd copies known to survive are of finer paper. A small number of copies have an additional half sheet of two pages containing 126 errata headed by Fitzer's apology for the large number of errors in such a short work. Most copies have been cut down and are bound in volumes with other tracts. The text was not printed separately again until the twentieth century.

Harvey's small book aroused a large protest. One of the earliest opponents of Harvey's theory, Emilio Parisano (1567–1643), printed most of *De motu cordis* in alternate paragraphs with his refutations, in the second volume of his work *Nobilium exercitationum de subtilitate*, published in 1635. Johannes Maire of Leyden reprinted this dual argument in 1639, adding the sections of Harvey's work which Parisano had omitted and a treatise by James Primerose (1580–1659), the most vociferous English critic of the circulation theory. In 1647 Maire reissued this with other works relevant to the debate, including his 1640 edition of the first account of the lacteal vessels by Gaspare Aselli (1581–1625); Aselli's *De lactibus* was first published in 1627. In the scarce duodecimo edition printed in Padua in 1643, *De motu cordis* is accompanied for the first time by the two letters of Jan de Wale (Walaeus) (1604–49) of Leyden, approving Harvey's work.

It is slightly surprising, in view of the number of errors in the first edition, that the first corrected text appeared 20 years after it. This revised text was produced not by Harvey but by two doctors of Rotterdam, Zacharias Sylvius (van den Bossche) and Jacobus de Back, who contributed a pro-Harveian treatise *Dissertatio de Corde*. Subsequent editions usually followed this text and incorporated De Back's dissertation. In 1649 Harvey finally joined in the debate which his first book had engendered, with his *Exercitatio anatomica de circulatione sanguinis*, two essays addressed to Jean Riolan, professor of anatomy at Paris and perhaps the most eminent of his opponents. *De circulatione sanguinis* was first published in Cambridge in 1649; it evidently took three attempts to get the title-page of this edition right, as the original was cancelled and the first substitute found in some copies has a word scratched out from the imprint. In the same year an edition was published in Rotterdam and another in Paris in 1650 but thereafter it was usually printed with *De motu cordis*. The earliest translation of *De motu cordis* was a Dutch translation printed in Amsterdam in 1650; the translator added verses on the death of Harvey, somewhat prematurely. The first English translation was published in 1653 and includes both *De circulatione sanguinis* and De Back's *Discourse*. This translation was reprinted in 1673 and was used by Sir

Geoffrey Keynes for the Nonesuch Press edition of 1928 and as the basis for Gweneth Whitteridge's translation published in 1976. Kenneth J. Franklin produced new translations of both *De motu cordis* and *De circulatione sanguinis*. An early English abridged version of *De motu cordis* was printed in volume three of *Bibliotheca anatomica, medica, chirurgica*, a work based on Daniel Leclerc and Jacques Manget's *Bibliotheca anatomica*, which was published in monthly parts from November 1709, with general title-pages dated 1711 to 1714. This version was first described by F. N. L. Poynter, and Richard Durling provided details of other eminent writers translated into English for the first time as part of this collection.

The publication of Harvey's work on embryology, *Exercitationes de generatione animalium*, London, 1651, was due to the persuasion of Sir George Ent (1604–89), Harvey's friend and supporter, who prepared the book for the press. An English translation of this work was published in 1653, and a revised and annotated version of this was published by Gweneth Whitteridge in 1981. There are only two separate editions of Harvey's collected works in Latin; an edition of the three major works was printed in two parts at Leyden, 1737 and an authoritative corrected edition was prepared by Mark Akenside for the Royal College of Physicians and published by the College in 1766. This includes various miscellaneous writings, such as Harvey's account of the anatomy of Thomas Parr and Harvey's letters. The only English translation of the collected works, by Robert Willis, was published by the Sydenham Society in 1847.

Three early unpublished works by Harvey exist in two manuscripts among the Sloane collection in the British Library, MSS. 230 and 486. Gweneth Whitteridge published the first transcription and translation of *De motu locali animalium*, 1627, in a volume sponsored by the Royal College of Physicians of London. A facsimile of the manuscript of *Prelectiones anatomiae universalis*, 1616, was published in 1886 with an inaccurate transcription, and a translation based on this version was published in 1961. Gweneth Whitteridge retranscribed the manuscript and published the Latin text with an English version which is not likely to be superseded. It includes the short work *De musculis*, 1619. Numerous books and articles on Harvey have appeared, particularly in response to the tercentenary of his death and the quatercentenary of his birth, and some of the more significant are listed in the notes.[12]

Harvey's demonstration of the circulation of the blood came to be almost universally accepted in his lifetime. Its authority was gradually endorsed by other eminent medical writers. Perhaps the most significant of these was René Descartes (1596–1650), who adopted the theory of the circulation immediately on the appearance of Harvey's book and made it central to his view of human physiology. Descartes, although French by birth, lived in Holland for much of his life, and his *Discours de la méthode*, part four of which has a detailed account of the physiology of circulation, was published in Leyden in 1637. Although Descartes rejected Harvey's description of the heart as a muscle which pumps blood, believing instead that the blood was heated in the heart, his approval of the circulatory system was influential. The *Discours* was translated into English in 1649. Other of Descartes's writings are concerned in part with physiology, especially *Des passions de l'âme*, Amsterdam, 1649, and the posthumous *De homine*, Leyden, 1662, which was translated into French (1664) and Dutch (1695).

Descartes is primarily important in the history of medical thought for his mechanistic view of the human body; Descartes's exposition of this idea is the best known but it was widely adopted in the seventeenth century and the school known as iatro-physicists applied the laws of mechanics to physiological processes in the same way that the iatro-chemists explained them from chemical principles.[13] Another landmark in the dissemination of Harvey's discovery was the incorporation of it into the revised version of the anatomical textbook by Caspar Bartholin (1585–1629), first published as *Anatomicae institutiones*, Wittenberg, 1611. This was revised by Caspar's son, Thomas Bartholin (1616–80); his first version was published at Leyden in 1641, a second was published from Padua in 1645, and a completely revised text was published at Leyden in 1651 with the title *Anatomia, ex Caspari Bartholini parentis Institutionibus ... tertium ad sanguinis circulationem reformata*; this edition adds the two letters of Jan de Wale on the motion of the chyle and the blood. This was followed by a further edition published at The Hague in 1655 which added an appendix containing Thomas Bartholin's observations on the lymph vessels and the thoracic duct. There were many subsequent editions and an English translation, *Bartholinus anatomy*, translated by Nicholas Culpeper was printed in 1663. The Bartholins were a Danish family and, although Thomas Bartholin travelled widely in Europe, he returned to Copenhagen and was appointed professor of mathematics and subsequently, in 1649, professor of medicine. His writings were published from various countries; the early works in Italy, *Anatomica aneurysmatis dissecti historia*, Palermo, 1644 and *De unicornu observationes novae*, Padua, 1645. Bartholin's doctoral thesis *De pleuritide* was printed at Basle in 1645. His interest in medicine and the bible is evidenced in the early *De latere Christi aperto dissertatio*, Leyden, 1646. Bartholin's most important works are *De lacteis thoracicis in homine brutisque nuperrime observatis*, Copenhagen, 1652, which contains his account of his discovery of the human thoracic duct, following Pecquet's discovery of this organ in dogs, and the two works *Vasa lymphatica, nuper Hafniae in animantibus inventa*, Copenhagen, 1653, and *Vasa lymphatica in homine nuper inventa*, 1654, which announce and confirm Bartholin's discovery of the lymphatics as a separate system. Thomas's son Caspar Bartholin (1655–1738) in turn edited some of his father's works, and was the author of *De ovariis mulierum et generationis historia*, Rome, 1677, which contains a description of the vulvovaginal glands.[14] The increasing tendency of scholars to view Harvey in the context of his contemporaries rather than in isolation has produced some new insights. Robert Frank Gregg's *Harvey and the Oxford physiologists, a study in scientific ideas* (Berkeley, 1980) has traced the influence of Harvey on the Oxford based group which included Richard Lower, John Mayow and Thomas Willis.

Richard Lower (1631–91) and John Mayow (1641–79) were Cornishmen, friends and respectively assistant to and pupil of Thomas Willis. A joint bibliographical study of their writings was published by John Fulton. Lower's first published work, *Diatribae Thomae Willisii ... de febribus vindicatio adversus Edmundum Meara*, London, 1665 (two issues) is a defence of the theories of his mentor. Lower is remembered for his pioneering experiments in blood transfusion. His account of the first transfusion, performed on dogs, was published in the *Philosophical Transactions* of the Royal Society in 1665 and on 23 November 1667, Lower and Edmond King publicly demonstrated at Arundel House the first transfusion with a human subject made in England; this operation had first been successfully performed in Paris by Jean Denis on 15 June 1667. Lower's most important work is the *Tractatus de corde*, London, 1669. It has been suggested by K. J. Franklin that the first edition was actually published in 1668, since a copy in the British Library annotated by Walter Charleton is thus dated by him. Franklin produced the first translation into English of *De corde* and noted some textual changes in successive editions. The second edition, which is bibliographically complex, was published in London, 1670, a third edition appeared in Amsterdam, 1671 and a fourth in London in 1680. A French translation was published in Paris in 1679 and has been discussed by R. Rullière. There were also editions printed in Geneva in 1685 and 1699 and in Leyden 1708, 1722, 1740 and 1749.

In his 1935 bibliography, Fulton listed *De catarrhis*, 1672, as a separate tract although no copy was then known; it appears as an extra chapter in later editions of *De corde*. Richard Hunter and Ida Macalpine discovered that there are three different versions of the second edition of *Tractatus de corde*; the one which they had acquired and of which they located another copy in Dr Williams's Library, consists of the original sheets of the first edition with *De catarrhis* as a separate pamphlet without a full title-page, evidently issued as an addendum; they reproduced this in facsimile with a translation. The description of the lancet, *De venae sectione*, which was added with *De catarrhis*, was translated into English in 1674 as an addition to a translation of *Cista militaris* by Hildanus. Two works were published under Lower's name but are of doubtful authenticity; *Bromographia* had several continental printings; the popular *Dr. Lower's and several other eminent physicians receipts*, London, 1700, was published nine years after his death.[15]

John Mayow graduated in law and medicine and became a Fellow of All Souls in 1660. He made original contributions to both physiology and chemistry, particularly in the areas of respiration and combustion. He published on respiration and rickets in his *Tractatus duo*, Oxford 1668, reprinted with a new title-page in 1669 and twice subsequently, in Leyden, in 1671 and 1708. Mayow's *Tractatus quinque medico-physici*, Oxford, 1674, had several continental editions and was translated into French, Dutch and German. An English translation was published in 1907 as Alembic Club Reprint, No. 17. The tract on rickets, *De rachitide*, which was included in both Mayow's earlier works, was translated into English as ραχιτιδολογια, *or a tract of the disease rhachitis commonly called the rickets*, Oxford, 1685.[16]

The most eminent of the circle of Oxford medical men was Thomas Willis (1621–75), who graduated from Christ Church College and after an interval of military service obtained a medical degree and was licensed to practise in 1646. Willis's academic career was interrupted by the Commonwealth, during which he practised medicine and pursued his anatomical and chemical researches. In 1660 he obtained an MD and was appointed Sedleian Professor of Natural Philosophy; some of his lectures are preserved in the notebooks of John Locke and have been edited by Kenneth Dewhurst, as has a casebook of Willis's dating from this period. Willis retained his Chair when, at the invitation of the Archbishop of Canterbury, he moved to Westminster in 1667. He was elected a Fellow of the Royal Society and is buried in Westminster Abbey. Willis's first book was *Diatribae duae medico-philosophicae*, London, 1659; John Aubrey's copy in the Bodleian Library has an inscription dated 1658 but may have been an advance copy. It contains tracts on fermentation, on fevers and a dissertation on urine. A second edition appeared in 1660, a third in 1662 and a fourth in 1677. It was also printed at The Hague, 1662 and Amsterdam, 1663 and 1669 and a French translation was made of the last part, *Dissertation sur les urines*, Paris, 1683 and 1687. Willis's major work, *Cerebri anatome: cui accessit nervorum descriptio et usus*, London 1664, contains an accurate description of the nervous system and describes the 'nerve of Willis' and the 'circle of Willis'. It also has the distinction that some of the original drawings for the fine plates were made by Sir Christopher Wren, who, with Thomas Millington, had worked with Willis on preparing the book (see Plate 6).[17] Willis merits a full published bibliography, but the lack of this is partly met by the unpublished study by H. J. R. Wing, 1962, and the bibliographical survey of *Cerebri anatome*, by H. R. Denham, published with the tercentenary edition of Samuel Pordage's English translation. The latter gives much information on the editions of *Cerebri anatome*; the first edition, in quarto, was followed in the same year by an octavo edition printed in London and two issues from different printers in Amsterdam, one of which, printed by Commelin, adds William Croone's *De ratione motus musculorum*, first published in London, 1664. *Cerebri anatome* was reprinted in Amsterdam in 1666 (two issues), 1667, 1676 and 1683. Willis moved from the anatomy of the nervous system to its pathology in his *Pathologiae cerebri*, Oxford 1667. In 1668 an edition was published by Allestry in London and Daniel Elzevir in Amsterdam, with the device and imprint altered accordingly; a further Amsterdam edition appeared in 1670 and a fourth edition in London in 1678. In answer to Nathaniel Highmore's attack on this work, Willis published his description of hysteria, *Affectionum quae dicuntur hystericae et hypochondriacae pathologia spasmodica vindicata*, London, 1670 and 1678, also printed at Leyden, 1671 (two issues). Willis regarded *De anima brutorum*, Oxford, 1672, as his greatest work. It is mainly concerned with the nervous system, arthritis, mental diseases and contains a chapter on general paralysis. The section on mental deficiency contains a description of schizophrenia, and myasthenia is also described. The first printing in quarto was followed by a series of octavo editions, London, 1672 (two issues from different booksellers), Amsterdam, 1672 and 1674. An English translation, *Two discourses concerning the soul of brutes*, by Samuel Pordage was published in London in 1683. Willis's last work was *Pharmaceutice rationalis*, an epitome of the materia medica, the second part of which was published posthumously; Part I, Oxford, 1674, Part II, 1675 (two issues); Part I, The Hague, 1675 (engraved title-page dated 1674), Part II, 1677. The third edition was printed at Oxford in 1679, although the title-page of Part II is dated 1678. Willis's collected writings were printed several times on the continent; *Opera medica & physica*, two volumes, Lyons, 1676, and *Opera omnia*, Geneva, 1676–7 (two issues, one with 'Coloniae Allobrogum' in place of 'Genevae' in the imprints), and 1680 (similarly in two issues); other editions appeared at Lyons, 1681, Amsterdam, 1682 (edited by Gerard Blasius and usually counted the best edition), Geneva, 1695 and in folio at Venice, 1708 and 1720. An English work dating from 1666, *A plain and easie method for preserving those that are well from the infection of the plague*, was edited by J. Hemming from Willis's manuscript and published in 1691; there are two issues of the first edition. Various selections and translations of Willis's works have been published; Samuel Pordage translated *Pharmaceutice rationalis*, London, 1679, which forms the second part of the collected edition of Willis's works published as *The remaining medical works*, 1681. A new version of this was published in 1684 as *Dr. Willis's practice of physick*, which includes a new translation of Part I of *Pharmaceutice rationalis* and Pordage's English version of *De anima brutorum*. *The London practice of physick*, a selection of Willis's writings on clinical subjects was printed at London in 1685, 1689, 1692 and 1695.[18]

Willis's circle at Oxford included Sir William Petty (1623–87), Reader in Anatomy, who, with Willis, resuscitated a servant maid, Anne Greene, who had been hanged for murdering her child. Petty was subsequently appointed to survey and superintend the redistribution of land in Ireland for the Commonwealth and went on to write treatises on political economy. He was one of the original Fellows of the Royal Society. Because of Petty's interest in statistics, he was regarded as the author of *Natural and political observations upon the Bills of Mortality*, 1662. The real author, John Graunt (1620–74), also a Fellow of the Royal Society, was the first to examine this source of medical statistics. Sir Geoffrey Keynes has published a bibliography of Petty's works which includes Graunt's book.[19] The Bills of Mortality, compiled by the Company of Parish Clerks, were criticized by Graunt for their inaccuracy, but, despite their limitations, they remain a unique record of causes of death in the capital city. They were published weekly and the most complete series is held by the Guildhall Library in London. The most visually dramatic record of the Great Plague is surely the collection *London's dreadful visitation, or a collection of all the Bills of Mortality for the present year*, 1665.

A survey of diseases in London which parallels this statistical record was conducted by Thomas Sydenham (1624–89), although he actually left the city during the plague, as did many of his colleagues. Sydenham also held academic office in Commonwealth Oxford. He entered Magdalen Hall in 1642 but his studies were interrupted by the Civil War, during which he joined his family in fighting on the side of the Parliamentarians. Although he returned to Oxford and was appointed a Fellow of All Souls in 1648, he remained scornful of the value of academic study as opposed to clinical fieldwork. He resigned his fellowship in 1655 and moved to Westminster. His skill in the field of clinical medicine was recognized in his lifetime, particularly on the continent, and he was known as the 'English Hippocrates', though his Puritan sympathies and antagonism to the methods of his contemporaries hindered his advancement at home. Sydenham's early writings were translated from his original English into Latin for publication, with a consequent loss of vigour and individuality. Fortunately some of his English prose is preserved in manuscripts and these have been edited by Kenneth Dewhurst, with a biographical study. Sydenham's first published work, *Methodus curandi febres*, London and Amsterdam, 1666, second edition 1668, was redeveloped and enlarged as *Observationes medicae circa morborum acutorum historiam et curationem*, London, 1676, which was reprinted several times on the continent. Sydenham's *Dissertatio epistolaris ...*, London, 1682, with a second edition in 1685, on hysteria, is a landmark in psychological medicine. A sufferer from gout, Sydenham wrote a classic account of the disease in his *Tractatus de podagra et hydrope*, London, 1683, reprinted Leyden, 1684 and Geneva, 1686. His differentiation of chorea minor is contained in the last work to be published in his lifetime, *Schedula monitoria de novae febris ingressu*, 1685; *Processus integri* ... was published posthumously in 1693. There were various editions of his collected works, *Opuscula*, Amsterdam, 1683 and *Opera universa*, London, 1685. The Sydenham Society, dedicated to bringing out translations of important medical works, published the works in Latin edited by William Alexander Greenhill in 1844 and 1846 and in an English translation by R. G. Latham in two volumes, 1844–50.[20]

Sydenham's reputation was eagerly promoted by his friend and colleague, John Locke (1632–1704), who began his study of medicine at Oxford, assisted Richard Lower's experiments and attended the lectures of Thomas Willis. Locke's clinical training was done under Sydenham, who was frequently called in to advise on Locke's patients, including his patron Lord Shaftesbury, and when Locke gave up medicine Sydenham seems to have taken over most of his practice. Locke's extensive papers have been mined for medical material by Kenneth Dewhurst, who has published a biography with an edition of the medical notes from Locke's journals from 1675 to 1698. Locke acted as Sydenham's amanuensis and some of Sydenham's manuscript works are in his hand.[21]

Richard Morton (1637–98) was an admirer of Sydenham and contributed an important account of tuberculosis to medical literature, *Phthisiologia, seu exercitationes de phthisi*, London, 1689, which includes an account of anorexia nervosa. This was translated into English in 1694.

Cambridge also of course produced eminent medical men during this period apart from William Harvey. Francis Glisson (1598–1677), like Harvey, graduated from Gonville and Caius College and was Regius Professor of Physic at Cambridge for forty years. A founder member of the Royal Society, Glisson was also President of the College of Physicians from 1667 to 1669. His classic monograph on rickets arose from the efforts of a group of medical men to write a treatise on the subject. Glisson's contribution was so original that he was invited to complete the work himself, though his colleagues George Bate, author of a popular pharmacopœia, and Ahasuerus Regemorter are credited as co-authors. The work, *De rachitide, sive morbo puerili, qui vulgo 'The rickets' dicitur*, London, 1650 was immediately translated into English by Philip Arnim. This translation was published in 1651 and another issue appeared in the same year with the preliminary leaves reset and an altered title-page, adding that Nicholas Culpeper had 'enlarged, corrected and amended' the work. This was reprinted in 1668. Editions of the Latin text were printed in London 1660, Leyden 1671 and The Hague 1682. Glisson's treatise on the liver, *Anatomia hepatis*, London, 1654 is important for his description of the fibrous sheath of the liver which is known as Glisson's capsule. His other works were *Tractatus de natura substantiae energetica*, London, 1672 and *Tractatus de ventriculo et intestinis*, London, 1677, second edition Amsterdam, 1677. His collected works, *Opera medico-anatomica*, three volumes in one, were printed at Leyden in 1691. Twelve volumes of Glisson's manuscripts are in the Sloane collection in the British Library and his unpublished work on the theory of circulation (1662) has been edited by Jeffrey Boss.[22]

Glisson's book was regarded as the first book devoted to rickets, but Daniel Whistler (1619–84) had anticipated it with his thesis *De morbo puerili Anglorum, quem patrio idiomate indigenae vocant The Rickets*, Leyden 1645, reprinted 1684. The theory that Whistler's claim to priority was false was disproved when a copy of the original edition was discovered at the Royal College of Physicians in 1883. This small quarto of 18 pages contains an account which has been found clinically sound. A translation into English was published by G. T. Smerdon in 1950, with biographical information on Whistler. An early English work on rickets, John Bird's *Ostenta Carolina. Or the late calamities of England with the authors of them. The great happiness and happy government of K. Charles II ensuing, miraculously foreshewn by the finger of God in two wonderful diseases, the Rekets and Kings-evil*, London, 1661, promotes the Royal Touch as the only remedy. Bird's account of the disease has been shown to be based on Glisson's.[23]

The Royal Touch assumed a considerable political importance at the Restoration confirming as it did the divine authority of the monarch, and Charles II touched an amazing number of the sick. An account of his healing powers is contained in the treatise *Adenochoiradelogia: or, an anatomick-chirurgical treatise of glandules and strumaes, or King's-Evil swellings*, London, 1684, the frontispiece of which shows the ceremony at which the touching was performed. The author of this work, John Browne (1642–1702) was born and educated in Norwich, to which he returned after a period of naval service and where he became acquainted with Sir Thomas Browne. In 1683 he joined the staff of St Thomas's Hospital as surgeon, retaining this position for eight years. His works were largely compilations and he has been described as a plagiarist by K. F. Russell, who has written several papers on Browne and his writings. Browne's first book, *A compleat treatise of preternatural tumours*, London, 1678, was followed in the same year by his *A compleat discourse of wounds*. Browne's most popular work, *A compleat treatise of the muscles as they appear in humane body, and arise in dissection*, London, 1681, was printed by T. Newcombe for the author. It was subscribed for by proposals for printing issued on 28 August 1680. The text was taken from William Molins's Μυσκοτομια: *or, the anatomical administration of all the muscles of an humane body*, 1648. The plates for Browne's book were mostly copied from the *Tabulae anatomicae* of Julius Casserius (1561–1616), with alterations, and even the title-page is reproduced from the engraved title-page of the 1632 edition of Casserius. Despite criticism, notably from James

Yonge, Browne's book went into several editions. The sheets of the first edition were reissued in 1683 with a new title-page. In 1697 a new edition was published entitled *Myographia nova*, with an additional section on the heart by Richard Lower. A further edition was published in 1698 and a 'second edition' in 1705. Latin editions were published in London, 1684; Leyden, 1687 and 1690 and Amsterdam, 1694. A German translation by Christian Maximilian Spener appeared in Berlin in 1704. Browne's *Somatopolitia: or, the city of humane body artificially defended from the tyranny of cancers and gangreens*, London, 1702, was reissued in 1703 with the title *The surgeons assistant*. The Royal College of Surgeons of England holds the manuscript of Browne's work on muscles and the Hunterian Collection of Glasgow University has a manuscript of an unpublished work on 'The anatomy of the eye'. A syllabus exists among the Sloane manuscripts in the British Library and the Royal Society possesses a three-page article in Browne's handwriting containing the first description of cirrhosis of the liver, probably the author's most original contribution to medical literature.[24]

Plagiarism, particularly of illustrations, was a common feature of medical literature in this period. Even the single plate in William Harvey's *De motu cordis* was copied from an illustration to a work by Fabricius, but borrowing was not usually on such a grand scale as that of William Cowper (1666–1710), who adopted all the anatomical plates from Bidloo's *Anatomia humani corporis*. Govert Bidloo (1649–1713) was professor of anatomy at The Hague from 1688 and held the same position at Leyden from 1694. The 105 anatomical plates illustrating his work were drawn by Gerard de Lairesse (1640–1711), and 300 impressions of them were given by the publisher to Cowper, who published them with his introductory text as *The anatomy of humane bodies*, Oxford, 1698. Christian Bernhardt Albinus published a revised edition, Leyden 1737, and another edition with the text translated into Latin by William Dundas was printed at Leyden in 1739. William Cowper was a surgeon who served his apprenticeship to a London surgeon, William Bignall, and practised in London from 1691. In 1696 he became a Fellow of the Royal Society and published in the *Philosophical Transactions*, November 1699, 'An account of two glands and their excretory ducts lately discover'd in human bodies'. A Latin version of this was published in 1702 with an additional work, Εὐχαριστια. Cowper's other anatomical folio, *Myotomia reformata; or a new administration of all the muscles of humane bodies*, was first published in 1694 and reprinted in 1724, edited by Richard Mead and published at his expense.[25]

A contemporary of Cowper's, also a Fellow of the Royal Society, was Edward Tyson (1650–1708). Tyson was educated at Oxford and took his medical degree at Cambridge in 1680. He was a Fellow of the College of Physicians, physician to Bridewell and Bethlem hospitals and reader in anatomy at Surgeons Hall. Tyson is noted for his work on comparative anatomy and published several papers in the *Philosophical Transactions*. His major work was *Orang-outang, sive homo-sylvestris: or, the anatomie of a pygmie compared with that of a monkey, an ape, and a man. To which is added a philological essay concerning the pygmies ... of the ancients*, London, 1699. The orang-outang was in reality a chimpanzee. A facsimile reprint was published in 1966 with an introduction by M. F. Ashley Montagu, who has also written a separate study of Tyson. The drawings for Tyson's book were made by William Cowper, who also contributed the section on the muscles. A second edition entitled *The anatomy of a pygmy*, London, 1751, appears to be a reissue of the 1699 edition with another title-page and some of Tyson's papers from the *Philosophical Transactions* added. Tyson's *Philological essay* was edited by Bertram C. Windle and issued in a limited edition of 550 copies in 1894. Tyson's *Opera omnia*, 1751 consists of the 1699 *Orang-outang* with reprints of his other works.[26]

The development of the microscope was one of the most important advances of the seventeenth century. The first English work on microscopy was the *Experimental philosophy* of Henry Power (1623–68), which was published in 1664, a year earlier than the much more famous book on the subject by the polymath, Robert Hooke (1635–1703). Hooke made notable contributions to many branches of knowledge, and his interests ranged through the sciences from physics to biology. A graduate of Christ Church College, Oxford, he assisted Thomas Willis and subsequently Robert Boyle with experiments, designing and constructing the air-pump which Boyle used in experiments on combustion and respiration. In 1662 Hooke was appointed curator of experiments to the Royal Society, was elected a Fellow the following year and appointed Secretary in 1677. From 1679 to 1682 Hooke edited the *Philosophical Collections* which temporarily replaced the *Philosophical Transactions*. Sir Geoffrey Keynes's bibliography of Hooke's writings gives full details of his many publications, the most significant being *Micrographia: or some physiological descriptions of minute bodies made by magnifying glasses*, London, 1665. This appeared in April of that year, the imprimatur of the Royal Society being dated 23 November 1664. A reissue with a new title-page was published in 1667 and contains some slight alterations. *Micrographia* is illustrated with very fine and justly famous plates; a facsimile was produced by Dover Books, New York, 1961. Hooke's *Diary* in the Guildhall Library has been edited, and there have been several studies of his life and writings.[27]

The *Philosophical Transactions* of the Royal Society provided a forum for the exposition of discoveries made by an international community of scientists and natural philosophers. Antoni van Leeuwenhoek (1632–1723) was by profession a civil servant, occupying various civic posts in his native town, Delft, but began in 1671 in his spare time to experiment with

.grinding lenses and constructing and improving microscopes. At the suggestion of Regnier de Graaf, a Dutch correspondent of the Royal Society, Leeuwenhoek was invited by the Society to communicate his discoveries. Leeuwenhoek's first letter was received in 1673 and during the next fifty years he sent about 200 more, many of which appeared in the *Philosophical Transactions*. Translations of various of Leeuwenhoek's letters appeared in other similar learned journals such as the *Journal des Sçavans* and *Acta Eruditorum*. Leeuwenhoek observed micro-organisms in 1674 and his letter to the Royal Society of 9 October 1676, containing the first description of bacteria, was published in facsimile in 1937; he also conducted research on spermatozoa, the optic nerve, the skin, muscle and insects. Elected a Fellow in 1680, Leewenhoek bequeathed 26 of his microscopes to the Royal Society, none of which have survived. The history of the publication of Leeuwenhoek's writings is immensely complicated; some of his many letters were published both in the original Dutch and in Latin, with various locations and dates; the Dutch *Brieven* or *Werken* were published from Leyden and Delft, 1684–1718; the Latin versions appeared under the title *Arcana naturae*, in four volumes. A complete edition of his collected letters, edited from the originals rather than the often inaccurate printed translations, began publication in 1939. Leeuwenhoek's *Select works*, translated by Samuel Hoole, were published by subscription and printed for the translator. The first part of Volume I was dated 1798 but appeared in 1797; this rare issue has the misprint 'miscroscopical' on the title-page. A second issue, with the misprint corrected, was published in 1798. The second part is dated 1799 and Volume II appeared in 1807. Hoole used only the Dutch and Latin editions and did not incorporate material published solely in the *Philosophical Transactions*; he also bowdlerized the text, omitting passages dealing with spermatozoa and reproduction. The book by Clifford Dobell, first published in 1932, is still an important source on Leeuwenhoek. More recent studies of Leeuwenhoek include biographies by A. Schierbeek and Alma Smith Payne and a volume commemorating the 350th anniversary of his birth.[28]

Leeuwenhoek was partially cut off from the world of contemporary scholarship because of his lack of languages; in 1674 he observed corpuscles in the blood, unaware that they had already been observed by another associate of the Royal Society, Malpighi, who had described them, though identifying them wrongly, in 1665. Marcello Malpighi (1628–94) attended the University of Bologna from 1646, graduating in medicine and philosophy in 1653. In 1656 he was appointed professor of medicine at the University of Pisa where he stayed for three years before returning to Bologna. In Pisa Malpighi met Giovanni Alfonso Borelli (1608–79), the mathematician whose posthumous *De motu animalium* is a classic of physiology. Two letters of Malpighi addressed to Borelli, announcing his discovery of the structure of the lungs and observation of the capillaries, were published with the title *De pulmonibus observationes anatomicae*, Bologna, 1661. This is very rare, the only copy in Great Britain being held in the Medical Society of London collection at the Wellcome Institute. Malpighi interrupted his time at Bologna for a short interval at the University of Messina but continued his microscopical investigations and published two important works, *Epistolae anatomicae de cerebro, ac lingua ... quibus Anonymi accessit exercitatio de omento, pinguedine, et adiposis ductibus*, Bologna, 1665 and *De viscerum structura exercitatio anatomica*, Bologna, 1666, which had as appendix *De polypo cordis*. Editions of *De viscerum structura* appeared at Amsterdam, 1669, and London in the same year; a French translation was published in Paris in 1683 and reprinted in 1687; an Italian translation is included in *Celebrazione Malpighiane: discorsi e scritti*, 1966. In 1677 Malpighi was invited to correspond with the Royal Society and many of his communications were published thereafter in the *Philosophical Transactions*. Malpighi's later works were published in London under the auspices of the Royal Society and these include his detailed study of the silkworm, *Dissertatio epistolica de bombyce*, 1669 and his embryological work, *Dissertatio epistolica de formatione pulli in ovo*, 1673. In 1684 Malpighi's house was burned and all his microscopes and manuscripts destroyed. He was appointed personal physician to Pope Innocent XII in 1691, three years before his death. Malpighi's writings were collected in the *Opera omnia* published in London in 1686, reprinted Leyden, 1687, and *Opera posthuma*, London, 1697, reprinted at both Amsterdam and Venice in 1698. The bibliography of Malpighi's works by Carlo Frati, 1897, has not been superseded; the major contribution to Malpighi scholarship has been that of Howard B. Adelmann, who published a study in five volumes, covering Malpighi's life, embryological thought before Malpighi and his contribution to embryology, and his writings. Adelmann has also edited Malpighi's correspondence.[29]

Regnier de Graaf (1641–73), a physician of Delft and a friend of Leeuwenhoek, made important contributions to medical knowledge, despite his early death. De Graaf studied at Leyden and his thesis was an important first study of the pancreas and its secretions; *De succi pancreatici natura et usu, exercitatio anatomico-medica*, Leyden, 1664, was republished as *Tractatus anatomico-medicus de succi pancreatici natura et usu*, Leyden, 1671. A French edition with revised text, and the addition of a new section, was published at Paris in 1666 and an English translation appeared in 1676. De Graaf's classic account of the testicle, *De virorum organis generationi inservientibus de clysteribus et de usu siphonis in anatomia*, Leyden and Rotterdam, 1668, included an essay on clysters which was translated into French with the title, *L'instrument de Molière*, Paris, 1878; an English translation was published in 1954. De Graaf's account of the structures which became known as the Graafian follicles is contained in his work on the ovary, *De mulierum organis generationi inservientibus tractatus novus*, Leyden, 1672. A facsimile edition of this was published in Holland in 1965 and an English translation of both de Graaf's works on the human reproductive organs was published in 1972. His *Opera omnia* was first published at Lyons, 1677, and reprinted in the following year; a new edition was printed at Amsterdam, 1705 and a Dutch translation was published at Amsterdam, 1686.[30]

The change in obstetric practice with the advent of the man-midwife into a traditionally female domain began in the seventeenth century. The leading obstetrician in the later part of the century was François Mauriceau (1637–1709), author of *Traité des maladies des femmes grosses et celles qui sont accouchées*, Paris, 1668. This was translated into English by Hugh Chamberlen, of the Huguenot family which guarded their invention, the obstetric forceps, as a secret for many years. Chamberlen's translation, *The accomplisht midwife, treating of the diseases of women with child and in childbearing*, London, 1673, went into numerous editions. Mauriceau's other works were *Observations de la grossesse et l'accouchement des femmes*, Paris, 1694 and *Aphorismes touchant la grossesse, l'accouchement, les maladies et les autres indispositions des femmes*, 1694.[31]

Developments in practical surgery were often the result of experience gained in naval or military service. John Woodall (1569/70?–1643) had a varied career, beginning with his appointment as military surgeon in Lord Willoughby's regiment in 1591. He was admitted as a member of the Barber-Surgeons' Company in 1599 and was Master of the Company in 1633. For most of his life, Woodall was surgeon to St Bartholomew's Hospital in London, but he was created surgeon-general to the East India Company in 1612 and was responsible for fitting out chests for ships' surgeons. Woodall wrote *The surgion's mate*, 1617, with a section on scurvy, which Woodall, though not the first to use citrus fruits in the prevention of this condition, treated with lime-juice. The additional material in *Woodalls viaticum: the path-way to the surgions chest*, London, 1628, was incorporated into the enlarged *The surgeons mate, or military and domestique surgery*, 1639, which added a treatise of the cure of the plague which was also published separately in 1640. *The surgeons mate*, 1639, was printed at three presses; all sea-surgeons were obliged to possess a copy and there were four editions, the last in 1655.[32]

Richard Wiseman (1622?–76) was an innovative and skilful surgeon who learned his trade in service with the Dutch navy, with the Royalist army in the Civil War and afterwards with the Spanish navy. His first book was *A treatise of wounds*, London, 1672 and his subsequent collection, *Severall chirurgicall treatises*, London, 1676, is dedicated to Charles II. It contains treatises on tumours, of ulcers, of diseases of the anus, of the King's Evil, of wounds, gunshot wounds, of fractures and luxations and of lues venerea. A facsimile of Books V, VI and VII was produced in 1977. Wiseman described the first case of external urethrotomy for stricture and called tuberculosis of the joints 'tumor albus' for the first time. The work was reprinted under the title *Eight chirurgical treatises* in 1686, 1696, 1705, 1719, and 1734. A spurious second edition was published in 1692 by Samuel Clement; it consists of copies of the 1686 edition with a new title-page.[33]

James Yonge (1647–1721) started his career before the age of eleven as apprentice to a ship's surgeon. His several voyages are recorded in his Journal, which with other of his manuscripts is preserved in the Plymouth Institution, and edited by F. N. L. Poynter. Yonge settled in his native Plymouth and was surgeon to the naval hospital there. He contributed papers to the *Philosophical Transactions* and was elected a Fellow of the Royal Society in 1702. His published books include *Wounds of the brain, proved curable*, 1682, and two controversial works, *Medicaster medicatus*, 1685, attacking John Browne and *Sidrophel vapulans: or the quack-astrologer toss'd in a blanket*, 1699, against William Salmon. Yonge's most important work, *Currus triumphalis e terebintho. Or an account of the ... vertues of oleum terebinthinae*, 1679, contains a description of the use of turpentine in arresting haemorrhage, describes the flap operation in amputation, and mentions a device similar to a tourniquet.[34]

Most of the most learned and important medical and scientific works of the seventeenth century were published in Latin, which continued to be the major language of international scholarly communication. At the same time, there was an increasing movement towards translation into the vernacular for an audience of medical practitioners and laymen whose knowledge of the classical languages was elementary, and writers in all fields, aiming at a national rather than an international readership, were content with using the vernacular. Translation between vernacular languages increased, as a study of Anglo-Dutch translation has shown.[35] Two works written in this period and associated with medicine have entered the canon of English literature; they are, of course, Thomas Browne's *Religio medici* and Robert Burton's *The anatomy of melancholy*. Robert Burton (1577–1640) spent his life in Oxford, as tutor and librarian of Christ Church College. Possibly influenced by Bright's *Treatise of melancholy*, 1586, *The anatomy of melancholy* appeared first in 1621 in a quarto edition with the words 'by Democritus Junior' on the title-page. The author's name is revealed in the appendix. An enlarged folio edition was published in 1624 and there were several further editions, in 1628, 1632, 1638, 1652, 1660 and 1676. The vogue for Burton began in the nineteenth century, which saw over 40 editions and reissues of this work.[36]

Sir Thomas Browne (1605–82), after a period of study on the continent, obtained his doctorate in physic from Leyden in 1633 and was incorporated MD at Oxford in 1637. He settled in Norwich, where he practised successfully until his death and was knighted there in 1671, during a royal visit. *Religio medici* was not intended for publication, but after two unauthorized editions had been printed by Andrew Crooke in 1642, Browne bowed to the inevitable and an amended authorized edition appeared in 1643, from the same publisher and with the same title-page. The work was immediately popular, with two editions in 1645, a 'fourth' edition in 1656 and five subsequent printings before the end of the century. The book provides a neat example of the usual pattern in reverse, being translated into Latin, by John Merryweather; the Latin edition was printed at Leyden, 1644 and 1650, and editions appeared from Strasbourg, Paris, Zurich and Leipzig. It was also translated in the seventeenth century into Dutch (Leyden, 1665 and 1683) and French (1668); a German translation was published in 1746. Browne's *Pseudodoxia epidemica*, 1646, on popular superstitions, went into several editions and was also translated into Dutch, German, French and Italian. His antiquarian work, *Hydriotaphia, urne-buriall, or, a discourse of the sepulchrall urnes lately found in Norfolk. Together with The garden of Cyrus*, London, 1658 and his *Christian morals*, Cambridge, 1716, were also frequently reprinted.

Browne's son Edward (1642–1708) was a physician, and became president of the College of Physicians in 1704. He published only an account of his travels, but some unpublished notes for a lecture on the skin, probably written in 1676 with the help of his father, survive in manuscript. These have been edited by Geoffrey Keynes, who also edited Sir Thomas Browne's *Works*, 1928–31, reprinted 1964, and published a bibliography of his writings.[37]

Several popular manuals of anatomy were published in English during the seventeenth century. Helkiah Crooke (1576–1635), Fellow and Reader in Anatomy of the College of Physicians, was the author of perhaps the best known of these, *Mikrokosmographia, a description of the body of man*, 1616, which was largely based on Bauhin's *Theatrum anatomicum*.[38] An epitome of this was published in 1616 with the title Σωματογραφια ανθρωπινη. *Or a description of the body of man*, with a preface by Alexander Read (1580?–1641). Another edition in 1634 epitomized the expanded second edition of Crooke's work which had appeared in 1631. These compilations are notable for ignoring Harvey's discovery, although it must have been known to both authors. The successive revisions of Alexander Read's *The manuall of the anatomy or dissection of the body of man*, first published in 1634, demonstrate that he came to accept Harvey's theories in part; he revised a second edition of 1638 and the third of 1642. Read owned and annotated a copy of *De motu cordis* which survives among the books which he gave to Kings College, Aberdeen. Read also published *The chirurgicall lectures of tumors and ulcers delivered ... 1632, 1633 and 1634*, London, 1635; *A treatise of all the muscles of the whole body*, 1637 and *A treatise of the first part of chirurgerie*, 1638. Collected editions of his writings were published in 1650, 1652 and 1659.[39]

A determined antagonist of professional elitism, Nicholas Culpeper

(1616–54) aimed to make medical knowledge accessible to the layman. Culpeper was educated at Cambridge and apprenticed to an apothecary in London. He began practising as a physician and astrologer in about 1640 in Red Lion Street, Spitalfields. Most of the writings which appeared under his name were published after his early death; he was supposed to have left many manuscript works. It is probable that some at least of these translations and texts were given Culpeper's name in order to benefit from his undoubted popularity. Culpeper's first publication, *A physicall directory*, 1649, was an unauthorized and critical translation of the College of Physicians' *Pharmacopœia Londinensis* of 1618, which made Culpeper very unpopular with that body. A second edition was published in 1650 and a third in 1651 with new prefaces, the latter with the addition of a *Key to Galen's Method of physick*. In 1650 a second edition of the *Pharmacopœia Londinensis* was published and Culpeper's translation of this was published with the title, *Pharmacopœia Londinensis: or, the London dispensatory further adorned by the studies and collections of the Fellows, now living*; this appeared first in 1653 and was reissued by the original publisher, Peter Cole, several times before 1661 when he published an enlarged version. Editions from other publishers continued to appear into the early eighteenth century; the last edition, published in Boston, Massachusetts, in 1720 was probably the first full-length medical work to be published in America. Culpeper's *A directory for midwives*, 1651, was reprinted many times, the last edition being published in 1777; the popular work on the same topic known as 'Aristotle's masterpiece', which has nothing to do with Aristotle, appeared as *Culpepper's compleat and experienc'd midwife* in 1718. Culpeper has become a household name because of his herbal, which was first published with the title *The English physitian: or an astrologo-physical discourse of the vulgar herbs of this nation*, 1652. The first edition, like all Culpeper's works, was published by Peter Cole, and two other editions came out in the same year, one from W. Bentley and another, repudiated by Culpeper as a piracy, was 'printed for the benefit of the Commonwealth of England'. Cole published further editions until 1662 and the work has hardly been out of print since, with over one hundred recorded editions. Ebenezer Sibly produced an annotated version in 1789, on which most later editions are based. *Culpeper's last legacy*, 1655, was published by N. Brooke, who reprinted *Semeiotica uranica*, 1651, with the title *Culpeper's astrologicall judgment of diseases*, 1655. Several posthumous works were apparently authenticated by Culpeper's wife, and her 'Testimony' was printed with some of these, including *Culpeper's school of physick*, 1659; *Mr. Culpeper's treatise of aurum potabile*, 1656, was also said to be published by his wife. This latter is discussed by F. N. L. Poynter.

The number of translations published under Culpeper's name stretches belief, even given that he was provided with an amanuensis. Culpeper's publisher, Peter Cole, produced a series of translations of important medical works under the umbrella title of 'The Rationall Physician's Library'. Culpeper's translation of Galen's *Ars medica, Galen's Art of physick*, appeared in 1652; his translation of Johann Vesling's *Syntagma anatomicum* was published as *The anatomy of the body of man*, 1653, reprinted 1677. Jean Riolan's *Encheiridium anatomicum et pathologicum*, was translated as *A sure guide; or the best and nearest way of physick and chyrurgery*, 1657, with a 'third' edition in 1671; Thomas Bartholin's *Anatomia ex Caspari Bartholini parentis Institutionibus*, translated as *Bartholinus anatomy; made from the precepts of his father*, 1663 and 1668. Other writers whose work appeared in translation under Culpeper's name include Jean Fernel, John Jonston, Lazare Rivière, and Martin Ruland. Two authors in the tradition of chemical medicine, George Phaedro and Simeon Parlitz, also appear in translations assigned to Culpeper.[40]

Chemistry in seventeenth-century England is dominated by the figure of Robert Boyle (1626–91), a son of the Earl of Cork, who established a laboratory first at Oxford and later in London and devoted his life to scientific research. John Fulton has explored Boyle's bibliography, which is a minefield of variant issues, and his total contributions to science have been discussed elsewhere. However much of Boyle's writing was concerned with medicine, particularly the following: *Memoirs for the natural history of humane blood*, London, 1684, with a Latin edition of the same year and subsequent printings in Geneva, 1685 and 1686; *Experiments and considerations about the porosity of bodies*, 1684, which also had Latin editions from London, 1684, and Geneva; *Short memoirs for the natural experimental history of mineral waters*, 1684/5; *An essay of the great effects of even languid and unheeded motion*, 1685 (two issues) and 1690; *Of the reconcileableness of specifick medicines to the corpuscular philosophy*, 1685, with Latin editions from London, 1686, and Geneva, 1687. Boyle's most popular medical work was *Medicinal experiments; or, a collection of choice remedies*, 1692, volume 2, 1693 and volume 3, 1694; there were several subsequent editions. *Medicina hydrostatica: or hydrostaticks applyed to the materia medica*, 1690, with a Latin edition from Geneva, 1693, was among the last works of Boyle's life, and *The general history of the air*, 1692, was seen through the press by John Locke after Boyle's death.[41]

Robert Boyle represents the rational or sceptical side of chemistry in this period, but the medical world also encompassed proponents of chemical medicine in the Paracelsian tradition, who aroused the hostility of the 'Galenists', represented by the College of Physicians, who followed orthodox medical teaching. An attempt to consolidate the opposition to the College of Physicians was begun in 1665, when a 'Society of Chymical Physitians' was founded and applied to erect a headquarters, but the patent for this being refused and the plague reducing the numbers of supporters, the society failed to establish itself.[42]

The work of Walter Pagel and Allen Debus in particular has brought to light this more obscure aspect of early modern medical thought. Although the writings of Robert Fludd (1574–1637) had little influence, he is interesting as an English example of the mystical physician. Fludd had an ambivalent relation with the College of Physicians but was finally admitted a Fellow in 1609 and served as a Censor from 1618. He knew William Harvey and, like Harvey, bequeathed his library to the College; both libraries were destroyed in the Great Fire. Most of Fludd's works were published by Johann Theodor de Bry in Oppenheim and later Frankfort. Fludd possibly influenced William Harvey's decision to publish his *De motu cordis* in Frankfort; William Fitzer, its publisher, was the son-in-law of De Bry and subsequently published Fludd's *Medicina catholica*, 1629 and *Clavis philosophiae*, 1633. In the former work, Fludd devoted a section to the pulse which cited Harvey's book and is the first reference to it in print. The circulation of the blood fitted in with Fludd's theories of the relation of the microcosm of the human body to the macrocosm and in his *Anatomiae amphitheatrum*, 1623, he advanced the theory but without any physiological evidence.[43] Only one of Fludd's Latin works, *Philosophia Moysaica* was translated into English, and he published only one work in the vernacular. This was *Doctor Fludd's Answer unto M. Foster*, London, 1631, defending himself against a charge of witchcraft laid by William Foster, a parson, in a book called *Hoplocrisma-Spongus: or a sponge to wipe away the weapon-salve*, 1631.

The weapon-salve, with which the weapon which caused the wound was anointed in order to cure the wound by sympathetic attraction, was always a controversial idea and the argument over its efficacy continued for some time. Johann Baptista van Helmont (1579–1644) was persecuted by the ecclesiastical authorities for most of his life because of his defence of the theory of the magnetic cure of wounds in *De magnetica vulnerum naturali et legitima curatione*, Paris, 1621. Van Helmont was the major influence on the chemical medicine of the period. He published *Febrium doctrina inaudita*, Antwerp, 1642 and *Opuscula medica inaudita*, 1644, in four parts, including the second edition of his work on fevers and a part on urinary calculi. After Van Helmont's death, his son collected together his unpublished works with the title, *Ortus medicinae*, Amsterdam, 1648; of the later editions of this, from Venice, 1651, Lyons, 1655 and 1667, Frankfort, 1682, the best is traditionally that printed at Amsterdam in 1652. An English translation of this was published with the title *Oriatrike or physick refined*, London, 1662 and reissued with a new title-page in 1664. Van Helmont's *Opera omnia* was published at Frankfort in 1682 and 1707.[44]

English translations of some of Van Helmont's works were made by Walter Charleton and published in 1650, including in *A ternary of paradoxes*, the work on the magnetic cure of wounds. Walter Charleton (1619–

1707) is noted for producing the first work in English on atomism and for his contribution to zoology, but his medical works are not negligible. Charleton was physician to both Charles I and Charles II and held the office of President of the College of Physicians. A prolific author, Charleton wrote a work on physiology, *Exercitationes physico-anatomicae de œconomia animali*, Amsterdam, 1659; the second edition of this appeared in English as *Natural history of nutrition, life and voluntary motion*, London, 1659. A third edition with the title *Oeconomia animalis*, London, 1659, was followed by several further editions. A rewritten version appeared as *Enquiries into human nature, in IV anatomic praelections*, 1680. Charleton's own annotated copy of his *Three anatomic lectures*, 1683, on the heart, survives in the Wellcome Institute Library. His other medical writings include *Natural history of the passions*, 1674, which was published anonymously and is not merely a translation of J. F. Sénault's *De l'usage des passions*, 1641, as had been thought.[45]

By the end of the seventeenth century the revolution in scientific thought had established itself and such arcane notions as the sympathetic cure of wounds became the preserve of charlatans. The ideas of the iatrochemists were rejected by Georg Ernst Stahl (1660–1734) whose espousal of vitalism was to have great influence on eighteenth-century medical thought. Towards the end of the century, in 1694, the new university of Halle was founded and a strong medical faculty was created under Friedrich Hoffmann and Stahl. Stahl stayed at Halle until 1715, when he was appointed court physician to Frederick William I of Prussia. Stahl's publications overlap the turn of the century; the major medical works include *Observationum chymico-physico-medicarum*, Frankfort and Leipzig, 1697–8, which consists of a collection of essays published at monthly intervals; *Medicinae dogmatico-systematicae*, Halle, 1707; and *Theoria medica vera*, Halle, 1708 and 1737, a three-volume German translation of which was published in Berlin, 1831–2. Stahl's *Oeuvres médico-philosophiques et pratiques* was published at Paris, 1859–64, in six volumes.[46]

The writings of Bernardino Ramazzini (1633–1714) were largely published in the later years of his life and belong to the early eighteenth century. Ramazzini was professor of medicine at Modena and later at Padua. He wrote on artesian wells and on the health of the ruling classes in *De principium valetudine tuenda commentatio*, 1710 and 1712. His principal work, which proved immensely popular, with numerous editions and translations, was on occupational diseases: *De morbis artificum diatriba* was first published in Modena in 1700. It covers the hazards of almost every profession of the time and the 1713 edition has an essay on the health hazards of nuns; this section was translated into French by Etienne Coulet in 1724. An English version of Ramazzini's work, *Diseases of workers*, was published in 1705; a new translation by W. C. Wright appeared in 1940 with the Latin text.[47]

Anatomical studies were assisted by the development of techniques to preserve specimens. Both Jan Swammerdam (1637–80) and De Graaf had experimented with injecting vessels with coloured substances; their compatriot Frederik Ruysch (1638–1731) developed a method of preserving anatomical preparations and his collection became famous; it was catalogued in the work *Museum anatomicum Ruyschianum*, Amsterdam, 1691; further editions in 1721 and 1737. Ruysch served as demonstrator in anatomy to the surgeons guild of Amsterdam and as city obstetrician; he was the author of various works on anatomy: *Observationum anatomicochirurgicarum centuria*, Amsterdam, 1691, four volumes; *Thesaurus anatomicus, i-x*, Amsterdam, 1701–16, and *Opera omnia anatomico-medicochirurgico*, 1737. His first published work was an important account of the valves in the lymph vessels, *Dilucidatio valvularum in vasis lymphaticis et lacteis*, The Hague, 1665 (facsimile reprint, Nieuwkoop, 1964, in Dutch Classics on the History of Science, vol. II). The often bizarre arrangements of the exhibits in Ruysch's collection are preserved in the plates to his works. The collection was bought by Peter the Great in 1717 and some specimens are still in the Museum of the Academy of Sciences in Leningrad.[48]

As an icon of seventeenth-century anatomical teaching, Rembrandt's painting of the anatomy lesson of Dr Tulp occupies the same place as the frontispiece to Vesalius's *De humanae corporis fabrica* for the previous century. Its subject, Nicolaas Tulp (1593–1674), was the author of *Observationum medicarum libri tres*, Amsterdam, 1641, which went into new editions in 1652, 1672, 1685, and Leyden, 1716 and was translated into Dutch and French. Tulp notably described spina bifida but he has been mainly studied in relation to the most famous painting with a medical subject.[49]

Notes

1. For the background to the scientific renaissance see Thornton–Tully; Webster, Charles, *The Great Instauration: science, medicine and reform 1626–1660* (New York, 1976); Webster, Charles (ed.), *The intellectual revolution of the seventeenth century* (1974); Boas, Marie, *The scientific renaissance 1450–1630* (1962); and Hall, A. Rupert, *From Galileo to Newton 1630–1720* (1963).

2. *A catalogue of printed books in the Wellcome Historical Medical Library*, vol. 1, Books printed before 1641 (1962); Vol. 2, Books printed from 1641–1850, A–E (1966); Vol. 3, F–L (1976).

3. See Austin, Robert B., *Early American medical imprints: a guide to works published in the United States, 1668–1820* (Washington, 1961); Viets, Henry R., 'The first American medical publications', *New England J. Med.*, 268 (1963) pp.600–1; and *A brief rule to guide the common-people of New England how to order themselves and theirs in the small pocks, or measels. By Thomas Thacher. Facsimile reproductions of the three known editions, with an introductory note by Henry R. Viets* (Baltimore, 1937); (Publications of the Institute of the History of Medicine, the Johns Hopkins University, 4th ser. Bibliotheca Medica America. Vol. 1).

4. Ornstein, Martha, *The role of scientific societies in the seventeenth century*, 3rd edn (Chicago, 1938); Middleton, W. E. Knowles, *The experimenters: a study of the Accademia del Cimento* (Baltimore and London, 1971); Armytage, W. H. G., 'An early medical society: the Imperial Leopoldine Academy', *Br. Med. J.* (1960) I, pp.272–3.

5. Hunter, Michael, *Science and society in Restoration England* (Cambridge, 1981). See also the series of articles on the intellectual origins of the Royal Society by P. M. Rattansi, Christopher Hill, and A. R. and M. B. Hall in *Notes Rec. Roy. Soc. Lond.*, 23 (1968) pp.129–43, 144–56, and 157–68; Hall, Marie Boas, 'Sources for the history of the Royal Society in the seventeenth century', *History of Science*, 5 (1966) pp.62–76; Purver, Margery, *The Royal Society: concept and foundation* (1967); McKie, Douglas, 'The origins and foundation of the Royal Society of London', *Notes Rec. Roy. Soc. Lond.*, 15 (1960) pp.1–37; Hartley, Sir Harold, *The Royal Society – its origins and founders* (1960); *The correspondence of Henry Oldenburg, edited and translated by A. Rupert Hall and Marie Boas Hall*, 13 vols (Madison, Milwaukee and London, 1965–86).

6. Rostenberg, Leona, 'John Martyn, printer to the Royal Society', *Pap. Bib. Soc. Amer.*, 46 (1952) pp. 1–32 and 'The will of John Martyn, printer to the Royal Society', *Pap. Bib. Soc. Amer.*, 50 (1956) pp.279–84.

7. Hahn, Roger, *The anatomy of a scientific institution: the Paris Academy of Sciences, 1666–1803* (Berkeley, Los Angeles, 1971); McKie, Douglas, 'The early years of the Académie des Sciences', *Endeavour*, 25 (1966) pp.100–3; Faure-Fremiet, E., 'Les origines de l'Académie des Sciences de Paris', *Notes Rec. Roy. Soc. Lond.*, 21 (1966) pp.20–31.

8. Clark, Sir George *A history of the Royal College of Physicians*, Vol. 1 (Oxford, 1964); Urdang, George, *Pharmacopœia Londinensis of 1618* (Madison, 1944); (Hollister Pharmaceutical Library, No. 2).

9. Wall, Cecil *et al.*, *A history of the Worshipful Society of Apothecaries of London. Volume I, 1617–1815. Abstracted and arranged from the manuscripts of Cecil Wall by H. Charles Cameron. Revised, annotated and edited by E. Ashworth Underwood* (1963); (Publications of the Wellcome Historical Museum, No. 8); Scouloudi, I., 'Sir Theodore Turquet de Mayerne, royal physician and writer, 1573–1655', *Proc. Huguenot Soc. Lond.*, 16 (1940) pp.301–37.

10. Castiglioni, Arturo, *La vita e l'opera di Santorio Santorio Capodistriano, 1561–1636* (Bologna, 1920); Allegria, Ceferino, 'Santorio Santorio y su "Commentaria in artem medicinalem Galeni" ', *Archivo de Siluetas de Antano*, Publicacion occasional (1966) no. 13.

11. Fabricius, Hieronymus, *De venarum ostiolis, 1603 ... Facsimile edition with introduction, translation and notes by K. J. Franklin* (Springfield, Baltimore, 1933). *The embryological treatises of Hieronymus Fabricius of Aquapendente. The formation of the egg and of the chick. The formed foetus. A facsimile edition, with an introduction, a translation and commentary by Howard B. Adelmann* (Ithaca, New York, 1942). This is based on the texts of the first editions, contains a life of Fabricius (pp.6–35) and a bibliographical note (pp.122–34). See also König, Klaus G., 'Die Stellung der Anatomen unter den medizinischen Lehrern in Padua im 16. Jahrhundert (Vesal und Fabrizio d'Acquapendente)', *Centaurus*, 7 (1960–1) pp.1–5; Zen Benetti, Francesca, 'La libreria di Girolamo Fabrici d'Acquapendente', *Quad. Storia Univ. Padova*, 9–10 (1976–7) pp.161–83.

12. Keynes, Sir Geoffrey Langdon, *A bibliography of the writings of Dr. William Harvey, 1578–1657*. Third edition revised by Gweneth Whitteridge and Christine English (Winchester, 1989); also *The life of William Harvey* (Oxford, 1966) reprinted with corrections 1978.
    Translations of Harvey's works include the following: *Movement of the heart and blood in animals. An anatomical essay by William Harvey. Translated ... by Kenneth J. Franklin* (Oxford, 1957); *The circulation of the blood. Two anatomical essays by William Harvey, together with nine letters written by him. The whole translated ... by Kenneth J. Franklin* (Oxford, 1958) collected in *The circulation of the blood and other writings. Translated by K. J. Franklin*, 1963 (Everyman's Library, No. 262); *An anatomical disputation concerning the movement of the heart and blood in living creatures. Translated with introduction and notes by Gweneth Whitteridge* (Oxford, 1976); *De motu locali*

animalium, 1627. Edited, translated and introduced by Gweneth Whitteridge (Cambridge, 1959); *Lectures on the whole of anatomy: an annotated translation of Prelectiones anatomiae universalis 1616–1626? by C. D. O'Malley, F. N. L. Poynter and K. F. Russell* (Berkeley, Los Angeles, 1961), superseded by *The anatomical lectures. Prelectiones anatomie universalis. De musculis. Edited, with an introduction, translation and notes by G. Whitteridge* (Edinburgh, London, 1964).

Secondary works on Harvey include the following: Webster, C. *et al., William Harvey and his age* (Baltimore, 1979); (Henry E. Sigerist Suppl. to *Bull. Hist. Med.*, N.S.2); Whitteridge, Gweneth, *William Harvey and the circulation of the blood* (1971); Pagel, Walter, *New light on William Harvey* (Basle, 1976) and *William Harvey's biological ideas* (Basle, 1967); Weil, Ernst. 'William Fitzer, the publisher of Harvey's *De motu cordis*, *Lib. Trans. Bib. Soc.*, N.S.24 (1943–4) pp.142–64; Russell, K. F. 'The English translations of Harvey's works', *Australian N.Z. J. Surg.*, 27 (1957) pp.70–4; Poynter, F. N. L., 'An unnoticed English version of Harvey's "De motu cordis" London, 1714', *J. Hist. Med.*, 12 (1957) pp.256–8; Durling, Richard, 'Some unrecorded English versions of foreign seventeenth–eighteenth-century works', *Med. Hist.*, 5 (1961) pp.396–401.

13. Descartes, René, *Oeuvres, publiées par Charles Ernest Adams et Paul Tannery, sous les auspices du Ministère de l'Instruction Publique*, 12 vols, (Paris, 1897–1910); (index volume published 1913; Vol. 12 contains a biography of Descartes by Charles Adams). See also Sebba, Gregor, *Bibliographia Cartesiana. A critical guide to the Descartes literature 1800–1960* (The Hague, 1964); the periodical *Studia cartesiana*, which began publication in 1979; Lindeboom, Gerrit A., *Descartes and medicine* (Nieuwe Nederlandse Bijdragen tot de Geschiedenis der Geneeskunde, No. 1.); (Amsterdam, 1979); Carter, Richard B., *Descartes' medical philosophy: the organic solution to the mind–body problem* (Baltimore and London, 1983); Armitage, Angus, 'René Descartes (1596–1650) and the early Royal Society', *Notes Rec. Roy. Soc. Lond.*, 8 (1950–1) pp.1–19.

14. Porter, Ian Herbert, 'Thomas Bartholin (1616–1680) and Niels Steensen (1638–1686), master and pupil' *Med. Hist.*, 7 (1963) pp.99–125; Garboe, Axel, 'Thomas Bartholin' 2 pts, *Acta Hist. Sci. Nat. Med.*, Vols. 5–6 (1949–50); (in Danish with English summary in Pt 2, pp.188–96); Speert, Harold, 'Caspar Bartholinus and the vulvovaginal glands', *Med. Hist.*, 1 (1957) pp.355–8.

15. Fulton, John Farquhar, 'A bibliography of two Oxford physiologists, Richard Lower, 1631–1691, John Mayow, 1643 [sic]–1679', *Oxford Bib. Soc. Proc. Pap.*, Vol. 1, Pt1, i (1934) 62pp. (Oxford, 1935); (Figure 2 is a facsimile of the title-page of Walter Charleton's copy of *De corde*, with inscription dated 1668); Gunther, R. T., *Early science in Oxford. Vol. IX. De corde, by Richard Lower, London, 1669. With introduction and translation by K. J. Franklin* (Oxford, 1932); Franklin, K. J., 'Some textual changes in successive editions of Richard Lower's *Tractatus de corde item de motu & colore sanguinis et chyli in eum transitu'*, *Ann. Sci.*, 4 (1939) pp.283–94; Lower, Richard, *De catarrhis, 1672. Reproduced in facsimile and translated for the first time from the original Latin, together with a bibliographical analysis by Richard Hunter and Ida Macalpine* (1963); Rullière, R., '*Le Tractatus de corde item de motu et colore sanguinis de Richard Lower* (1669)', *Hist. Sci. Med.*, 8 (1974) pp.85–98, and 'La version française (1679) du Tractatus de corde (1669) de Richard Lower', *Int. Congr. Hist. Med.*, 27th, Barcelona, 1980 (Actas, 1981) vol. 1, pp.331–5.

See also Hall, A. Rupert and Marie Boas, 'The first human blood transfusion: priority disputes', *Med. Hist.*, 24 (1980) pp.461–5; Keynes, Sir Geoffrey, 'The history of blood transfusion', *Br. J. Surg.*, 31 (1943–4) pp.38–50.

16. Boehm, Walter, 'John Mayow and his contemporaries', *Ambix*, 11 (1963) pp.105–20; Patterson, T. S., 'John Mayow in contemporary setting; a contribution to the history of respiration and combustion', *Isis*, 15 (1931) pp.47–96, 504–46 (criticised by Partington, J. R., 'The life and work of John Mayow (1641–1679). Part I[–II]', *Isis*, 47 (1956) pp.217–30, 405–17; also his 'Some early appraisals of the work of John Mayow', *Isis*, 50 (1959) pp.211–26.

17. For Wren's medical interests see Gibson, William, 'The bio-medical pursuits of Christopher Wren', *Med. Hist.*, 14 (1970) pp.331–41; and Anson, Barry J, 'Doctor Thomas Willis and Sir Christopher Wren', *Surg. Gynec. Obstet.*, 87 (1948) pp.625–36.

18. Wing, H. J. R., 'A bibliography of Dr. Thomas Willis (1621–1675). Submitted in part requirement for the University of London Diploma in Librarianship, 1962' (typescript); Willis, Thomas, *The anatomy of the brain and nerves. W. Feindel, editor. Tercentenary edition* (Montreal, 1965); *Willis's Oxford casebook (1650–52). Introduced and edited by Kenneth Dewhurst* (Oxford, 1981); and *Thomas Willis's Oxford lectures* (Oxford, 1980). See also Isler, Hansruedi, *Thomas Willis, 1621–1675, doctor and scientist* (New York, 1968); Hierons, Raymond, and Alfred Meyer, 'On Thomas Willis's concepts of neurophysiology. Part I [–II]', *Med. Hist.*, 9 (1965) pp.1–15, 142–55; 'Willis's place in the history of muscle physiology', *Proc. Roy. Soc. Med.*, 57 (1964) pp.687–92; and their 'Observations on the history of the "Circle of Willis" ', *Med. Hist.*, 6 (1962) pp.119–30; Cranefield, Paul F., 'A seventeenth-century view of mental deficiency and schizophrenia: Thomas Willis on "stupidity or foolishness" ', *Bull. Hist. Med.*, 35 (1961) pp.291–316, which reprints the chapter on mental deficiency; and Alafovanine, Th. and A. Bourguignon, 'La première description de la myasthénie', *Presse Méd.*, 62 (1954) pp.519–20.

19. Keynes, Sir Geoffrey Langdon, *A bibliography of Sir William Petty F.R.S. and of Observations on the Bills of Mortality by John Graunt F.R.S.* (Oxford, 1971); Groenewegen, P. D., 'Authorship of the "Natural and political observations upon the Bills of Mortality" ', *J. Hist. Ideas*, 28 (1967) pp.601–2; Glass, D. V., 'John Graunt and his "Natural and political observations" ', *Notes Rec. Roy. Soc. Lond.*, 19 (1964) pp.63–100.

20. Dewhurst, Kenneth, *Dr. Thomas Sydenham (1624–1689): his life and original writings*, (1966); Boss, Jeffrey M. N., 'The 17th century transformation of the hysteric affection, and Sydenham's Baconian medicine', *Psychol. Med.*, 9 (1979) pp.221–34; Bates, Donald George, *Thomas Sydenham: the development of his thought, 1666–1676* (Ph.D. thesis, 1975, Johns Hopkins University); Poynter, F. N. L., 'Sydenham's influence abroad (Sydenham Lecture, 1972)', *Med. Hist.*, 17 (1973) pp.223–34; Sydenham, Thomas, *Methodus curandi febres ...*, ed. Geoffrey Guy Meynell (Folkestone, Kent, 1987).

21. Dewhurst, Kenneth, *John Locke (1632–1704), physician and philosopher; a medical biography. With an edition of the medical notes in his journals*, (1963) (Publications of the Wellcome Historical Medical Library. N.S. Vol. II.). See also the following papers by Dewhurst: 'Locke's Essay on respiration', *Bull. Hist. Med.*, 34 (1960) pp.257–73; 'Locke's midwifery notes', *Lancet* (1954) II, pp.490–1; and 'A review of John Locke's research in social and preventive medicine', *Bull. Hist. Med.*, 36 (1962) pp.317–40; 'An essay on coughs by Locke and Sydenham', *Bull. Hist. Med.*, 33 (1959) pp.366–74; and 'Locke and Sydenham on the teaching of anatomy', *Med. Hist.*, 2 (1958) pp.1–12. Wolfe, David E., 'Sydenham and Locke on the limits of anatomy', *Bull. Hist. Med.*, 35 (1961) pp.193–220.

22. Milnes Walker, R., 'Francis Glisson and his capsule', *Ann. Roy. Coll. Surg. Engl.*, 38 (1966) pp.71–91, and the paper in *Cambridge and its contribution to medicine*, 7th British Congress on the History of Medicine (1971) pp.35–47; Boss, Jeffrey M. N., ' "Doctrina de circulatione sanguinis haud immutat antiquam medendi methodum": unpublished manuscript (1662) by Francis Glisson', *Physis*, 20 (1978) pp.309–36, and 'An unpublished manuscript of Francis Glisson (1662) on the relation of the Harveian circulatory theory to medicine', *J. Physiol.*, 293 (1979) p.34P.

23. Clarke, Edwin, 'Whistler and Glisson on rickets', *Bull. Hist. Med.*, 36 (1962) pp.45–61; Smerdon, G. T., 'Daniel Whistler and the English disease: a translation and biographical 'note''', *J. Hist. Med.*, 5 (1950) pp.397–415 (translation on pp.401–15); Hunter, Richard, and Ida Macalpine, 'John Bird on "Rekets" (London, 1661)', *J. Hist. Med.*, 13 (1958) pp.397–403.

24. Russell, K. F., 'John Browne, 1642–1702, a seventeenth-century surgeon, anatomist and plagiarist', *Bull. Hist. Med.*, 33 (1959) pp.393–414, 503–25; 'A list of the works of John Browne (1642–1702)', *Bull. Med. Lib. Assn*, 50 (1962) pp.675–83.

25. Beekman, Fenwick, 'Bidloo and Cowper, anatomists', *Ann. Med. Hist.*, N.S.7 (1935) pp.113–29; Dumaître, Paule, *La curieuse destinée des planches anatomiques de Gérard de Lairesse, peintre en Hollande – Lairesse, Bidloo, Cowper* (Nieuwe Nederlandse Bijdragen tot de Geschiedenis der Geneeskunde en der Natuurwetenschappen, No. 6) (Amsterdam, 1982).

26. Montagu, M. F. Ashley, *Edward Tyson, M.D., F.R.S., 1650–1708, and the rise of human and comparative anatomy in England; a study in the history of science*, (Philadelphia, 1943), (Memoirs of the American Philosophical Society, Vol.XX.) and 'Tysoniana', *Isis*, 36 (1945–46) pp.105–8; Russell, K. F., 'Edward Tyson's "Orang-outang" [1699.] An essay review [of Ashley Montagu's facsimile reprint, 1966]', *Med. Hist.*, 11 (1967) pp.417–23.

27. Keynes, Sir Geoffrey Langdon, *A bibliography of Dr. Robert Hooke* (Oxford, 1960); (contains lists of MSS, which are mostly in the Royal Society, the British Library, the Bodleian Library and Trinity College, Cambridge, pp.75–84; letters from printed sources, pp.85–6; and a section on biography and criticism, pp.87–96); *The Diary of Robert Hooke, M.A., M.D., F.R.S., 1672–1680. Transcribed from the original in the possession of the Corporation of the City of London (Guildhall Library). Edited by Henry W. Robinson and Walter Adams* (1935); Gunther, R. T., *Early science in Oxford, Vols. 6–7. The life and work of Robert Hooke, Parts I–II* (Oxford, 1930); (vol. 8, 1931, consists of a facsimile of Hooke's *Cutler Lectures*, and vol. 13, 1938, of his *Micrographia*); Espinasse, Margaret, *Robert Hooke* (London, 1956); (Contemporary Science Series); Hall, A. Rupert, *Hooke's Micrographia 1665–1965. A lecture in commemoration of the tercentenary of the publication of Micrographia … delivered at the Middlesex Hospital Medical School* (1966); Bennett, J. A., 'Robert Hooke as mechanic and natural philosopher', *Notes Rec. Roy. Soc. London*; 35 (1980) pp.33–48.

28. *The Leeuwenhoek letter; a photographic copy of the letter of the 9th October, 1676, sent by Antony van Leeuwenhoek to Henry Oldenburg, Secretary of the Royal Society of London; and a translation into English by Barnett Cohen* (Baltimore, 1937). The original letter is still preserved by the Royal Society. See also *On the circulation of the blood. Latin text of his 65th letter to the Royal Society (Sept. 7, 1688); Facsimile, with an introduction by A. Schierbeek* (Nieuwkoop, 1962); (Dutch classics in the History of Science, 2); *The collected letters of Antoni van Leeuwenhoek* published under the auspices of the Leeuwenhoek Commission of the Royal Netherlands Academy of Sciences, Vols 1–8 (Amsterdam, 1939–67); (text in parallel Dutch and English). Dobell, Clifford, *Antony van Leeuwenhoek and his 'little animals'; being some account of the father of protozoology and bacteriology, and his multifarious discoveries in these disciplines* (1932; rev. edn, New York, 1958 and 1960); 'Samuel Hoole, translator of Leeuwenhoek's *Select works*: with notes on that publication', *Isis*, 41 (1950) pp.171–80; Palm, L. C. and H. A. M. Snelders (eds), *Antoni van Leeuwenhoek 1632–1723. Studies on the life and work of the Delft scientist commemorating the 350th anniversary of his birthday* (Amsterdam, 1982); (Nieuwe Nederlandse Bijdragen tot de Geschiedenis der Geneeskunde en der Natuurwetenschappen, No. 8); Payne, Alma Smith, *The cleere observer; a biography of Antoni van Leeuwenhoek* (1970); Schierbeek, A., *Antoni van Leeuwenhoek: zijn leven en zijn werken*, 2 vols (Lochem, 1950–1). Concise English version published as *Measuring the invisible world: the life and works of Antoni van Leeuwenhoek. With a bibliographical chapter by Maria Rooseboom* (London, New York, 1959).

29. Frati, Carlo, *Bibliografia Malpighiana, Catalogo discritivo delle opere a stampa di Marcello Malpighi e degli scritti che lo riguardano* (Milan, 1897); (reprinted London, 1960); Adelmann, Howard B., *Marcello Malpighi and the evolution of embryology*, 5 vols (Ithaca, New York, London, 1966); *The correspondence of Marcello Malpighi*, 5 vols (Ithaca, New York, 1975); 'A supplement to "The correspondence of Marcello Malpighi"', *J. Hist. Med.*, 33 (1978) pp.53–73; Anzalone, Michele, *Marcello Malpighi e suoi scritti sugli organi del respiro* (Bologna, 1966); *Celebrazione Malpighiane: discorsi e scritti* (Bologna, 1966); Toffoletto, Ettore, *Discorso sul Malpighi* (Bologna, 1965); Hayman, J. M., 'Malpighi's "Concerning the structure of the kidneys"; a translation and introduction', *Ann. Med. Hist.*, 7 (1925) pp.242–63.

30. Brockbank, William and O. R. Corbett, 'De Graaf's "Tractatus de clysteribus" ', *J. Hist. Med.*, 9 (1954) pp.174–90 (translation on pp. 177–89); De Graaf, *On the human reproductive organs. An annotated translation of Tractatus de virorum organis generationi inservientibus (1668) and De mulierum organis generationi inservientibus tractatus novus (1672) by H. D. Jocelyn and B. P. Setchell* (Oxford, 1972), and *De mulierum organis generationi inservientibus 1672*–facsimile with introduction by *J. A. von Dongen,*

(Nieuwkoop, 1965). See also Klein, Marc, 'Histoire et actualité de l'iconographie de l'ouvrage: De mulierum organis generationi inservientibus (1672) de R. de Graaf', *Bull. Soc. Int. Hist. Med.*, Special number, *Comptes Rendus 16e Congr. Hist. Med.*, 1 (1959) pp.316–20; Barge, J. A. J. 'Reinier de Graaf, 1641–1941', *Mededeelingen der Nederlandse Akademie van Wetenschappen*, Afdeeling Letterkunde 5, no.5 (1942) pp.257–81; Catchpole, Hubert R., 'Regnier de Graaf, 1641–1673', *Bull. Hist. Med.*, 8 (1940) pp.1261–1300.

31.   Robb, Hunter, 'The writings of Mauriceau', *Bull. Johns Hopkins Hosp.*, 6, (1895) pp.51–7; Speert, Harold, 'Obstetric-gynecologic eponyms. François Mauriceau and his maneuver in breech delivery', *Obstet. Gynec.*, 9 (1957) pp.371–6.

32.   Appleby, J. H., 'New light on John Woodall, surgeon and adventurer', *Med. Hist.*, 25 (1981) pp.251–68; Keynes, Sir Geoffrey Langdon, 'John Woodall, surgeon, his place in medical history', *J. Roy. Coll. Phycns Lond.*, 2 (1967) pp.15–33; Debus, Allen G., 'John Woodall, Paracelsian surgeon', *Ambix*, 10 (1962) pp.108–18; McDonald, D., 'Dr John Woodall and his treatment of the scurvy', *Trans. Roy. Soc. Trop. Med. Hyg.*, 48 (1954) pp.360–5.

33.   Wiseman, Richard, *Of wounds, of gun-shot wounds, of fractures and luxations. A facsimile of Books V, VI and VII from 'Severall chirurgicall treatises' first published 1676 with introduction, appendix and glossary by J. Kirkup* (Bath, 1977); Kirkup, J. R., 'The tercentenary of Richard Wiseman's "Severall chirurgicall treatises" ' (Vicary Lecture, 1976) *Ann. Roy. Coll. Surg. Engl.*, 59 (1977) pp.271–83; Smith, Alan DeForest, 'Richard Wiseman: his contributions to English surgery', *Bull. N.Y. Acad. Med.*, 46 (1970) pp.167–82; Longmore, Sir T., *Richard Wiseman, surgeon and sergeant-surgeon to Charles II; a biographical study* (London, New York, 1891).

34.   *The journal of James Yonge, Plymouth surgeon. Edited by F. N. L. Poynter* (1963); (contains, pp.25–6, 'A catalogue of the books I have writ and published'); Tubbs, F. A., 'A "Dick Whittington" of surgery: James Yonge, 1646 [*sic*]–1721', *St Thomas's Hosp. Gaz.*, 59 (1961) pp.35–42; Dewhurst, Kenneth, 'Three letters from James Yonge', *Med. Hist.*, 7 (1963) pp.381–2.

35.   Schoneveld, Cornelis W., *Intertraffic of the mind. Studies in Anglo-Dutch translation with a checklist of books translated from English into Dutch, 1600–1700* (Leyden, 1983).

36.   Babb, Lawrence, *Sanity in Bedlam. A study of Robert Burton's Anatomy of Melancholy* (Michigan, 1959); Jordan-Smith, Paul, *Bibliographia Burtoniana: a study of Robert Burton's The Anatomy of melancholy with a bibliography of Burton's writings* (Stanford, Calif., London, 1931); Osler, Sir William *et al.*, 'Robert Burton and the Anatomy of melancholy', *Proc. Pap. Oxford Bib. Soc.*, 1, iii (1926).

37.   Donovan, Denis G. *et al.*, *Sir Thomas Browne and Robert Burton. A reference guide* (Boston, 1981); Keynes, Sir Geoffrey Langdon, *A bibliography of Sir Thomas Browne, Kt., M.D ... Second edition, revised and augmented* (Oxford, 1968) and 'Notes for a lecture on the skin. By Sir Thomas Browne', *St Barts Hosp. Rep.*, 57, i (1924) pp.108–13; Batty Shaw, A., 'Sir Thomas Browne, the man and the physician' (Vicary Lecture, 1977) *Ann. Roy. Coll. Surg. Engl.*, 60 (1978) pp.336–44; Nathanson, Leonard, *The strategy of truth. A study of Sir Thomas Browne* (Chicago, London, 1967); Merton, Stephen, 'Old and new physiology in Sir Thomas Browne: digestion and some other functions', *Isis*, 57 (1966) pp.249–59; Huntley, Frank Livingstone, *Sir Thomas Browne: a biographical and critical study* (Ann Arbor, 1962).

38.   O'Malley, C. D., 'Helkiah Crooke, M.D., F.R.C.P., 1576–1648', *Bull. Hist. Med.*, 42 (1968) pp.1–18.

39.   French, R. K., 'Alexander Read and the circulation of the blood', *Bull. Hist. Med.*, 50 (1976) pp.478–500; Menzies, Walter, 'Alexander Read, physician and surgeon, 1580–1641: his life, works and library', *The Library*, 4th ser., 12 (1932) pp.46–74.

40.   Poynter, F. N. L., 'Nicholas Culpeper and his books', *J. Hist. Med.*, 17 (1962) pp.152–67, and 'Nicholas Culpeper and the Paracelsians', *Science, medicine and society in the Renaissance. Essays presented to Walter Pagel* (New York, 1972) vol. 1, pp.201–20; Cowen, David L., 'The Boston editions of Nicholas Culpeper', *J. Hist. Med.*, 11 (1956) pp.156–65; Russell, K. F., 'Nicholas Culpeper: his translations of Bartholin, Riolan and Vesling', *Australian N.Z. J. Surg.*, 26 (1956) pp.156–9.

41.   See Thornton–Tully, pp.101–6; Fulton, John Farquhar, *A bibliography of the Honour-*

able Robert Boyle ... Second edition (Oxford, 1961); (a new edition is in progress); Maddison, R. E. W., *The life of the Honourable Robert Boyle* (1969) and 'The first edition of Robert Boyle's *Medicinal experiments*', *Ann. Sci.*, 18 (1962) pp.43–7; Dewhurst Kenneth, 'Locke's contribution to Boyle's researches on the air and on human blood', *Notes Rec. Roy. Soc. Lond.*, 17 (1962), pp.198–206.

42. Webster, Charles, 'The English medical reformers of the Puritan revolution. A background to the Society of Chymical Physitians', *Ambix*, 14 (1967) pp.16–41; Thomas, Sir Henry, 'The Society of Chymical Physitians: an echo of the Great Plague of London, 1665', *Science, medicine and history*, Vol. 2 (1953) pp.56–71. See also Rattansi, P. M., 'The Helmont-Galenist controversy in Restoration England', *Ambix*, 12 (1964) pp.1–23; and Debus, Allen G., *The English Paracelsians* (1965) and *The chemical philosophy* (1977).

43. Godwin, Joscelyn, *Robert Fludd*, (1979); Hutin, Serge, *Robert Fludd (1574–1637), alchumiste et philosophe rosicrucien* (Paris, 1971); Debus, Allen G., 'Renaissance chemistry and the work of Robert Fludd', *Ambix*, 14 (1967) pp.42–59.

44. H. de Waele, *J. B. van Helmont* (Brussels, 1947); Pagel, Walter, *The religious and philosophical aspects of van Helmont's science and medicine* (Baltimore, 1944); Vandevelde, A. J. J. *Helmontiana. Verslagen en Mededeelingen K. Vlaamsche Academie voor Taal- en Letterkunde*, Pt 1 (1929) pp.453–76; Pt 2 (1929) pp.715–37; Pt 3 (1929) pp.857–79; Pt 4 (1932) pp.109–22; Pt 5 (1936) pp.339–87.

45. Rolleston, Sir Humphrey Davy, 'Walter Charleton, D.M., F.R.C.P., F.R.S.', *Bull. Hist. Med.*, 8 (1940) pp.403–16; Hunter, Richard A. and Emily Cuttler, 'Walter Charleton's "Natural history of the passions" (1674) and J. F. Senault's "The use of passions" (1649). A case of mistaken identity', *J. Hist. Med.*, 13 (1958) pp.87–92.

46. King, Lester S., 'Stahl and Hoffmann: a study in eighteenth-century animism', *J. Hist. Med.*, 19 (1964) pp.118–30; Strube, Irene, 'Die Phlogistonlehre Georg Ernst Stahls (1659–1734) in ihrer historischen Bedeutung', *Z. Gesch. Naturw. Techn. Med.*, 1 (1961) pp.27–51.

47. DePietro, Pericle, *Bibliografia di Bernardino Ramazzini* (Rome, 1977), and 'Le fonti bibliografiche nella "De morbis artificium diatriba" di Bernardino Ramazzini', *Hist. Philos. Life Sci.*, 3 (1981) pp.95–114; 'De virginium vestalium valetudine tuenda dissertatio. Introduced by A. Meiklejohn and A. P. Curran', *Med. Hist.*, 8 (1964) pp.371–5; Pazzini, Adalberto, 'Bernardino Ramazzini', *Scientia Medica Italica*, 4 (1956) pp.335–67.

48. Luyendijk-Elshout, Antonie M., 'Death enlightened. A study of Frederik Ruysch', *J. Amer. Med. Assn*, 212 (1970) pp.121–26; Mann, Gunter, 'Museums: the anatomical collection of Frederik Ruysch at Leningrad', *Bull. Cleveland Med. Lib.*, 11 (1964) pp.10–13.

49. Goldwyn, Robert M., 'Nicolaas Tulp (1593–1674)', *Med. Hist.*, 5 (1961) pp.270–6; Rickham, Peter P., 'Nicolaas Tulp and spina bifida', *Clinical Pediatrics*, 2 (1963) pp.40–2; Heckscher, William S., *Rembrandt's Anatomy of Dr. Nicolaas Tulp: an iconographical study* (New York, 1958); Schupbach, William, *The paradox of Rembrandt's 'Anatomy of Dr. Tulp'*, *Med. Hist.*, Supplement No. 2 (1982).

5 Medical books from 1701 to 1800
Patricia C. Want

If we try to find, in Hunter's mental character, the facts to which may be ascribed his great influence in the promotion of medicine and surgery, I think it may justly be assigned to the degree in which he introduced the exercise of the observant scientific mind into the study and practice of surgery.

(Sir James Paget)

Characteristic of this century was the general pursuit of enlightenment. In the subject field of medicine such a spirit of enquiry was very evident; new discoveries were more likely to be substantiated by scientifically-based research, possibly owing to the example set by William Harvey a century earlier. The growth of periodical literature and the increase in the number of medical and scientific societies at this time facilitated the dissemination of information and greatly contributed to the progress of medical science.

Surgical knowledge steadily advanced, and techniques improved, in the wake of a new and greater understanding of the intricacies of human anatomy. In this respect, the comparative studies of John Hunter (1728–93) remain one of the great achievements of the century. Giovanni Battista Morgagni, often regarded as the Father of Morbid Anatomy, was born in Forli on February 25 1682. At the age of sixteen he went to Bologna University from where he graduated in medicine and philosophy in 1701. He became prosector of anatomy under Antonio Maria Valsalva, whose anatomical works he later edited, and succeeded him as demonstrator when the latter moved to Parma. His first work was the *Adversaria anatomica*, containing a number of original observations. This was published in six parts between 1706 and 1723, reaching several editions. In 1711 he was appointed professor of theoretical medicine at Padua and, three years later, to the Chair in anatomy. When he died on 6 December 1771, Morgagni had held the professorship for 60 years. He was the author of *Epistolae anatomicae duae*, Leyden, 1728, and of a diversity of non-medical works on such subjects as archaeology, history, literature and philology. His greatest work, *De sedibus et causis morborum per anatomen indagatis libri quinque*, was printed in Venice in 1761 when he was 79 years of age. Based on his study of 640 post-mortems, it was the product of a long and diligent search for the causative factors of a number of diseases, bringing the two disciplines of pathology and anatomy to bear on the practice of clinical medicine. *De sedibus* went into many editions and was translated into French, German and Italian. A three-volume English version by Benjamin Alexander was printed in London in 1769 and a facsimile introduced by P. Klemperer was published in New York, 1980. Morgagni's collected works were incorporated in a set of five volumes, Padua, 1762–5. An interesting collection of 100 consultation documents, compiled by Morgagni from a vast collection of his clinical records, were entrusted, in 1771, to a favourite pupil, Michele Girardi, supplementing an earlier collection of 12 volumes previously given to him. In 1935 these reports were edited and published with annotations by Enrico Benassi in a limited edition of 500 copies, attracting little attention at that time. In 1984 this volume was translated and revised, with a detailed preface, by Saul Jarcho, and provides some insight into Morgagni's work as a practising clinician. Conditions range from sexually transmitted diseases and difficult births to asthma and tumours; in each case the possible cause is examined, symptoms described and proposed treatment outlined.[1]

William Cheselden (1688–1752) was born at Burrow on the Hill, Somerby, Leicestershire. He became a pupil of William Cowper at the age of 15 and was eventually appointed surgeon to St Thomas's Hospital. He achieved fame as a lithotomist, publishing *A treatise on the high operation for the stone*, London, 1723, which was dedicated to Richard Mead, but he later abandoned this technique for the lateral operation for which he is best known. His anatomical publications are noteworthy and his popular *Anatomy of the humane body*, London, 1713, was published when he was only 25 years of age, the text simply written and beautifully illustrated. Later editions appeared in 1722, 1726 (in which 'human' was substituted in the title for 'humane'), 1730, 1740, 1741, 1750, 1763, 1768, 1773, 1778, 1783 and 1792, the thirteenth and last. American editions were published in 1795 and 1806 and a German translation by August Ferdinand Wolff was published in Göttingen in 1790. Cheselden intended his greatest work, *Osteographia, or the anatomy of the bones*, London, 1733, to appear in three volumes, but it was never completed. Issued by subscription at four guineas, only 97 of the 300 copies printed were sold. The original copies were issued with two sets of plates, one set lettered and with text on the verso, the other unlettered and blank on the verso. An apparently unique copy of a trial issue printed in 1728 is in the Hunterian Library at Glasgow and bears the title *The anatomy of the bones*, London, 1728. It is without text or letterpress. A variant issue of the 1733 edition has the vignette on the title-page and the broken column on the last page printed in red, and an undated issue has no frontispiece, the title-page being engraved, not printed. This issue probably consisted of 183 sets of unlettered plates, and Cheselden also broke up 83 copies to offer sets of plates separately in an attempt to recover some of his expenditure. Most of the drawings for *Osteographia* were by Gerard Vandergucht, the others by Jacobus Schijnvoet (1685–1723). The original drawings were discovered in the Royal Academy, and were deposited on loan in the Royal College of Surgeons in

England. W. R. LeFanu[2] has contributed a paper on the artist Schijnvoet (called Shinevoet by Cheselden), indicating the plates for which he was responsible. LeFanu[3] has also noted that three engravings included by Charles Bell in his book on *The Hand* (1833) are based, without acknowledgement, on engravings of animal skeletons copied from the *Osteographia*. Cheselden devised a 'camera obscura' for his artists to obtain exact proportions, and the instrument is featured on the title-page of his book. In addition to these publications Cheselden was the author of five papers published in the *Philosophical Transactions*. Sir Zachary Cope[4] has produced a biographical study of Cheselden, and K. F. Russell[5] has provided bibliographical information regarding the *Osteographia*.

The anatomical atlases of Bernhard Siegfried Albinus (1697–1770) are outstanding for the beauty and quality of the figures, largely drawn and engraved by John Wandelaer (1690–1759). None was drawn free-hand, each being measured and brought down to scale. It has been stated that Albinus spent 24 000 florins on illustrations. A native of Frankfort-on-the-Oder, Albinus studied at Leyden under Boerhaave, and then in Paris. He returned to Leyden in 1719 to lecture on anatomy and surgery and from 1721 held these two Chairs at that University, following in the footsteps of his father. Albinus edited the works of Harvey, Fabricius and Eustachius, and wrote a large number of books, including: *Oratio inauguralis de anatome comparata*, Leyden, 1719; *Index supellectilis anatomicae*, Leyden, 1725; *De ossibus corporis humani ad auditores suos*, Leyden, 1726; *Historia musculorum hominis*, Leyden, 1734; *Dissertatio de arteriis et venis intestinorum hominis*, Leyden and Amsterdam, 1736; *Dissertatio secunda. De sede et causa coloris Aethiopum et caeterorum hominum*, Leyden and Amsterdam, 1737; *Icones ossium foetus humani; Accedit osteogeniae brevis historia*, Leyden, 1737, which is his principal work; *Tabulae sceleti et musculorum corporis humani, cum explanatio*, Leyden, 1747, of which extracts appear in a recent book by Punt[6] containing a biographical study (pp.3–13) and notes on his approach to anatomical illustration; an English translation appeared as *Tables of the skeleton and muscles of the human body*, London, 1749, and Edinburgh, 1777; *Explicatio tabularum anatomicarum Bartholem. Eustachii, anatomici summi*, Leyden, 1744; *De sceleto humano liber*, Leyden, 1762; and *Index supellectilis anatomicae*, Leyden, 1771. A number of letters written from Albinus in Leyden to a friend in London, Dr Robert Nesbitt, have been preserved and reported in the literature.[7]

Another excellent draughtsman was Antonio Scarpa (1752–1832), a former pupil of Morgagni. He became a leading anatomist and surgeon and was appointed professor of anatomy first at Modena, and then at Pavia. In *Tabulae neurologicae ad illustrandam historiam anatomicam cardiacorum nervorum*, Pavia, 1794, Scarpa's command of Latin was combined with his artistic skill to produce his finest work, the beautiful anatomical drawings being engraved by Faustino Anderloni. This book demonstrates the nerves of the heart, and Scarpa also made important observations on aneurysm, hernia, the ear and diseases of the eye. His writings include *De structura fenestrae rotundae auris, et de tympano secundario anatomicae observationes*, Modena, 1772, in which Scarpa first described the cul-de-sac of the scala tympani. This has been translated into English by Lyle M. Sellers and Barry J. Anson.[8] Scarpa was also the author of *Anatomicarum annotationum liber primus (et secundus)*, 1779; *Anatomicae disquisitiones de auditu et olfactu*, Padua, 1789; *Saggio di osservazioni e d'esperienze sulle principali malattie degli occhi*, Pavia, 1801, of which there were several editions and translations into English, French, German, and Spanish; *Riflessioni ed osservazioni anatomico chirurgiche sull'aneurisma*, Pavia, 1804, which was translated into English and French. *Sull'ernie, memorie anatomico-chirurgiche*, Milan, 1809–10, also translated into English and French; *Ospuscoli di chirurgia*, three volumes in one, Pavia, 1825–32; and *De anatome et pathologia ossium commentarii*, Pavia, 1827. His collected works were published in Florence, 1836–8. Scarpa formed a large art collection, and when he came to London in 1780 he met Percivall Pott, the Hunter brothers, and William Cruikshank.[9]

Samuel Thomas Soemmerring was born in Thorn, East Prussia, on 18 January 1755 and studied at Göttingen before travelling to England, Scotland and the Netherlands. In the course of his career he was taught by Albinus at Leyden and later became friendly with William Hunter and Peter Camper. In 1779, Soemmerring became professor of anatomy at the Collegium Carolinum in Cassel and, five years later, professor of medicine at Mainz. He established himself as a physician at Frankfort-on-Main in 1797. Soemmerring was an admirer of Albinus, and aimed at perfect accuracy in anatomical illustration. He was a good artist, endeavouring to represent the parts as they appeared in the living body, and he trained Christian Köck to draw his plates. Soemmerring's publications include *De basi encephali et originibus nervorum cranio egredientium libri quinque*, Göttingen, 1778, his inaugural dissertation containing plates drawn by himself, and engraved by Carl Christian Glassbach, Jr; *Von Hirn- und Rückenmark*, Mainz, 1788; *Über die Wirkungen der Schnürbrüste*, Berlin, 1793, his treatise on corsets containing one copper-plate drawn by Köck, and engraved by Daniel Berger; *Vom Baue des menschlichen Körpers*, three volumes, Frankfort-on-Main, 1791–6, also published in four volumes, 1800, and in eight volumes, 1839–45; *Tabula sceleti feminini juncta descriptione*, Frankfort-on-Main, 1797, which is especially noted for anatomical accuracy; *Icones embryonum humanorum*, Frankfort-on-Main, 1799; and *Abbildungen des menschlichen Auges*, Frankfort-on-Main, 1801, containing sixteen copper-plates drawn by Köck. A Latin edition of the latter by Bernhard Nathanael Gottlob Schreger was printed as *Icones oculi humani*, Frankfort-on-Main, 1804, containing the same plates. Soemmerring is often erroneously credited with the first description of the substantia nigra, sometimes known as 'Soemmerring's substance', but he, in fact, accords priority in its description to Vicq d'Azyr.[10] An account of his life and work appeared in *Annals of Medical History* in 1924.[11] Soemmerring died on 2 March 1830.

Johann Friedrich Blumenbach (1752–1840) was internationally recognized for his expertise in many fields of scientific endeavour, which included natural history and palaeontology as well as medicine. These diverse interests are reflected in his publications and correspondence[12] but he is perhaps best known for his studies on anthropology, to which his knowledge of comparative anatomy contributed. He was appointed professor of medicine at Göttingen in 1776, a year after the publication of his first major work, *De generis humani varietate nativa*, Göttingen, 1775. His other writings include *Ueber den Bildungstrieb und das Zeugungsgeschäft*, Göttingen, 1781, translated into English as *An essay on generation*, London, 1792; *Medicinische Bibliothek*, three volumes, Göttingen, 1783–88; *Geschichte und Beschreibung der Knochen des menschlichen Körpers*, Göttingen, 1786; *Institutiones physiologicae*, Göttingen, 1786; *Handbuch der vergleichenden Anatomie*, Göttingen, 1805, his most important work on comparative anatomy; and *Collectio craniorum diversarum gentium illustrata, Decas i-vi, Göttingen*, 1790–1820, Blumenbach's invaluable anthropological treatise, which earned for him the title of 'founder of modern anthropology'. He wrote several other books, and many of his writings were translated into English, including the *Anthropological treatises*, London, 1865.

Several important contributions to surgical literature were made by Percivall Pott,[13] who was born in London on 6 January 1714. In 1729 he was apprenticed to one Edward Nourse (1701–61), a surgeon at St Bartholomew's Hospital, and continued to work with him after qualification. Pott occupied several prominent posts in the Corporation of Surgeons, eventually becoming Master in 1765. He was elected assistant surgeon to St Bartholomew's Hospital in 1745, and four years later became full surgeon, which position he held until 1787. His career was eminently successful but, apart from a communication to the Royal Society in 1744, he wrote nothing until confined to bed following an accident in 1756. He subsequently produced the many books and papers, which have ensured his fame to posterity: *A treatise on ruptures*, London, 1756, of which further editions followed in 1763, 1769, and 1775; *An account of a particular kind of rupture frequently attendant upon new-born children*, London, 1756, of which a second edition appeared in 1765, and a third in 1775; *Observations on that disorder of the corner of the eye, commonly called fistula lachrymalis*, London, 1758, which was also printed in 1763, 1769, 1772 and 1775; *Observations on the nature and consequences of wounds and contusions of the head*, London, 1760; *Practical remarks upon the hydrocele or watery rupture,* London, 1762 and 1767, which was translated into German; *Remarks on the disease, commonly called a fistula in ano,* London, 1765, with later editions in 1767, 1771 and 1775; *Observations on the nature and consequences of those injuries to which the head is liable from external violence,* London, 1768,[14] 1771 and 1773; *Some few general remarks upon fractures and dislocations,* London, 1768, and 1773, of which Italian editions appeared in 1777 and 1784, and French editions from Paris in 1771 and 1788; *An account of the method of obtaining a perfect or radical cure of the hydrocele,* London, 1771, 1773 and 1775; *Chirurgical observations relative to the cataract,* London, 1775, with a German edition from Berlin in 1776; *Remarks on the necessity and propriety of amputation,* London, 1777; *Remarks on that kind of palsy of the lower limbs, which is frequently found to accompany a curvature of the spine,* London, 1779, which was also translated into Dutch (Leyden, 1779); French (Brussels, 1779; Paris, 1783 and 1785) and German (Leipzig, 1786); and *Further remarks on the useless state of the lower limbs, in consequence of a curvature of the spine ...,* London, 1782. His writings were collected together and published as *Chirurgical works,* two volumes, London, 1771, with a quarto edition in 1775, and three-volume editions published in 1779, 1790 and 1808, the last two being edited by Sir James Earle. There were numerous other editions and translations of these writings published both in this country and abroad.[15] Pott's name is connected eponymously with a number of descriptions, and he was the first to describe chimney sweepers' cancer of the scrotum.[16] His writings on head injuries, and his works in general can still be read with great interest since, as well as reflecting contemporary surgical knowledge through the interpretation and opinions of an eminent practitioner, they also reveal much about the social conditions of the time. Pott died on December 22 1788, leaving numerous pupils to continue his work.

There is some confusion between contemporary surgeons bearing the surname Douglas and the initial J. There was, for example, a John Douglas (*c.*1690–1743), brother of James, and another John Douglas (died 1758), author of *Treatise on the hydrocoele,* 1755. It was the former who attacked Cheselden in *Animadversions on a late pompous work entitled Osteographia,* 1735, and the blame is often placed on James Douglas (1675–1742). Born at Baads, near Edinburgh, little is known of his life in subsequent years but he is known to have been in Utrecht where his library of some 72 volumes was catalogued in 1698. There is, however, no record of his attendance at that University and it is known that he obtained his degree of Docteur de la Faculté de Médecine from the University of Rheims in July 1699. Shortly afterwards, probably in 1700, he arrived in London, and extant case histories suggest that in the course of his career he was well acquainted with Paul Chamberlen, of the family so closely associated with the early history of midwifery forceps. He was elected a Fellow of the Royal Society on 4 December 1706, and an Honorary Fellow of the Royal College of Physicians in 1720, for which privilege he paid the sum of £100. He was a versatile scholar, whose interests ranged from anatomy, zoology and botany to phonetics and Horace. Amongst his manuscripts in the Hunterian Collection of Glasgow University are more than 60 pamphlets written by him, mostly unpublished. Several hundred more papers in that collection are also attributable to James Douglas, these having been acquired by William Hunter and sent to Glasgow with his own collections after his death in 1783. Much of this material has been neglected and would obviously repay careful investigation. K. Bryn Thomas,[17] in his biographical study of James Douglas, incorporates an annotated catalogue of the manuscripts and drawings attributed to Douglas, and many of the documents have been photographed and made available in the Wellcome Historical Medical Library. James Douglas was lecturing at least as early as 1706. He left many unpublished manuscripts on a variety of subjects but a number of works appeared in print, including several papers published in the *Philosophical Transactions*. He was the friend of Sir Hans Sloane, Cowper and Mead, and was visited by Haller. William Hunter lived in his house after staying with Smellie, and became assistant to James Douglas and tutor to his son. Douglas's publications include: *Myographiae comparatae specimen: or, a comparative description of all the muscles in a man and in a quadruped*, 1707, which went into a second edition, Edinburgh, 1750, and a third edition, Edinburgh, 1775. Other printings include Dublin, 1755 and 1777; and London and Edinburgh, 1763. It was also translated into Latin by J. F. Schreiber, Leyden, 1729, and into Dutch, Leyden, 1732. *Bibliographiae anatomicae specimen, sive catalogus omnium pene auctorum qui ab Hippocrate ad Harveum rem anatomicam ... scriptus illustrarunt*, London, 1715, consists of a chronological list of authors, with biographical and bibliographical notes, of which a second edition was produced in Leyden, 1734. Further publications were *Index materia medicae or a catalogue of simple medicines that are fit to be used in the practice of physick and surgery*, London, 1724; *The history of the lateral operation: or an account of the method for extracting a stone*, London, 1726 and reprinted in 1731, with a French translation, Paris, 1726, and a Latin translation, Leyden, 1753. His description of the pouch of Douglas is contained in *Description of the peritonaeum*, 1730, which was dedicated to Richard Mead, and translated into Latin by Lorenz Heister, Helmstadt, 1733. His botanical writings include *Lilium Sarniense: or a description of the Guernsay-Lilly*, London, 1725; and *Arbor Yemensis fructum Coféferens: or, a description of the coffee tree*, London, 1727; both of these publications are folios. An account of Douglas's botanical activities has been published by Helen Brock.[18] Of his unpublished work, of particular interest is his proposed publication on bones, an impressive undertaking intended to include within its comprehensive contents not only a set of some 60 osteological drawings, but also a history of osteology and its illustration. Had it appeared in print it may well have been one of the most outstanding anatomical atlases of the period. A short commentary on the career of James Douglas, his unpublished writings and two rare published works, is provided by Brock in *The Bibliothek*.[19]

The most outstanding man-midwife of this period, and a pioneer of modern obstetrics, was William Smellie (1697–1763). Born in the parish of Lesmahagow in 1697, he attended the Grammar School in Lanark and later became apprenticed to a prominent apothecary of the town, William Inglis. He then elected to join the Royal Navy as a Surgeon's mate and served at sea for a period of 20 months between 1720 and 1721. After this he returned to Lanark and slowly built up his own practice, gradually taking over from the elderly Inglis who died in 1727. Smellie's early life has been researched in some detail by Butterton,[20] who has published an interesting account of his life and career prior to his migration to London in or around 1739. In London Smellie built up a flourishing practice and established himself as a teacher, giving 280 courses of lectures and training some 900 pupils. During this time he took the opportunity to visit Paris. In 1745 Glasgow University conferred an MD upon him, and finally he retired to Lanark in 1759. He died on 5 March 1763. Smellie was the author of *A course of lectures upon midwifery*, 1742, which was followed by *A treatise on the theory and practice of midwifery*, London 1752 (reprinted London, 1974). This went into several editions, and was translated into French (Paris, 1754 and 1771), German (Altenburg, 1755), and Dutch (Amsterdam, 1765). This book was followed by *A collection of cases and observations in midwifery*, London, 1754, and *A collection of preternatural cases and observations in midwifery*, London, 1774 these being called volumes two and three respectively. These three volumes were edited by Smellie's friend Tobias Smollett. The New Sydenham Society printed a three-volume edition, London, 1876–8. The work is still of interest for the rules it contains regarding the safe use of obstetric forceps, and for its remarkable collection of case-histories. Smellie also produced *A sett* [*sic*] *of anatomical tables with explanations*, London, 1754, which contains 39 plates, 26 from originals by Jan van Rymsdyk,[21] and the others by Smellie 'assisted by a pupil called Camper'. The volume was reprinted in 1971 in Auckland, New Zealand. A second edition of the *Tables* was published in 1761, and others include printings in Edinburgh in 1785 and 1792. The life and work of Rymsdyk has been researched by John L. Thornton and further information can be found in the small volume which appeared in 1982.[22] R. W. Johnstone[23] has produced an interesting study of William Smellie and numerous articles published over the years detail his many outstanding contributions to the teaching and practice of midwifery in Britain.[24] The classic biography by John Glaister[25] published in 1894 remains, however, the definitive work, and could usefully be reprinted with a new introduction.

Pieter Camper was born in Leyden on 11 May 1722. He studied medicine at the University, where he was greatly influenced by Albinus, and in 1746 obtained his doctorate. After this he travelled on the continent and by the end of 1748 had reached London where, on 5 January 1749, he enrolled on one of the midwifery courses run by William Smellie. He then journeyed to Paris, Lyons and Geneva before returning again to England in 1752 in order to make some drawings for Smellie. By this time, on 17 January 1751, he had been elected a Fellow of the Royal Society, although he was not formally admitted until a few years later. On 24 April 1755 he was appointed professor of anatomy at the Athenaeum Illustre in Amsterdam and from 1763–73 he occupied the chair of theoretical medicine, anatomy, surgery and botany at Gröningen. He died on 7 April 1789. His reputation as an anatomist was established with the publication of his *Demonstrationum anatomico-pathologicarum liber primus* [-*secundus*], Amsterdam, 1760–2. It is written in two parts and contains a fine series of plates. A list of his publications and essays, in chronological order, is appended to a biographical paper by Kaplan[26] and a comprehensive bibliography is to be found on pages 178–99 of a volume by Visser[27] concerning his zoological contributions; this also contains a good biographical introduction. Camper paid a third visit to England in 1785 and his diary records his meetings with many distinguished men. It is preserved in Amsterdam University and was published in Dutch and English in *Opuscula selecta neerlandicorum de arte medica, Fascicule XV*, Amsterdam, 1939.[28]

Another person greatly influenced by Smellie was William Hunter (1718–83), a figure often overshadowed as a result of the prominence gained over the years by his younger brother John. This results, perhaps, from the fact that John Hunter's museum has been exploited to the full in the Royal College of Surgeons of England, whilst William Hunter's magnificent collection in Glasgow has been somewhat neglected. However the balance has been redressed to some extent with the opportunity afforded by the bicentenary of William Hunter's death to re-examine his contributions to anatomy and obstetrics.[29] Hunter attended Glasgow University from 1732 to 1736, from which centre he also obtained his MD in 1750. At the end of 1740 Hunter left Glasgow for London and there gained a great reputation as a teacher and man-midwife. He became a Fellow of the Royal Society in 1767. His most outstanding publication was the monumental *Anatomia uteri humani gravidi tabulis illustrata*, printed by the Baskerville Press in Birmingham and published in London in 1774.[30] It is an elephant folio with Latin and English titles on the same page, and contains 34 plates, each with facing text. The life-size plates were engraved by several artists from drawings by Jan van Rymsdyk. A reprint, on a rather reduced scale, appeared in 1980 with an accompanying booklet of editorial notes.[31] Another edition was printed in London in 1815, with a preface signed by Thomas Denman, and the Baskerville sheets were reissued in 1818. This is known as Ballantyne's edition and is rare, the only known copies being at King's College Hospital Medical School and the Royal College of Physicians and Surgeons of Glasgow. An undated London edition was published by Edward Lumley and a further edition appeared in 1851 produced by the Sydenham Society. Another rare item is *Lectures on the gravid uterus and midwifery: as taught and practised by the late Dr. Hunter (With the medical terms in midwifery explained for the benefit of female practitioners.) By one who studied under him*, London, 1783. A copy is housed in the Royal College of Physicians and Surgeons of Glasgow. Hunter was the first scientist to see the folio volume of anatomical drawings by Leonardo da Vinci housed in Windsor Castle,[32] which opportunity was doubtless afforded as a consequence of his office as physician to the Queen. His impressions of the drawings are a feature of his *Two introductory lectures*, London, 1784, prepared by him for printing but published after his death, and which relate to the history and study of anatomy. Another posthumous publication was *An anatomical description of the human gravid uterus and its contents*, London, 1794. This has a preface signed by Matthew Baillie and was originally intended to accompany Hunter's great atlas. A second edition was produced by Edward Rigby, London, 1843, later translated into German by L. F. Froriep, Weimar, 1802 and into Portuguese, Lisbon, 1813. Contributions to the *Philosophical Transactions, Medical Observations and Inquiries,* and other papers and fragments are recorded by W. R. LeFanu.[33] A facsimile edition of two notebooks of a series of anatomical lectures given in Manchester, written by C. White, presumably Charles White (1728–1813), has now been published.[34] As yet no definitive biography of William Hunter has appeared, but certain short appraisals of his life and career are available.[35] In 1970 Illingworth drew attention to a hitherto unrecorded paper published in *Archaeologia*, three years after Hunter's death, consisting of his observations on a lead-filled human femur.[36] Hunter's unique collections are housed in the University of Glasgow, where the Hunterian Library contains much manuscript material,[37] including a paper in William Hunter's hand, describing a foetus, with drawings presumably by Nicholas Blakey (died 1758)[38] and another on William Harvey consisting of 18 pages of notes, the subject of a paper by K. Bryn Thomas.[39] The history of Hunter's Museum has been surveyed by Helen Brock in a paper published in 1980.[40]

Another distinguished midwifery practitioner of the period was Thomas Denman (1733–1815). His contributions to contemporary obstetric practice and to the literature are now often overlooked in favour of those of Smellie and Hunter, whose great atlases have ensured their immortality. Denman also published an atlas, entitled *A collection of engravings tending to illustrate the generation and parturition of animals and of the human species*, London, 1787, which contains nine plates which had been separately published between 1783 and 1787. Eight plates dating from 1788–1801 were later added and all were published in the third, quarto, edition of Denman's *Introduction to the practice of midwifery*, London, 1801. The plates were also published in another quarto volume, *Engravings, representing the generation of some animals; some circumstances attending parturition in the human species; and a few of the diseases to which the sex is liable*, London, 1815. Denman also employed Jan van Rymsdyk as one of his illustrators.[41] He wrote numerous other books and papers, his major work being the textbook *Introduction to the practice of midwifery*, first published in London in 1782. The title-page bears the misprint '*Part the fisrt*', and no second part appeared at that time. Later, a two-volume set was published, the parts dated in 1788 and 1798 respectively, but only the latter has 'second edition' on the title-page. A further two volumes were published, dated 1794 and 1795, and other editions, not always clearly designated, appeared in 1801, 1805 (two), 1816, 1824 and a seventh and last in 1832. American editions were published in New York in 1802, 1821 and 1825 and in Vermont in 1807. The London editions of 1824 and 1832 are of particular interest in that they both contain an introductory memoir of Denman, largely autobiographical. It has been pointed out by W. E. Snell[42] that extracts from the diaries of one John Knyveton, a fictitious naval surgeon, which were edited by Ernest Gray, closely resemble the account of the career of Denman himself as outlined in his memoir. A popular small volume, *Aphorisms on the application and use of the forceps and vectis*, appeared in seven editions in England, and was also published in America as well as being translated into French. Other publications include a series of *Essays* on natural, difficult and preternatural labours, respectively; also, on uterine haemorrhages and puerperal fever. The last work was also translated into French and German.

Born in Bakewell, the son of an apothecary, Denman assisted in the practice but at the age of 21 decided to go to London to gain further experience and attended a series of anatomical lectures at St George's Hospital. He then joined the Navy as a ship's surgeon, in which occupation he remained for nine years, until 1763. He began to take an interest in midwifery as a potential career, studying under William Smellie, but was unable to establish himself until the year 1770 when he joined forces with William Osborn to present a series of lectures. At this time he was also elected one of the man-midwives to the Middlesex Hospital. Upon the death of William Hunter in 1783 Denman became the capital's leading accoucheur and in that same year, on 22 December, he was admitted by the College of Physicians as its first Licentiate in Midwifery. His twin daughters, Sophia and Margaret, were married to the physician Matthew

Baillie and the obstetrician Sir Richard Croft respectively, the latter taking over Denman's practice until his untimely death following the loss of his royal patient, the Princess Charlotte of Wales, in childbirth, in 1817. Denman died on 26 November 1815.

The most distinguished of Percivall Pott's pupils was undoubtedly John Hunter, who was largely responsible for placing surgery on a scientific basis. John Hunter was born at Long Calderwood, near Glasgow, on 13 February 1728, the youngest of a family of ten. He paid little attention to education during his schooldays and, in the hope that he would settle down to follow the same career, was sent to London in 1748 to assist his elder brother. William Hunter was well-educated, and had already established himself as an anatomist and surgeon. He set John to dissecting, at which the latter soon excelled. His surgical education was completed under Cheselden and Pott, and at St George's Hospital, where he was later appointed surgeon. An attempt to further John's general education by sending him to Oxford failed miserably, for John was anxious to continue practical work. Following an attack of pneumonia, John Hunter was advised to lead an outdoor life, upon which he enlisted as an army surgeon, serving from 1761 to 1763 with the British expedition to Belle Isle.[43] He benefited from this extensive experience of surgery, particularly in respect of knowledge of gunshot wounds. On his return to London John settled down to surgery, and to teaching, and he purchased a country house at Earls Court, where he maintained numerous animals. He collected any rarity relating to natural history, thus establishing the wonderful Hunterian Collection, later housed in the Royal College of Surgeons. Much of this collection was destroyed during the Second World War but the remainder has been handsomely housed in the rebuilt College. John Hunter wrote several books and numerous papers, and at his death left an extensive collection of manuscripts, many of which were destroyed by his brother-in-law, Sir Everard Home, after using much of the material in his own writings. John Hunter published three books in his lifetime, and a fourth appeared posthumously in 1794. He died on 16 October 1793. A handlist of his writings has been prepared by W. R. LeFanu,[44] and the following information is derived from that work. A full-scale bibliography would be welcomed by all interested in John Hunter and his writings.

Hunter's first book, *The natural history of the human teeth*, London, 1771, was followed by a second part entitled *A practical treatise on the diseases of the teeth*, London, published in 1778, the two parts being issued in a second edition the same year. The third followed in 1803. A Dutch and Latin translation was published at Dordrecht in 1773, a German translation in 1780, printed in Leipzig, and an Italian translation from Milan in 1815. Following the publication of this book, Hunter set up a printing press in his house at No. 13, Castle Street, and printed the following books: *A treatise on the venereal disease*, London, 1786, which enjoyed great popularity, but was inaccurate, largely owing to a faulty experiment. This book was reissued in 1787, a second edition appearing in 1788, while several others were published in London, and also Philadelphia, up to 1859. Several French translations were printed between 1787 and 1859, while a German version was published at Leipzig in 1787. Hunter's *Observations on certain parts of the animal oeconomy* was first printed at his house in 1786, a second edition following in 1792. A German translation was published at Braunschweig in 1813. The material collected by Hunter while serving as an army surgeon was not published until after his death, and probably represents his most important book. This appeared as *A treatise on the blood, inflammation and gunshot wounds*, London, 1794,[45] and contains a short biography of Hunter by Everard Home. Other editions of this appeared from Philadelphia, 1796 (in two volumes); London, 1812 (in two volumes); Philadelphia, 1817; London, 1818 (in two volumes); Philadelphia, 1817; and London, 1828. A French translation was published in Ostend, An VII [1799], which was reissued from Paris, without date. A German version in two volumes bound in three was printed in Leipzig, 1797–1800. There are numerous editions and translations of Hunter's *Works*, edited by James F. Palmer, printed in four volumes with a volume of plates, 1835–7.[46] John Hunter also wrote *Observations and reflections on geology*, London, 1859; *Essays and observations on natural history, anatomy, physiology, psychology, and geology*, which was edited by Richard Owen in two volumes, London, 1861; also several smaller works, and numerous papers printed in the *Philosophical Transactions* of the Royal Society.

John Hunter conducted detailed investigations into the structure of the body in man and in the lower animals, and his researches on comparative anatomy caused him to raise the craft of surgery to a scientific level. His lack of general education precluded a full appreciation of the work of his predecessors, yet his diligent researches ensured that his name would long be honoured as one of the great benefactors of mankind. It has been noted by K. Bryn Thomas[47] that Hunter amputated a leg after John Carrick Moore (1763–1834) applied a tourniquet for the compression of nerves, an early example of amputation under analgesia recorded in a pamphlet published in 1784.

The beginning of experimental surgery is associated with John Hunter, and this aspect of his work was stressed by Sir Cecil Wakeley[48] in his Hunterian Oration for 1955. Hunter employed collectors, and artists such as Rymsdyk, William Bell, J. St Aubin, and the incomparable William Clift drew the specimens for him.[49] During the last few years of his life John Hunter was Surgeon-General and Inspector of Regimental Hospitals in the British Army, and this neglected episode has been investigated by Lloyd G. Stevenson.[50] Many others have written books and articles on his life and on various aspects of his career, yet these generally fail to appreciate the full significance of the man and his work as seen by his contemporaries, and in perspective.[51]

It is impossible to mention John Hunter without giving thought to William Clift, for it was his industry that led to the preservation of Hunter's specimens and of some of his manuscripts after his death. William Clift was born at Burford Mill, Bodmin, Cornwall on 14 February 1775, and when John Hunter was in need of an amanuensis in 1791 Clift was recommended, and became Hunter's apprentice and artist. Clift arrived at Leicester Square on 14 February 1792, his seventeenth birthday and Hunter's sixty-fourth. He worked diligently with Hunter until the latter's death, after which Clift looked after the museum until it was purchased in 1799. He then became Conservator and, having taught himself French and German, he built up a library, attended scientific meetings and visited Paris and Italy. The outstanding achievements of this largely self-taught man were recognized by election to the Fellowship of the Royal Society on 8 May 1823. William Clift prepared illustrations for many authors, including Everard Home, William Long, Astley Cooper, James Earle and Matthew Baillie. He retired in 1842 and was succeeded by Richard Owen, who had married his daughter, Caroline, in 1835. Clift died on 20 June 1849, but he left behind numerous monuments to his memory, including a fascinating diary preserved at the Royal College of Surgeons of England. A comprehensive biography of this remarkable man has been written by Jessie Dobson,[52] who additionally wrote a short biographical paper in the *Annals of the Royal College of Surgeons of England*.[53] Clift's correspondence has also provided some interesting subject matter.[54]

Charles White, the Manchester obstetrician, was born on 4 October 1728, the same year as his friend and respected colleague, John Hunter. Both studied under John's brother, William, and a series of notes made by White from one of these courses held in Manchester in 1752, have been published.[55] Charles was the son of one Thomas White, a medical practitioner skilled in midwifery. He is best known for his contribution to the early history of puerperal fever, but is often overlooked as a result of the prominence given to the later work of Semmelweis. He was instrumental in founding the Publick Infirmary, later the Manchester Royal Infirmary, which had its origins in the small hospital into which his home had been converted. His name is also associated with the beginnings of the St Mary's Hospitals and with the College of Arts and Sciences where he lectured on anatomy. He contributed several important papers to journals, including a description of the first recorded excision of the head of the humerus.[56] His *An inquiry into the nature and cause of that swelling in one or both of the lower extremities which sometimes happens to lying-in women*, Warrington, 1784, was the first accurate description in English of the condition later known as 'phlegmasia alba dolens'. A second edition followed, London, 1792, and a separate second part also appeared, Manchester, 1801. His *Account of the regular gradation in man*, London, 1799 was an early English work on anthropological measurement, the introduction containing an acknowledgement to John Hunter, to whom is dedicated White's most important work, *A treatise on the management of pregnant and lying-in women, and the means of curing, but more especially of preventing, the principal disorders to which they are liable*, London, 1773, a second edition appearing four years later. The book reached five editions within 20 years, was translated into French and German, and was reprinted at Worcester, Mass. in 1793. A reprint, with a new introduction by Lawrence D. Longo, was published in Canton, Maryland in 1987. White was elected a Fellow of the Royal Society on 18 February 1762. He died in February 1813.[57]

Arguably the most eminent physician of the period, and described as the 'greatest clinical teacher of the eighteenth century', Herman Boerhaave was born in Voorhout, near Leyden on 31 December 1668, the son of a minister in whose footsteps it was hoped he would follow. After a period pursuing his studies in divinity and philosophy, it was suggested to him that he turn his attention to the field of medicine. This was not incompatible with his other interests and within a remarkably short space of time he obtained his degree from the University of Leyden. He was appointed to the chair of medicine and botany there in 1709, and to that of chemistry in 1718. He became famed throughout Europe as a physician, orator and teacher, and soon attracted students from all over the world. He was still giving occasional lectures at the age of 69, in the spring of 1738, but his health was failing rapidly and he died on 23 September that same year. His publications were eagerly received and a number of these ran into several editions. He also edited various works by other authors, including Vesalius, Aretaeus and Swammerdam, in addition contributing to volumes edited by colleagues. The following represent his more important books, but many were pirated and some published after spurious editions had been produced by pupils and other opportunists. A bibliography of his publications is provided by G. A.Lindeboom in his excellent biography of Boerhaave.[58] His *Institutiones medicae*, Leyden, 1708, went into later editions in 1713, 1720 and 1721, with several others published in Holland, including editions by Haller from Amsterdam, 1751 and 1755, and editions from various other countries, including translations into Dutch, German, French, English and Italian. This was followed by *Aphorismi et cognoscendis et curandis morbis in usum doctrinae domesticae*, Leyden, 1709 and 1713, with a second edition in 1715, a third in 1721 and 1722, and several other editions, including translations into Dutch, German, French and English. Commentaries on the *Aphorisms* include the best known, by Gerard van Swieten (1700–72), five volumes, Leyden, 1741–72, of which there were several editions and translations, including one into English in 18 volumes, 1744–73, with a second edition 1771–3. *Libellus de materie medica*, Leyden, 1719 and 1721, followed an unauthorized edition published in 1714 and went into numerous editions and translations, as did *Tractatus de viribus medicamentorum*, Leyden, 1719 and 1725, with two editions from Paris in 1723 and 1726. Boerhaave wrote *Atrocis, nec descripti prius, morbi historia*, Leyden, 1724[59] and 1740 (two editions), and Frankfort and Leipzig, 1771, which has been translated into English by V. J. Derbes and R. E. Mitchell;[60] *Atrocis, rarissimique morbi historia altera*, Leyden, 1728; *Tractatus medicus de lue venerea praefixus aphrodisiaco*, Leyden, 1728 and 1731; *Tractatus medico-practicus de lue venerea*, Leyden, 1751; *Praelectiones academicae de morbis nervorum*, two volumes, Leyden, 1761, Frankfort, two volumes, 1762, Berne, 1762, and Venice, 1762 and 1763; *De comparando certo in physicis*, Leyden, 1715; *Praxis medica*, five volumes, Padua, 1728; *Praelectiones academicae in proprias institutiones rei medicae*, six volumes in four, Göttingen, 1740–4; *Consultationes medicae*, Göttingen, 1744; *Praelectiones publicae de morbis oculorum*, Göttingen, 1746; and *Methodus studii medici*, two volumes, Amsterdam, 1751, the English translation of which (London, 1719) was from an unauthorized edition. Boerhaave also wrote on botany and chemistry, including *Index plantarum*, Leyden, 1710, 1718, 1720, etc.; *Historia plantarum quae in hortoacademico Lugduni Batavorum crescunt*, Rome, 1727; and *Elementa chemiae*, two volumes, Leyden, 1732, which went into numerous editions, translations and abridgements. An English translation (second edition) in two volumes, 1741 was preceded by an English translation from the spurious *Institutiones et experimenta chemiae*, two volumes, Paris, 1724, published as *A new method of chemistry*, London, 1727. His collected writings appeared as *Opera omnia medica*, Venice, 1722, 1731, 1735, 1742, etc.; and as *Opuscula omnia*, The Hague, 1733 and 1738. Several editions and translations of Boerhaave's letters have been published, including *Consultationes medicae*, The Hague, 1734, 1744, and Leyden, 1744; and a modern series by G. A. Lindeboom.[61] Boerhaave collected books to form a good library, a catalogue of which was compiled for auction purposes as *Bibliotheca Boerhaavinia*, Leyden, 1739. Samuel Johnson wrote a short life of Boerhaave of which a brief résumé has been printed by D. A. K. Black.[62]

One of Boerhaave's many prominent pupils, whose writings were published in London, Edinburgh, Amsterdam, Bremen, Munich, Paris, Venice, Naples and Lisbon, was John Huxham (1692–1768), the son of a Devonshire butcher. Having completed his schooling he enrolled as a medical student at Leyden on 7 May 1715. He completed his studies at Rheims, for financial reasons, and obtained his degree in 1717. He then returned to England, eventually to establish himself in practice in Plymouth. He is best remembered for his book *An essay on fevers and their different kinds*, London, 1750, of which a second edition appeared later in the year, and third and fourth editions in 1757 and 1764 respectively. Translations appeared in French, Latin and other languages. The second edition is of interest in that it contains the first use of the word 'influenza' by an English physician. He also wrote an account of Devonshire colic, *De morbo colico Damnoniensi*, London, 1739, and *Observationum de aëre et morbis epidemicis*, three volumes, London, 1752–70, of which the third appeared posthumously and the first two as second editions, the work having been first published in 1739. An English translation of volumes 1–2 appeared, Plymouth, 1759–67. Huxham's classical account of diphtheria was printed as *A dissertation on the maligant ulcerous sore throat*, London, 1757. His collected writings were issued posthumously as *Opera physico-medica*, Leipzig, 1784.[63]

The son of a Southwark innkeeper, the elder William Heberden (1710–1801) was educated at St John's College, Cambridge, gaining his MD in 1738. Whilst there he wrote, for his students, the pamphlet later published as *An essay on Mithridatium and theriaca*, London, 1745 which exposed the use of mithridatics as poison antidotes. In 1746 he was elected FRCP and on 25 January 1750, after moving to London, to the Fellowship of the Royal Society. He became an eminent physician, attending royalty in addition to a number of leading figures from the world of the arts, many of whom, William Cowper and Samuel Johnson among them, were also his friends. Benjamin Franklin, another associate, requested that he write a pamphlet on inoculation for the American colonies which appeared as *Plain instructions for inoculation in the small-pox*, London, printed at the expense of the author, to be given away in America, 1759. On 21 July 1768, he read a paper to the Royal College of Physicians of London entitled *Some account of a disorder of the breast*, describing for the first time a disease which he named angina pectoris. The paper was published in 1772.[64] In 1782 Heberden completed his *Commentaries on the history and cure of diseases*, London, 1802, published posthumously by his son. A Latin translation appeared that same year. The book contains an analysis of Heberden's 40 years' experience as a physician and went into several editions. His collective writings were published as *Opera medica*, Leipzig, 1831. Heberden is also remembered as the first to differentiate chickenpox from smallpox[65] and for his classic description of nyctalopia.[66] In 1927, LeRoy Crummer discovered in London an unpublished Heberden manuscript which appeared as *An introduction to the study of physic [Now for the first time published ... A prefatory essay by LeRoy Crummer] ... With a reprint of Heberden's Some account of a disorder of the breast*, New York, 1929.[67] The original, superior, manuscript of *An introduction*, is in the Francis A. Countway Library, Boston, where many books and documents from the personal collections of Heberden and his son, also William (1767–1845), now reside.[68]

John Fothergill was born at Wensleydale, Yorks, on 8 March 1712, of a

Quaker family, and was educated at a Grammar School at Sedbergh. At the age of 16 he was apprenticed to Benjamin Bartlett, a Bradford apothecary and, in 1734, entered Edinburgh University. Here Monro persuaded him to study medicine, and Fothergill graduated in 1736, his inaugural thesis being *De emeticorum usu*. He then came to London to enter St Thomas's Hospital and, after a visit to the continent, set up practice in the capital. Following an epidemic of malignant scarlatina he published *An account of the sore throat attended with ulcers*, London, 1748.[69] As many as 500 copies were sold in a few weeks, and the work went into six editions in Fothergill's lifetime, being translated into several other languages. He also wrote a four-page pamphlet entitled *A sketch of the late epidemic disease, as it appeared in London*, [London, 1775], and contributed many papers to *Medical observations and inquiries*, including two papers on angina pectoris, and to the Royal Society, of which he was elected a Fellow in 1763. To Fothergill's annoyance, a small book was published bearing his name, but for which he was not responsible. This was *Rules for the preservation of health by J. Fothergill*, London, 1762, which went into fourteen editions. His collected works were published in 1781 and 1782, and an edition by John Coakley Lettsom in three volumes in 1783.

John Fothergill collected books, corals, insects and shells, and he also maintained a botanical garden at Upton, Essex. He died on 26 December 1780, and the sale of his library occupied eight days, a copy of the printed catalogue existing in the Friends Reference Library. His collection of drawings of flowers by various artists was sold to the Empress Catherine of Russia; his shells and corals were purchased by William Hunter and are now in Glasgow; and his hothouses and tropical plants were bought by Lettsom and transferred to Camberwell. A collection of some 200 selected letters written by Fothergill, many addressed to friends in the colonies, have been published, with a substantial introduction, in a volume edited by Betsy C. Corner and Christopher C. Booth.[70] The correspondence, arranged chronologically, provides considerable insight into the life and work of this man, with his many diverse interests. The footnotes and references give additional information, and the book also contains a genealogical table and brief chronology of Fothergill's life.

William Cullen (1710–90) was renowned as a teacher and attracted students from all over the world to Edinburgh. He achieved fame as a chemist, physiologist, botanist and physician. A native of Hamilton, Lanarkshire, the son of a lawyer, he was educated at Hamilton Grammar School and at Glasgow University, before being apprenticed to a surgeon at Glasgow, and then to an apothecary in London. Cullen made a voyage to the West Indies as a ship's surgeon, and was a friend of William Hunter. He lectured at Glasgow on botany, chemistry, materia medica, and the practice of physic, and in 1751 was appointed professor of medicine there. In 1755 he was elected to the chair of chemistry at Edinburgh, and in 1766 added the chair of institutes or theory of medicine. William Cullen's first book, *Synopsis nosologiae methodicae*, Edinburgh, 1769, went into numerous editions and was first translated from Latin into English in 1792. He also wrote *First Lines of the practice of physic*, four volumes, Edinburgh, 1777–8, of which there were many editions and translations. This is rather confusing bibliographically, and Leonard Jolley[71] has stated that volume one was issued in 1777, with a second edition correction of this in 1778; volume two was printed in 1779 and volume three in 1781. Volumes one and two were apparently reissued, and this is sometimes called the third edition. Volume four was published in 1784, when the first three volumes were reissued, and Cullen appears to have regarded this as the second edition, even volume four being a so-called second edition. The first two volumes were revised, and at first Cullen refused to supply volumes three and four separately, John Murray remonstrated with Cullen, and in July 1784 published the correspondence on the subject. Cullen's *Lectures on the materia medica*, Dublin, 1773, was later expanded into *A treatise of the materia medica*, two volumes, Edinburgh, 1789.[72] Cullen's *Works* were edited by John Thomson in two volumes, Edinburgh and London, 1827.[73] A collection of his letters, in 20 quarto volumes covering the period 1755–90, are in the MSS collection of the Royal College of Physicians of Edinburgh.[74]

Also originating from Edinburgh was the eminent neurophysiologist, Robert Whytt. He was born on 10 September 1714 and began to study medicine in 1730. He left Edinburgh in 1734 and enrolled as one of Cheselden's pupils in London, after which he travelled for some time on the continent. He returned to Scotland and taught in Edinburgh for many years until failing health prevented him from continuing with his work. He died on 15 April 1766. Further details of his life and work can be found in the book by R. K. French published in 1969.[75] His writings on physiology and neurology in particular were very popular, and went into several editions. He wrote *An essay on the vital and other involuntary motions of animals*, Edinburgh, 1751; *Observations on the dropsy in the brain*, Edinburgh, 1762, which represents the earliest account of tuberculous meningitis in children; *An essay on the virtues of limewater in the cure of the stone*, London, 1752, of which several editions were printed; *Physiological essays*, Edinburgh, 1755, which also reached subsequent editions; and the first important British work devoted to neurology, *Observations on the nature, causes, and cure of those disorders which have been commonly called nervous, hypochondriac, or hysteric*, Edinburgh, 1764. Several editions of this appeared, including a German translation (Leipzig, 1766), a French translation in two volumes (Paris, 1767 and 1777), and a Swedish translation (Stockholm, 1786). Whytt's *Works* were first published in Edinburgh in 1768, and a German translation was printed in Leipzig in 1771.

John Brown (1735–88) was a pupil of Cullen, whom he later criticized, and was born at Buncle, Berwickshire, graduating from St Andrews in 1779. Brown formulated the Brunonian theory, which was popular in Europe for 25 years, especially in Germany and Italy, and also in America. He was the author of the anonymously published *Observations on the principles of the old system of physic, exhibiting a compend of the new doctrine*, Edinburgh 1787, which was translated into French, Paris, 1805. This was followed by his *Elementa medicinae*, Edinburgh, 1780, which was expanded into two volumes, Edinburgh, 1784, and which ultimately appeared in approximately 28 editions in six languages including translations into Spanish (Madrid, 1800); French (Paris, An XIII, [1805]); German (Frankfort-on-Main, 1795 and Vienna, [1796]); Danish (Copenhagen, 1798); Italian (Naples, 1796 and Venice, 1800); an American edition was printed at Philadelphia in 1790. A bibliographical study of the three London editions of 1788, 1795 and 1804, together with a description of Mexican, German and American editions, has been published by Judith A. Overmier.[76] John Brown's *Works* were published in three volumes in 1804, with a biography by W. C. Brown, a German translation being printed in Frankfort-on-Main, 1806–7.

William Withering was born in March (probably the 28th), 1741, at Wellington, Shropshire. The son of a physician, he studied medicine at Edinburgh, where he graduated doctor of physic in 1766. There, Alexander Monro *primus*, his son *secundus*, William Cullen and Robert Whytt were his teachers. Withering's thesis on sore throat was printed as *Dissertatio medica, inauguralis de angine gangraenosa*, Edinburgh, 1766. Few copies were printed and it is very rare, having never been reprinted or translated until an English translation with a facsimile of the original text was published by C. D. O'Malley.[77] The material is not included in Withering's *An account of the scarlet fever and sore throat or scarlatina anginosa, particularly as it appeared in Birmingham in 1778*, London, 1779, of which a second edition was printed at Birmingham in 1793. Withering toured the continent in 1766, and on his return settled in Stafford, being appointed the first physician of the Stafford Infirmary. In 1775 he removed to Birmingham, where he produced *A botanical arrangement of all the vegetables naturally growing in Great Britain, with descriptions of the genera and species according to Linnaeus*, two volumes, 1776–92. This contains twelve copperplates, and was the first complete flora of the British Isles in English. Three editions were published during Withering's lifetime, the second being in two volumes, 1787, with a third volume added in 1792, and the third edition was published in 1796. His son produced four editions in 1801,[78] 1812, 1818 and 1830; others followed, and the title varied in different editions. The use of the foxglove in dropsy was first called to Withering's notice in 1775, and he conducted numerous experiments with the drug, believing the profession was misusing it. He laid down the general principles of the use of digitalis in *An account of the foxglove, and some of its medical uses; with practical remarks on dropsy and on other diseases*, Birmingham, London, 1785, which is now a rare book. It contains 207 pages with 163 case reports, and the frontispiece of the foxglove is coloured in copies costing five shillings when published, and plain in those issued at four shillings. This frontispiece in some copies appears to be reversed, and it has been suggested by Estelle Brodman[79] that these may have been the original illustrations engraved by Sowerby for the *Flora Londinensis* published by William Curtis in 1777, and that these were bound into *An account of the foxglove* until supplies were exhausted. The plate was then re-drawn through the original. This book was reprinted in facsimile in 1949.

The 200th anniversary of the publication of this classic work has resulted in numerous recent contributions to the literature.[80] Withering also wrote several papers for the *Philosophical Transactions*, and *Chemical analysis of the water at Caldas da Rainha*, 1795, which is in English and Portuguese. His *Miscellaneous tracts*, edited by his son, were posthumously published in two volumes, London, 1822. A small collection of his letters is preserved in the Library of Birmingham University and an autograph letter dated 1795 has been noted elsewhere.[81] Withering died on 6 October 1799, and was buried in Edgbaston Church, Birmingham.

John Coakley Lettsom (1744–1815) was born into a Quaker family living in the West Indies, and at the age of six he came to England to be educated. In 1761 he was apprenticed to Abraham Sutcliff, a surgeon and apothecary at Settle, Yorks., before coming to London with letters of introduction to John Fothergill. Lettsom served as surgeon's dresser under Benjamin Cowell at St Thomas's Hospital, but returned to the West Indies in 1767, upon the death of his father. He immediately freed the slaves he had inherited, and set up in practice, making enough money in six months to enable him to return to England to complete his education. Lettsom studied at Edinburgh, Paris and Leyden, graduating MD at the latter in 1769, before settling down to practise in London. In this he was most successful, and he proceeded to make himself popular through his philanthropic activities. He was largely responsible for the founding of the Royal Humane Society, the Royal Sea-bathing Hospital at Margate, and the Medical Society of London.[82] Lettsom championed the cause of Jenner, and was a friend of Benjamin Franklin, Baron Dimsdale and Benjamin Rush. He collected together an extensive museum and library and was also a keen botanist.

Lettsom's thesis at Leyden was entitled *Observationes ad vires theae pertinentes*, Leyden, 1769, which was later extended in an English edition as *The natural history of the tea-tree, with observations on the medical qualities of tea, and effects of tea-drinking*, London, 1772, containing a coloured folding-plate of a tea-tree which flowered in the Duke of Northumberland's garden. A pirated edition was printed in Dublin the same year, and a French translation was published in Paris in 1775. Lettsom published anonymously the popular *Naturalist and traveller's companion,* 1772, which went into further editions in 1774 and 1779, and was translated into German, French (Paris, 1775), and Dutch (Amsterdam, 1775). Other anonymous publications by Lettsom include *Reflections on the general treatment and cure of fevers,* London, 1772, and *Observations preparatory to the use of Dr. Myerbach's medicines,* London, 1776. He also wrote *Some accounts of the late John Fothergill,* London, 1783; *Medical memoirs of the General Dispensary in London,* London, 1774; *History of the origin of medicine,* London, 1778, of which a French translation was published in 1787. He published many pamphlets and tracts, the more popular of which he reprinted in three volumes as *Hints designed to promote beneficence, temperance and medical science,* 1802, the imprint incorrectly stating 1801. These volumes contain material on a diversity of subjects such as poverty, female character, wills, the deaf and dumb, a monument to John Howard, humane societies, the cow pock, card parties, rabies and substitute for wheat bread. After Lettsom's death John Nichols bought the copyright of the *Hints,* which he reissued in 1816 with extra notes, illustrations, and a memoir. Correspondence and documents relating to Lettsom can be found in various repositories, but most of this material is the property of either the Medical Society of London or at the Wellcome Institute for the History of Medicine.[83]

The fame of Benjamin Rush (1746–1813) can be judged by the fact that he has been frequently alluded to as 'the Sydenham of America', 'the Fothergill of America', 'the American Hippocrates', or 'the Sydenham of Columbia'. He is also noted for the fact that he signed the Declaration of Independence. He was born on 4 January 1746, at Byberry, and attended the College of New Jersey before being apprenticed to John Redman, who was on the staff of Pennsylvania Hospital. After serving five and a half years, Rush went to Edinburgh for two years, studying under Monro, Cullen, Black, Gregory and Hope, and in 1768 took his doctorate of medicine with the thesis *De coctione ciborum in ventriculo.*[84] Rush later came to London, where he attended St Thomas's Hospital, and also John Hunter's lectures. After a visit to Paris he returned to America where he built up a substantial practice in Philadelphia. He was professor of chemistry at Philadelphia from 1769–91 where he also succeeded John Morgan as professor of practical and theoretical medicine, then, following the founding of the University of Pennsylvania, Rush was appointed to a similar post there. He was also a founder of the Philadelphia College of Physicians, 1787. He died on 19 April 1813, after a successful career, during which he had written extensively.

Rush translated Sydenham's works into English, and was the author of *Medical inquiries and observations,* two volumes, Philadelphia, 1789–93, which was later enlarged by the addition of two other volumes, *The account of the yellow fever epidemic of 1793* (the third volume, 1794), and a fourth in 1796. A second revised edition was published in four volumes, 1805, a third in 1809, a fourth in 1815, and a fifth in 1819. Rush also wrote *The new method of inoculating for the smallpox*, Philadelphia, 1781 (second edition, 1789; third edition, 1792); *Medical inquiries and observations upon the diseases of the mind*, Philadelphia, 1812, which was the first book published in the United States on mental diseases,[85] and went into later editions in 1818, 1827, 1830 and 1835, with a German translation by Georg König, printed in Leipzig in 1825; *Syllabus of a course of lectures on chemistry*, Philadelphia, 1770; a collection of Rush's non-medical articles was published as *Essays, literary, moral and philosophical*, Philadelphia, 1798, a second edition appearing in 1806. A selection from his writings was published in 1947,[86] and his autobiographical material appeared the following year.[87]

A pupil of John Hunter, Edward Jenner (1749–1823) was born at Berkeley, Gloucestershire, and was keenly interested in natural history. After serving with Daniel Ludlow, a surgeon of Sodbury, near Bristol, he came to London, where he lived in Hunter's house for two years. He then returned to Berkeley, where he built up a large practice. He continued to correspond with John Hunter, however, and conducted experiments for him in addition to sending him natural history specimens. Jenner, having heard a countrywoman mention that she could not take small-pox, having already contracted cow-pox, proceeded to make his first vaccination experiment in 1796. He received little support from friends whom he endeavoured to interest in the subject, but nonetheless published a memoir in June 1798.[88] This was entitled *An inquiry into the causes and effects of the variolae vaccinae, a disease discovered in some of the western countries of England, particularly Gloucestershire, and known by the name of the cow-pox*, London, 1798, and facsimile editions of this were published in 1923 (Milan) and 1949 (Denver). There was a second edition, London, 1800, and a third the following year. An American printing from the second London edition appeared at Springfield, 1802, while the book was translated into German (Hanover, 1799, and Leipzig, 1911), Latin (Vienna, 1799), French (Lyons, 1800, and Privas [ND.]), Portuguese (Lisbon, 1803), Italian (Pavia, 1800 and Modena, 1853), Dutch (Haarlem, 1801), Spanish (Madrid, 1801) and Russian (St Petersburg, 1896). A reprint of the second edition of 1880 was made in Australia in 1884 by the Government printer in Sydney for official distribution. It was made from a copy belonging to George Bennett (1804–93), and was intended to promote compulsory vaccination, following several epidemics. It contains several variations from the original second edition.[89]

Jenner wrote numerous articles and pamphlets on vaccination which went into many editions, some of which consisted of several items issued together, the following being the more important: *Further observations on the variolae vaccinae or cow-pox*, London, 1799, which was contained in the second edition of the *Inquiry*, was reprinted with most subsequent issues, and was also translated into several other languages; *A continuation of facts and observations relative to the variolae vaccinae or cow-pox*, London, 1800; *The origin of the vaccine inoculation*, London, 1801 (2 issues), of which a reprint with the sole exception of the title-page appeared in the *Columbian Centinal*;[90] this was also reprinted in 1867 (London) and translated into French in 1802 (Paris); *Facts, for the most part unobserved, or not duly noticed, respecting variolous contagion*, London, 1808, certain copies of which, including that in the Osler Library (Bib. Osler, 1263), contain an extra leaf, paged 17, which was printed later, quoting a letter written in 1809, and probably represent the reprint issued in 1811; *Instructions for vaccine inoculation*, [London,], consisting of a single sheet together with a coloured plate; and *A letter to Charles Henry Parry, M.D. ... on the influence of artificial eruptions in certain diseases incident to the human body*, London, 1822. This was reissued in Philadelphia, 1822, with translations into Dutch (Rotterdam, 1822) and French (Paris, 1824). A total of 500 copies of the *Letter* were printed in 1821 but were not published, the edition being cancelled. A trial proof copy of this date is in Edinburgh University Library. An alternative, controversial, view of Jenner's contribution to this whole subject has been presented by P. Razzell.[91] Jenner also wrote on the cuckoo, on migration of birds, and contributed several other articles to periodicals. W. R. LeFanu has recently produced a new, limited, edition of his indispensable *Bibliography of Edward Jenner* (formerly entitled 'biobibliography').[92] A biographical introduction is provided, but the volume lacks the location list of Jenner letters found in the original publication. A volume of Jenner letters from the Henry Barton Jacobs collection has been published, edited by Genevieve Miller, containing a commentary and notes.[93] Other letters have also recently been recorded.[94] A manuscript containing the substance of Jenner's *Inquiry* in his handwriting is preserved at the Royal College of Surgeons of England, and one in another hand, but with corrections by Jenner, is in the Wellcome Historical Medical Library.[95]

Caleb Hiller Parry (1755–1822), a native of Cirencester, became a life-long friend of Edward Jenner, with whom he attended a grammar school. He studied at Edinburgh then finally settled at Bath in 1779. Parry was the author of *An inquiry into the symptoms and causes of the syncope anginosa, commonly called angina pectoris*, Bath, London, 1799, which consists of a paper read in 1788, but not published until eleven years later. This classic work on angina was translated into French by A. Matthey and published in Paris, 1806. It was followed by *Cases of tetanus, and rabies contagiosa*, London, 1814; *Elements of pathology and therapeutics*, Volume I, London, 1815, which was republished with the unfinished second volume in 1825; *An experimental inquiry into the nature, cause, and varieties of the arterial pulse*, London, 1816, of which a German translation was published at Hanover, 1817. Caleb's son Charles Henry Parry issued his father's unpublished writings after his death as *Collections from ... unpublished medical writings*, two volumes, London, 1825. This contains his original description of exophthalmic goitre, first noted by Parry in 1786, and the first recorded cases of facial hemiatrophy.[96]

Matthew Baillie (1761–1823), whose mother was the sister of William and John Hunter, has been described as the 'father of medical pathology'. He was the last owner of the gold-headed cane.[97] After spending five years at Glasgow University, Baillie came to live in London with William Hunter, attending the latter's lectures, and also those of John. Baillie lectured at the Great Windmill Street School, and also practised, having graduated in medicine at Oxford. He was appointed physician at St George's Hospital in 1787, and became physician extraordinary to George III, but declined the baronetcy offered to him in 1810. Matthew Baillie wrote several papers for the *Philosophical Transactions*, and in 1793 published his best known work, *The morbid anatomy of some of the most important parts of the human body*, London, the material being mainly furnished from William Hunter's museum.[98] The book is beautifully illustrated with copperplates by William Clift, and went into many editions, being translated into German by S. T. Soemmerring (Berlin, 1794), into French by M. Farrell (Paris, 1803) and by M. Guerbois (Paris, 1815), and into Italian by Pietro Gentilini (Pavia, 1807). An American edition was published in Boston, 1795. Baillie then published *A series of engravings, accompanied with explanations, which are intended to illustrate the morbid anatomy of some of the most important parts of human body*, London, 1799–1802, consisting of ten separate fasciculi, which were issued in book form in 1803; a second edition of this followed in 1812. Baillie also wrote *Lectures and observations on medicine*, London, 1825, and his *Works* were published in two volumes in 1825, with an account of his life by James Wardrop. W. R. LeFanu has provided details of correspondence between Baillie and Laënnec.[99]

John Howard (1726–90), born in Clapton on 2 September 1726, was educated at the Dissenting School of Hertford and the Dissenting Academy, London. He was apprenticed to a wholesale grocer, but was enabled to buy himself out when his father's death left him a wealthy man. In 1773 he was appointed High Sheriff for Bedfordshire and an investigation into the state of prisons led him to spend the remaining years of his life endeavouring to improve the conditions endured by the inmates. He made three extensive tours in England and Wales, and seven tours abroad, during which he visited every European country. He found the prison buildings in a state of decay, a lack of sanitation and medical attention, the sexes were mixed, and young and old mingled together; drinking and gambling were common. Howard died on 20 January 1790, while on a visit to Russia to inspect military prisons, and was accorded a royal funeral in that country. He edited several works, and contributed a few articles to periodicals, but his three important books went into many editions and translations.[100] *The state of the prisons in England and Wales*, Warrington, 1777, was beautifully printed and produced and was sold at twelve shillings. It was also printed in 1780 and 1784 at Warrington, in London, 1792 (two issues), and New York and London, 1929; a French translation was issued in two volumes, Paris, 1788[101] and 1791, and a German translation, Leipzig, 1780. This book was followed by *Appendix to the state of the prisons in England and Wales*, Warrington, 1780, with a second edition in 1784, and *An account of the principal lazaretos in Europe*, Warrington, 1789. The second edition of this was published in London, 1791 (two issues), and the book was also translated into French (two volumes, Paris, 1799, and a second edition, 1801), German (Leipzig, 1791) and Italian (Venice, 1814).[102]

A pioneer in the care of children by modern methods was William Cadogan (1711–97), who was possibly born at Cowbridge rather than London as is usually suggested. He attended Oriel College, Oxford, before studying medicine at Leyden where he qualified MD in 1737 with a thesis entitled *De nutritione, incremento, et decremento corporis*. In 1747 Cadogan was elected physician to Bristol Infirmary, but resigned in 1752 and moved to London, becoming physician to the army at the age of 51. Cadogan was the author of *An essay upon nursing, and the management of children from their birth to three years of age*, London, 1748, which formed the 'foundation stone of modern child care', and in which he urged the value of breast-feeding. A reprint of the *Essay* has been incorporated into a biography of Cadogan written jointly by M. and J. Rendle-Short.[103] His book on gout was very popular, going into ten editions in two years. Entitled *A dissertation on the gout and all chronic diseases*, London, 1771, it was also reprinted in 1925.[104]

Military hygiene found an apostle in Sir John Pringle (1707–82). Born in Stichel House, Roxburghshire, he was to become a brilliant student at St Andrews, Edinburgh. He moved, in 1728, to Leyden, where he studied under Boerhaave, obtaining an MD in 1730. Pringle returned to Edinburgh as professor of moral philosophy, but in 1742 became Surgeon-General to the British Army, which position he held until 1758. At the Battle of Dettingen (1743), at Pringle's suggestion, both sides agreed to respect military hospitals; this was eventually to lead to the introduction of the Red Cross. Returning to England, Pringle served under the Duke of Cumberland and was present at the Battle of Culloden. His position in the history of military medicine has been considered in a paper by D. Hamilton.[105] He read a series of short papers before the Royal Society,

1750–2, as *Experiments upon septic and antiseptic substances*, using the word 'antiseptic' for the first time. He later served as President of the Society, and was also physician to George III and Queen Charlotte. Among other works, Pringle wrote *Observations on the nature and cure of hospital and jayl-fevers*, London, 1750, but his most important publication deals with the ventilation of hospitals, barracks and jails, and with military hygiene in general. Under the title *Observations on the diseases of the army*, London, 1752, it went into many editions, including translations into German (Altenburg, 1754), Italian (Naples, 1757), Dutch (Middelburg, 1763, and in three volumes, Amsterdam, 1785–8) and French (Paris, 1771). Pringle died on 18 January 1782, and was buried in Westminster Abbey.[106]

James Lind (1716–94) performed a similar service for the British Navy, and was instrumental in greatly improving the living conditions of sailors and in combating scurvy by the use of lime or lemon juice. He was not the first to write effectively on scurvy, Boyle, Clowes, Woodall and others[107] having preceded him, and in fact Lind's book was rather overshadowed by two others on the subject by better known, but less well-informed, authors, Anthony Addington (1713–90), and Charles Bisset (1717–91).[108] Lind was born and educated at Edinburgh, entering the Navy at the age of 23. He retired from the sea in 1748 and, after practising in Edinburgh for ten years, was appointed physician to the Haslar Hospital. Lind's writings on scurvy, naval hygiene, and on tropical medicine were all valuable contributions to medicine and went into several editions. His Edinburgh MD thesis was entitled *De morbis venereis localibus*, Edinburgh, 1748, and was followed by his *A treatise of the scurvy*, Edinburgh, 1753,[109] reprinted without change in 1754, with a second edition, London, 1757, and a third, London, 1772 in which the word *of* on the title-page was altered to *on*. A French translation was published in Paris, 1756, and yet another translation into French in two volumes, Paris, 1883. The book was also translated into Italian (Venice, 1766), and German (Leipzig, 1775). A reprint of the first edition was published in 1953.[110] Lind's next book was *An essay on the most effectual means of preserving the health of seamen in the Royal Navy*, London, 1757, with a second edition in 1762, and a third in 1779. A Dutch translation of this was published in Middelburg, 1760, which was also translated into French and German. This was followed by *De febre remittente putrida paludum quae grassabatur in Bengalia A.D. 1762*, Edinburgh, 1768, translated as *A treatise on the putrid and remitting marsh fever which raged in Bengal in the year 1762*, Edinburgh, 1776. Lind's *An essay on diseases incidental to Europeans in hot climates*, London, 1768, went into five editions in his lifetime and was also translated into German, Dutch and French. In his *Treatise of scurvy* Lind provides a list of published contributions to the subject from 1534, giving full credit to those whose observations preceded his own.[111]

Another pioneer of sanitary reform, Johann Peter Frank (1745–1821) has been described as the 'Father of Public Health'. He was a native of Rodalben, and studied medicine at Heidelberg and Strasbourg, later becoming a professor both in Pavia and Vienna. Frank spent his life preaching public health, and produced a monumental work of six volumes and three supplements, which was published as *System einer vollständigen medicinischen Polizey*, nine volumes, Mannheim, 1779– 1827.[112] His other contributions to the literature include *De curandis hominum morbis epitome*, three volumes, Vienna, 1810–21, and *Opuscula posthuma*, Vienna, 1824.[113]

Although chiefly recognized for his biological writings, and as being one of the earliest scientists to dispute the doctrine of spontaneous generation, Lazaro Spallanzani (1729–99) also made important experiments on respiration, on gastric juice, and on the circulation. His writings were very popular, most of them having been translated into English. They include *Saggio di osservazione microscopiche relative al sistema della generazione*, Modena, 1767; *Prodromi sulla riproduzione animale. Riproduzione della coda del girino*, Modena, 1768, which was translated into English, London, 1769; *De'fenomeni della circolazione osservata nel giro universale de'vasi*, Modena, 1773, translated into French (Paris, An VIII [1800]), and into English as *Experiments upon the circulation of the blood*, London, 1801; *Opusculi di fisica animale e vegetabile*, two volumes, Modena, 1776,[114] which contains his experiments on gastric juice; *Fisica animale e vegetabile*, three volumes, Venice, 1782; and *Mémoires sur la respiration*, Geneva, An XI [1803], translated into English, London, 1805. These *Mémoires* are translated from the author's manuscript, and not from an Italian edition. Spallanzani's letters were published in five volumes as *Espistolario*, Florence, 1958–64,[115] and his collected writings were issued as *Le opere*, five volumes in six, Milan, 1932–6.[116]

Erasmus Darwin (1731–1802) was a scientist, physician and poet who foreshadowed the theory later advanced by his grandson. His most important work, *Zoonomia; or, the laws of organic life*, two volumes, 1794–6, contains a system of pathology and a treatise on generation. It went into numerous editions, including printings at New York, 1796 (three volumes); Philadelphia, 1797 and 1818; Dublin, 1800 (two volumes); Boston, 1803 and 1809; a third English edition in four volumes, 1801, was translated into Italian, four volumes, Venice, 1803– 6. Erasmus Darwin also edited a book by his son, Charles Darwin (1758– 78), which contains a biography, the author having died at an early age as the result of a dissection wound. This volume was entitled *Experiments establishing a criterion between mucaginous and purulent matter, and an account of the retrograde motions of the absorbent vessels of animal bodies in some diseases*, Lichfield, 1780. Desmond King-Hele has recently edited a volume of his letters.[117]

William Hewson (1739–74), a native of Hexham, Northumberland, studied at London, Edinburgh and Paris. He was closely connected with John and William Hunter, setting up in partnership with William at the anatomical school in Litchfield Street. Later Hewson founded his own anatomical school in Craven Street, the Strand. A brilliant scientist, he was elected a Fellow of the Royal Society in 1770 and made several important contributions to the *Philosophical Transactions*. Although an outstanding teacher of anatomy, he was also a keen physiologist and practitioner. He died at an early age as the result of a dissection wound, thus cutting short a fine career. In addition to his contributions to periodical literature, Hewson wrote *An experimental inquiry into the properties of the blood*, London, 1771, which went into several editions, including German and Latin translations. The second edition bore the title *Experimental inquiries: Part the first*, and was published in 1772, to be followed by *Experimental inquiries: Part the second. Containing a description of the lymphatic system in the human subject and in other animals*, London, 1774. Hewson demonstrated the existence of lymph vessels in animals, explained their function, and also ascertained that the coagulation of blood was caused by a substance in the plasma. His co-worker was Magnus Falconar (1754–78), and their joint work on the morphology of blood cells was published after the death of Hewson by Falconar as *Experimental inquiries: Part the third. Containing a description of the red particles of the blood in the human subject, and other animals ... Being the remaining part of the observations and experiments of the late Mr. William Hewson*, London, 1777. In this it was shown that the red blood cells were discoid, but the fact that they were biconcave was overlooked and, due to inadequate microscopes, a nucleus was described.[118] Hewson's *Works*, edited by George Gulliver, were published by the Sydenham Society in 1846, and contain biographical information.[119]

The bibliographical works of Albrecht von Haller (1708–77) have been dealt with elsewhere,[120] but in addition he made important contributions to anatomy, physiology and medicine, as well as to botany.[121] He has been described as 'the most prodigious and versatile writer of all times', and is said to have been responsible for several thousand scientific papers. Haller's most important books appeared in various editions and translations, and include *Experimenta et dubia circa ductum salivalem novum Coschwizianum*, Leyden, 1727; *Icones anatomicae ...*, eight parts, Göttingen, 1743–56; *De respiratione experimenta anatomica*, Göttingen, 1746; *Disputationes anatomicae selectae*, seven volumes, Göttingen, 1746–52; *Primae lineae physiologicae in usum praelectionum acade-*

micarum, Göttingen, 1747;[122] *De aortae venaeque cavae gravioribus quibusdam morbis*, Göttingen, 1749; *Disputationes chirurgicae selectae*, five volumes, Lausanne, 1755–6; and *De partium corporis humani praecipuarum fabrica et functionibus*, eight volumes, Berne and Lausanne, 1778. One of the most important publications in the history of physiology was Haller's *Elementa physiologiae corporis humani*, eight volumes, 1757–66,[123] and his lesser works were collected together as *Opera minora emendata, aucta et renovata*, three volumes, Lausanne, 1762–8. Haller's letters to Morgagni, edited by Erich Hintzsche, have been published as *Briefwechsel 1745–1768*, Berne, Stuttgart, 1964. These are in their original Latin, and are followed by full abstracts in German with brief summaries of Morgagni's communications. Correspondence with Leopoldo Marco Antonio Caldani (1725–1813) between the years 1756 and 1776 has also been edited by Hintzsche and was published in Berne, 1966.[124]

The use of percussion in the diagnosis of diseases of the chest was introduced by (Joseph) Leopold Auenbrugger (1722–1809), who was born at Graz, Austria on 19 November 1722. He was an accomplished musician and studied medicine under Gerard Van Swieten in Vienna from which centre he graduated in 1752, and where he was eventually appointed physician to the Spanish Hospital. In 1754 he noted a difference in the sounds made by striking the wall of the chest, but delayed publishing the results of his experiments for seven years. His book was printed as *Inventum novum ex percussione thoracis humani ut signo abstrusos interni pectoris morbos detegendi*, Vienna, 1761, of which there were two issues, the first having the verso of page 95 blank, and the second bearing errata and corrigenda in that location. A second edition appeared in 1763, but is textually the same as the first two issues, although the title-page differs. A French translation by Rozière de la Chasagne was published in Paris, 1770, and later reached a second edition, but Auenbrugger's percussion theory was neglected until his book was re-translated and revised by Jean Nicolas Corvisart and published in Paris, 1808. The book was translated into Dutch by Lambertus Nolst (Dordrecht, 1788); into German by S. Ungar (Vienna, 1843); into Italian by Giovanni Piccardi, with the Latin original (Milan, 1844); and into English by John Forbes (1824). This translation was reprinted in Baltimore in 1936, and a facsimile of the first edition, with English, French and German translations, edited by Max Neuburger, was published in Vienna and Leipzig, 1922. P. James Bishop[125] has published a bibliography of this book, recording several other editions and extracts, and has also contributed a useful list of writings on Auenbrugger and the history of percussion.[126]

William Cumberland Cruikshank (1745–1800) originally intended to enter the Church but eventually developed a preference for medicine as a career. After serving an apprenticeship he came to London as assistant to William Hunter and also carried out some dissections for his brother, John. He conducted a series of experiments on the lymphatics and, in his *Experiments on the insensible perspiration of the human body*, 1779, which was privately printed and later republished, London, 1795, he proved that carbon dioxide is given off by the skin. Cruikshank also wrote *The anatomy of the absorbing vessels of the human body*, London, 1782, a second edition appearing in 1790; and *Remarks on the absorption of calomel from the internal surface of the mouth*, London, 1779. An important paper containing Cruikshank's observations on nerve regeneration was sent by John Hunter to the Royal Society in 1776, but was not finally published until 1795.[127]

A pioneer in the field of modern embryology, Caspar Friedrich Wolff (1733–94) was a native of Berlin, but spent the last 30 years of his life in St Petersburg after his theories had received a hostile reception in his own country. Wolff's 'De formatione intestionum' was first published in a journal in 1768–9,[128] but was translated into German by Johann Friedrich Meckel (1761–1833) as *Über die Bildung des Darmkanals in bebruteten Hühnchen*, Halle, 1812. His *Theoria generationis*, Halle, 1759 was translated into German by Wolff himself as *Theorie von der Generationen*, Berlin, 1764,[129] and it appeared, together with the published doctoral dissertation of 1759, in facsimile reprint, Hildesheim, 1966. A second edition of the Latin version was published in 1774. A new German translation by Paul Samassa appeared in 1896.[130]

Luigi Galvani (1737–98) of Bologna was the founder of electrophysiology, and his *De viribus electricitatis in motu musculari*, Bologna, 1791 was first published in the proceedings of the Bologna Academy that same year. Twice reprinted in 1791, two editions were printed in Modena in 1792, one having the plates printed in red. Numerous other printings and translations followed, including a facsimile edition (Berlin, 1925); German translations by Johann Mayer (Prague, 1793), and by Arthur John von Oettingen (Leipzig, 1894); an Italian translation (Bologna, 1937 and Brescia, 1983);[131] a Russian translation (Moscow, Leningrad, 1937); a French translation (Paris, 1939); and two English translations published in 1953, one by Robert Montraville Green[132] and the other by Margaret Glover Foley.[133] Galvani's collected writings were published as *Opere edite ed inedite*, two volumes, Bologna, 1841–2, and in 1937 appeared *Memorie ed experimenti inedite*, Bologna, containing the first Italian translation of *De viribus electricitatis*, and a description of Galvani's existing manuscripts.[134]

Robert Willan (1757–1812) was born at Marthwaite, near Sedbergh, Yorkshire.[135] In 1777 he went to Edinburgh to study medicine and graduated MD in 1780.[136] After postgraduate work in London, Willan became physician to the Public Dispensary in Carey Street, but resigned in 1803 to concentrate on private practice. Willan's book *On cutaneous diseases* was issued in four parts between 1798 and 1808, but this only completed the first volume. It was suggested that there was an earlier edition, as a German translation was published in four volumes, Breslau, 1799–1816. In fact there were not two editions of the volume, but only of the first three parts, which were issued as *The description and treatment of cutaneous diseases*, although the title-page gives *On cutaneous diseases*. F.M. Sutherland[137] has investigated the publication of the separate parts, and concluded that the earlier parts were not only reprinted to satisfy the demand, but were also revised by Willan. Order 1 was first published in 1798; order 2 in 1801; order 3, part 1 in 1805, and order 3, part 2 with order 4 in 1808. There was a second edition of order 3, part 1 in 1807, but amended versions of the first two fascicules were issued in their original wrappers. When bound, some volumes have complete sets of original issues, others have variations. Volume two of the work was not published, owing to the death of Willan in 1812, but the section on porrigo and impetigo was published posthumously as *A practical treatise on porrigo, or scalled head, and on impetigo, the humid, or running tetter, edited by Ashby Smith*, London, 1814. Willan also wrote *On vaccine inoculation*, London, 1806, in which he demanded compulsory vaccination; *Reports on the diseases in London*, London, 1801, which was translated into German (Hamburg, 1802); and his *Miscellaneous works*, London, were published in 1821.[138]

An early exponent of psychotherapy, Franz Anton Mesmer (1734–1815) studied medicine in Vienna. He attempted to establish his idea on a scientific basis, but his career was terminated by the holding of an inquiry into the activities of his clinic in Paris. His *Dissertatio physico-medica de planetarum influxu*, Vienna, 1766, contained ideas later incorporated in his theory of animal magnetism and it has been suggested by Frank A. Pattie[139] that these were plagiarized largely from Richard Mead's *De imperio solis ac lunae in corpora humana et morbis inde oriundis*, London, 1704. Mesmer's *Mémoire sur la découverte du magnétisme animal*, Geneva, Paris, 1779, was translated into German in 1781, and probably influenced the later development of hypnotism in medicine. An English translation by Gilbert Frankau, with an introduction, was published in London in 1948 and a collection of Mesmer's scientific and medical writings have been translated and compiled by George Bloch, Los Altos, California, 1980.[140]

Philippe Pinel (1745–1826) qualified in medicine at Toulouse in 1773. He spent five years at Montpellier, then moved to Paris in 1778. He translated Cullen's *Institutions of medicine*, and in 1787 began publishing articles on insanity. He was head of the Bicêtre for two years from 1793, and then went to the Salpêtrière. Pinel sought to humanize the general treatment of the insane and urged that mental patients be kept unchained. His authoritative book on the subject, *Traité médico-philoso-phique sur l'aliénation mentale, ou la manie*, Paris, 1801, went into a second edition in 1809. A German translation was published in Vienna, 1801; a Spanish translation, Madrid, 1804; and an English translation by D.D. Davies. Sheffield, 1806 and 1809, with possibly a third edition about 1818. The 1806 edition was also published in facsimile in New York, 1962, with an introduction by Paul F. Cranefield. A previously unpublished manuscript of 1793 on the clinical training of doctors has been edited and translated with an introductory essay, by D. B. Weiner,[141] who has also reported a new document relating to his period of apprenticeship.[142]

The author of the first book on mental disease to be written in England was William Battie (1704–76). Educated at Eton and King's College, Cambridge, he graduated DM in 1737, and became a Fellow of the Royal Society and President of the Royal College of Physicians. He was physician to St Luke's Hospital from 1751 to 1764. Battie's Lumleian lectures were published as *De principiis animalibus* in 1737, and he was also the author of *Aphorismi de cognoscendis et curandis morbis*. His most important book was *A treatise on madness*, London, 1758, which was reproduced in facsimile in 1962 with an introduction and annotations by Richard Hunter and Ida Macalpine,[143] and also reprinted in New York in 1969 with an introduction by J. A. Brussell.

A figure much admired by Pinel was John Haslam (1764–1844). He was born in London and, in 1795, became Apothecary to Bethlem, from which post he was to be dismissed in 1816. Haslam favoured restraint in some measure, and his views were set down in his publication *Observations on insanity*, London, 1798, which went into a second edition as *Observations on madness, and melancholy*, London, 1809; *Illustrations of madness*, London, 1810; *Considerations on the moral management of insane persons*, London, 1817; *Medical jurisprudence, as it relates to insanity*, London, 1817; *Sound mind*, London, 1819, and others. Haslam collected together a library, which he sold in 1816.[144]

A book on physiognomy, which went into numerous editions and translations, was written by Johann Kaspar Lavater (1741–1801), a Swiss poet and theologian who was born in Zurich. His *Physiognomische Fragmente zur Beförderung der Menschenkenntnis und Menschenliebe*, 1775–8 became popular and, by 1810, 16 German, 15 French, two American, two Russian, one Dutch, one Italian and 20 English versions had appeared.[145] It was translated by Henry Hunter as *Essays on physiognomy*, three volumes in five, 1789–98, and there was a four-volume edition in 1797, with numerous other editions, abridgements and translations.

American medical literature continued to increase, and the first medical publication from Canada was *Direction pour la Guérison du Mal de la*

Baie St. Paul, Quebec, 1785. The first American textbook on surgery was by John Jones (1729–91), entitled *Plain concise practical remarks on the treatment of wounds and fractures*, New York, 1775, of which a second edition was published at Philadelphia in 1776.[146] The earliest general medical treatise from America was Juan Manuel Venegas' *Compendio de la medicina: o medicina practica ...*, Mexico, 1788, which was republished in Philadelphia in 1827. Robert B. Austin[147] has produced a most useful list of works printed in the United States between 1668 and 1820.

Societies of many kinds were established and proliferated during this period.[148] They were a dominant feature in the social life of the upper classes, particularly during the second half of the century, the members often meeting in coffee-houses and clubs. The medical profession was no exception. The Royal Society, for example, included many eminent physicians and surgeons, such as the Hunter brothers, in its ranks, but there was a surge of interest in the creation of alternative forums for discussion and debate and the promotion of medical knowledge. An appendix to the first edition of this book provides a useful, though incomplete, list of medical societies, and a paper by C. E. Dukes[149] details the history of 12 of the more important London groups. A more recent paper by A. Batty Shaw[150] updates this information, concentrating on societies founded prior to 1850. A few of these eighteenth-century societies are described below, with emphasis on those which have particular relevance to the earlier contents of this chapter or which have gathered together notable libraries over the years.

A number of medical societies have been founded by students as a means of communicating and disseminating information to mutual advantage and many of these individuals rose to eminence in their profession in later years. The Royal Medical Society of Edinburgh, dating from 1737, was instituted as an association of students; members included such distinguished figures as John Fothergill (1712–80) and William Cullen (1710–90). The society was incorporated by Royal Charter in 1778 and, as early as 1834, possessed a Library of 11 000 volumes.[151]

In London, Guy's Hospital was opened in 1725 and the Guy's Hospital Physical Society was formed in 1771. The society soon collected together a Library, many of the original volumes being housed in the present Wills Library. Eminent members have included Edward Jenner (1749–1823), who addressed the Society on the subject of vaccination in 1802, and John Hunter (1728–93) who spoke on ligature of the femoral artery for popliteal aneurysm.[152]

The Medical Society of London was the first in England to draw together, in a single group, practising physicians, surgeons and apothecaries. John Coakley Lettsom published a pamphlet in 1773, entitled *Hints for the formation of a medical society of London*, and founded that same year, with the assistance of friends, the Medical Society of London, with John Millar as its first President.[153] In 1805 many members left the Medical Society to form the Medico-Chirurgical Society, which was later to become the Royal Society of Medicine. This was mainly owing to the fact that James Sims remained President for 22 years and otherwise upset certain members of the Medical Society.[154,155]

John Hunter and George Fordyce were jointly responsible for the formation of two medical societies, the first, founded in 1783, being the Society for the Improvement of Medical and Chirurgical Knowledge. It originally had nine members, with power to increase to 12, and met once a month at Slaughter's Coffee house to dine, and to discuss papers. Three volumes of *Transactions* were issued between 1793 and 1812. The Society was finally dissolved in 1818. The second society, the Lyceum Medicum Londinense, was established in January 1785, and had an extensive membership, a large proportion of which had not yet qualified. Members met every Friday evening in Hunter's lecture room from October to May, and the Society also possessed a Library.[156]

The Gloucestershire Medical Society held meetings at the Fleece Inn, Rodborough, near Bristol, and members referred to it as the Fleece Inn Medical Society. It was organized in 1788 by Edward Jenner, Caleb Hillier Parry and others, and Jenner's work on vaccination was first discussed there, with several other papers by him. Meetings were held from 1788 to 1793, and a minute book of the Society is housed in the Royal College of Physicians, London.[157]

Medical book societies were also responsible for the development of certain medical societies. The book-circulating clubs developed as a result of poor library provision, particularly in the provinces, but the foundation of numerous infirmaries and the formation of medical schools served to remedy the situation to some extent. The book clubs consisted of a few medical men banding together to purchase and circulate books among themselves, and these date from about 1770. W. J. Bishop[158] collected together the scanty information available regarding some of these, but most have left no records whatsoever.

Notes

1. *The clinical consultations of Giambattista Morgagni. The edition of Enrico Benassi (1935), translated and revised by Saul Jarcho* (Boston, Charlottesville, 1984). See also Cameron, G. R., 'The life and times of Giambattista Morgagni, F.R.S., 1682–1771', *Notes Rec. Roy. Soc. Lond.*, 9 (1951–2) pp.217–43; Tedeschi, C. G., 'Giovanni Battista Morgagni, the founder of pathologic anatomy: a biographic sketch, on the occasion of the 200th anniversary of the publication of his *De sedibus et causis morborum per anatomen indagatis'*, *Boston Med. Quart.*, 12 (1961) pp.112–25.
2. LeFanu, W. R., 'Anatomical drawings of Jacobus Schijnvoet', *Oud-Holland* (1960) pp.54–8.
3. LeFanu, W. R., 'Charles Bell and Cheselden', *Med. Hist*, 5 (1961) p.196.
4. Cope, Sir Zachary, *William Cheselden, 1688–1752* (Edinburgh, London, 1953); Cope, Sir Zachary, 'William Cheselden and the separation of the Barbers from the

Surgeons' (Thomas Vicary Lecture delivered at the Royal College of Surgeons of England on 30 October 1952), *Ann. Roy. Coll. Surg. Engl*, 12 (1953) pp.1–13.

5. Russell, K. F., 'The Osteographia of William Cheselden', *Bull. Hist. Med.*, 28 (1954) pp.32–49.

6. Punt, H., *Bernard Siegfried Albinus (1697–1770) on 'human nature': anatomical and physiological ideas in eighteenth century Leiden* (Amsterdam, 1983).

7. See Klaauw, J. C. van der, 'A letter of B. S. Albinus from Leiden to R. Nesbitt in London', *Janus*, 35 (1931) pp.217–20; LeFanu, W. R., 'More letters from B. S. Albinus to Robert Nesbitt', *Janus*, 36 (1932) pp.1–26.

8. Scarpa, A., 'Anatomical observations on the round window ...', Translated and edited by Lyle M. Sellers and Barry J. Anson', *Arch. Otolaryng.*, 75 (1962) pp.2–45.

9. See Bishop, W. J., 'Antonio Scarpa, 1752–1832', *Med. Biol. Ill.*, 4 (1954) pp.7–9; and Monti, A., *Antonio Scarpa in scientific history, and his role in the fortunes of the University of Pavia ... Translation by Frank L. Loria* (New York, 1957).

10. Faull, R. L. M., D. W. Taylor, and J. B. Carman, 'Soemmerring and the substantia nigra', *Med. Hist.*, 12 (1968) pp.297–9.

11. Bast, T. H., 'The life and work of Samuel Thomas von Sömmerring', *Ann. Med. Hist.*, 6 (1924) pp.369–86.

12. Dougherty, F. W. P., 'The correspondence of Johann Friedrich Blumenbach', *Hist. Anthrop. Newsl.*, 10(2) (1983) pp.6–9.

13. See Thornton, J. L., 'Percivall Pott (1714–1788)', *St Bart's Hosp. J.*, 68 (1964) pp.8–11. The January 1964 issue of this journal commemorates the 250th anniversary of Pott's birth, and contains the following articles: LeFanu, W. R., 'A background for Percivall Pott', pp.12–13; Seddon, H. J., 'Pott's disease', pp.14–15; Aston, J. N., 'Pott's fracture', pp.16–17; and Hanbury, W. J., 'Pott's puffy tumour', pp.18–19. See also Dobson, J., 'Percivall Pott', *Ann. Roy. Coll. Surg. Engl.*, 50 (1972) pp.54–65.

14. See Power, Sir D'Arcy, 'Eponyms. VII. Percivall Pott; his own fracture', *Br. J. Surg.*, 10 (1922–3) pp.313–15.

15. See bibliography of Pott's works (pp.334–6) in Lloyd, G. Marner, 'The life and works of Percivall Pott, 1714–1789 [*sic*]' *St. Bart's Hosp. Rep.*, 66 (1933) pp.291–336.

16. Kipling, M. D. and H. A. Waldron, 'Percivall Pott and cancer scroti', *Br. J. Industr. Med.*, 32 (1975) pp.244–50; Melicow, M. M., 'Percivall Pott (1713–1788): 200th anniversary of first report of occupation-induced cancer scrotum in chimney sweepers (1775)', *Urology*, 6 (1975) pp. 745–9.

17. Thomas, K. Bryn, *James Douglas of the pouch and his pupil William Hunter* (London, 1964). See also Brock, H., 'James Douglas of the Pouch', *Scott. Soc. Hist. Med. Rep. Proc.* (1972–3) in *Med. Hist.*, 18 (1974) pp.162–72.

18. Brock, C. H., 'James Douglas (1675–1742), botanist', *J. Soc. Bibliog. Nat. Hist.*, 9 (1979) pp.137–45.

19. Brock, C. H., 'The rediscovery of James Douglas', *Bibliotheck*, 8 (1977) pp.168–76.

20. Butterton, J. R., 'The education, naval service and early career of William Smellie' (William Osler Medical Essay), *Bull. Hist. Med.*, 60 (1986) pp.1–18.

21. Rymsdyk's original drawings are in Glasgow University, and Camper's are at the Royal College of Physicians, Edinburgh and Leyden University. See Thornton, J. L. and Patricia C. Want, 'Jan van Rymsdyk's illustrations of the gravid uterus drawn for Hunter, Smellie, Jenty and Denman, *J. Audiovisual Media Med.*, 2 (1979) pp.10–15.

22. Thornton, J. L., *Jan van Rymsdyk: medical artist of the eighteenth century* (Cambridge, 1982).

23. Johnstone, R. W., *William Smellie: the master of British midwifery* (Edinburgh, London, 1952).

24. See, for example, Cameron, S. J., 'William Smellie', *Scottish Med. J.*, 2 (1957) pp.439–44; and Wall, L. L., 'William Smellie (1697–1763), the father of scientific obstetrics', *Med. Heritage*, 2 (1986) pp.158–67.

25. Glaister, J., *Dr. William Smellie and his contemporaries: a contribution to the history of midwifery in the eighteenth century* (Glasgow, 1894).

26. Kaplan, E. B., 'Peter Camper 1722–1789', *Bull. Hosp. Joint Dis.*, 17 (1956) pp.371–85.

27. Visser, R. P. W., *The zoological work of Petrus Camper (1722–1789)* (Amsterdam, 1985).
28. See Guthrie, D., 'The travel journals of Peter Camper (1722–1789), anatomist, artist and obstetrician', *Edinburgh Med. J.*, 55 (1948) pp.338–53.
29. See Bynum, W. F. and R. Porter (eds), *William Hunter and the eighteenth-century medical world* (Cambridge, 1985) containing revised versions of papers presented at an International Symposium; Thornton, J. L. and Patricia C. Want, 'William Hunter (1718–1783) and his contributions to obstetrics', *Brit. J. Obstet. Gynaec.*, 90 (1983) pp.787–94; Simmons, S. F., *William Hunter, 1718–1783: a memoir, by Samuel Foart Simmons and John Hunter*, edited by C. H. Brock (East Kilbride, 1983) which contains a reassessment of Hunter on pp.43–81.
30. See Thornton, J. L. and Patricia C. Want, 'William Hunter's "The anatomy of the human gravid uterus" 1774–1974', *J. Obstet. Gynaec. Brit. Cwlth.* 81 (1974) pp.1–10; and, by the same authors, 'Artist versus engraver in William Hunter's "Anatomy of the human gravid uterus" 1774', *Med. Biol. Illus.*, 24 (1974) pp.137–9; and 'Jan van Rymsdyk's illustrations of the gravid uterus drawn for Hunter, Smellie, Jenty and Denman', op. cit. (no. 21 above); see also Ollerenshaw, R., 'Dr. Hunter's "Gravid uterus" – a bi-centenary note', *Med. Biol. Illus.*, 24 (1974) pp.43–57.
31. Reprinted Birmingham, Alabama, 1980 for the Classics of Medicine Library.
32. Russell, K. F., 'William Hunter sees the drawings of Leonardo da Vinci', *Med. Hist. Aust. Newsl.*, No.5 (1982) pp.1–2.
33. LeFanu, W. R., 'The writings of William Hunter, F. R. S.', *Bibliotheck*, I, iv (1958) pp.46–7.
34. Hunter, W., 'Lectures of anatomy' (Amsterdam, New York, 1972) prepared for publication by N. Dowd.
35. See Fox, R. H., *William Hunter, anatomist, physician, obstetrician (1718–1783), with notices of his friends Cullen, Smellie, Fothergill and Baillie* (London, 1901); and Oppenheimer, J. M., *New aspects of John and William Hunter* (New York, 1946).
36. Illingworth, Sir Charles, 'Dr. William Hunter's observations on lead-filled bones', *Med. Hist.*, 14 (1970) pp.390–6.
37. Illingworth, Sir Charles, 'William Hunter's manuscripts and letters: the Glasgow collection', *Med. Hist.*, 15 (1971) pp.181–6.
38. See Thomas, K. Bryn, 'A female foetus, drawn from nature by Mr. Blakey for William Hunter', *Med. Hist.*, 4 (1960) p.256.
39. Thomas, K. Bryn, 'William Hunter on William Harvey', *Med. Hist.*, 9 (1965) pp.279–86.
40. Brock. C. H., 'Dr. William Hunter's Museum, Glasgow University', *J. Soc. Bibliog. Nat. Hist.*, 9 (1980) pp.403–12.
41. Thornton, J. L. and Patricia C. Want, op. cit (no.21 above).
42. Snell, W. E., 'The diaries of John Knyveton, naval surgeon'. *Hist Med.*, 6 (1975) pp.23–7.
43. Drew, Sir Robert, 'John Hunter and the Army', *J. Roy. Army Med. Cps*, 113 (1967) pp.4–17.
44. LeFanu, W. R., *John Hunter: a list of his books*, for the Royal College of Surgeons of England, 1946. This provides more complete details of editions, translations, variants, etc.
45. See Russell, K. F., 'Hunter and his masterpiece', *Australian N.Z. J. Surg.*, 8 (1939) pp.335–9.
46. See LeFanu, W. R., op. cit. (no.44 above).
47. Thomas, K. Bryn, 'John Hunter and an amputation under analgesia in 1784', *Med. Hist.*, 2 (1958) pp.53–6.
48. Wakeley, Sir Cecil, 'John Hunter and experimental surgery', *Ann. Roy. Coll. Surg. Engl.* 16 (1955) pp.69–93.
49. Dobson, J., 'John Hunter's artists', *Med. Biol. Illus.*, 9 (1959) pp.138–49.
50. Stevenson, L. G., 'John Hunter, Surgeon-General, 1790–1793', *J. Hist. Med.*, 19 (1964) pp.239–66.
51. The following references are among the best sources available: Peachey, G. C., *A memoir of William and John Hunter* (Plymouth, for the author, 1924); Gloyne, S. R.,

John Hunter (Edinburgh, 1950); Paget, S., *John Hunter, man of science and surgeon, (1728–1793)* (London, 1897); Oppenheimer, Jane M., *New aspects of John and William Hunter* (New York, 1946); Qvist, G., *John Hunter 1728–1793* (London, 1981); Dobson, Jessie, *John Hunter* (Edinburgh, 1969); and Dobson, Jessie, 'John Hunter's anatomy', *Ann. Roy. Coll. Surg. Engl.*, 41 (1967) pp.493–501.

52. Dobson, Jessie, *William Clift* (London, 1954).
53. Dobson, Jessie, 'The conservators of the Hunterian Museum, I. William Clift', *Ann. Roy. Coll. Surg. Engl.*, 30 (1962) pp.46–52.
54. See Austin, F. and B. Jones 'William Clift: the surgeon's apprentice', *Ann. Roy. Coll. Surg. Engl.*, 60 (1978) pp.261–5; and Dobson, Jessie, 'William Clift to Philip Syng Physick', *Ann. Roy. Coll. Surg. Engl.*, 34 (1964) pp.197–203.
55. Hunter, W., op. cit. (no.34 above).
56. *Phil. Trans.*, 59 (1769) 1770, pp.36–46.
57. See Adami, J. G., *Charles White of Manchester (1728–1813), and the arrest of puerperal fever ... With which are reprinted Charles White's published writings upon puerperal fever* (Liverpool, London, 1922); Sheehan, D., 'Charles White, eighteenth-century surgeon', *Ann. Med. Hist.*, 4, series 3 (1942) pp.132–46; and Behr, G., 'Charles White of Manchester: the 250th anniversary of his birth', *Br. Med. J.* (1978) II, pp.1699–1700.
58. Lindeboom, G. A., *Herman Boerhaave: the man and his work* (London, 1968). See also Heniger, J., 'Some botanical activities of Herman Boerhaave, Professor of Botany and Director of the Botanic Garden at Leiden', *Janus*, 58 (1971) pp.1–78; and Lindeboom, G. A., 'Boerhaave: author and editor', *Bull. Med. Lib. Assn*, 62 (1974) pp.137–48.
59. A facsimile of the first edition and of the first French translation with an introduction by G. A. Lindeboom, has been published in the Dutch Classics on the History of Science series, 1964.
60. Derbes, V. J. and R. E. Mitchell, 'Hermann Boerhaave's *Atrocis, nec descripti prius, morbi historia.* The first translation of the classic case report of rupture of the esophagus, with annotations', *Bull. Med. Lib. Assn*, 43 (1955) pp.217–40.
61. Lindeboom, G. A., *Boerhaave's correspondence*, 3 vols (Leyden, 1962–79). See also Houtzager, H. L., 'A letter from Herman Boerhaave to Johan Philip Burgraf jr.', *Janus*, 67 (1980) pp.201–5.
62. Black, D. A. K., 'Johnson on Boerhaave', *Med. Hist.*, 3 (1959) pp.325–9.
63. See McConaghey, R. M. S., 'John Huxham', *Med. Hist.*, 13 (1969) pp.280–7; and Schupbach, W., 'The fame and notoriety of Dr. John Huxham', *Med. Hist.*, 25 (1981) pp.415–21.
64. *Med. Trans. Coll. Phycns Lond.*, 2 (1772) pp.59–67. See Bedford, D. E., 'William Heberden's contributions to cardiology', *J. Roy. Coll. Phycns*, 2 (1968) pp.127–35; and Silverman, M. E., 'William Heberden and *Some account of a disorder of the Breast*', *Clin. Cardiol*, 10 (1987) pp.211–13.
65. 'On the chicken-pox', *Med. Trans. Coll. Phycns Lond.* (1768) 1, pp.427–36.
66. 'Of the night-blindness or nyctalopia', ibid., pp.60–3.
67. This contains a bibliography of Heberden's writings (pp.60–1) consisting of 23 items, and a checklist of Heberden's manuscripts (pp.64–7), several of which are preserved at the Royal College of Physicians.
68. See Talbott, J. H., 'From the library of the William Heberdens', *Bull. Med. Lib. Assn*, 53 (1965) pp.438–41. See also Heberden, E., 'William Heberden the elder (1710–1801): aspects of his London practice', *Med. Hist.*, 30 (1986) pp.303–21; and Heberden, E., 'The correspondence of William Heberden FRS with the Reverend Stephen Hales and Sir Charles Blagden', *Notes Rec. Roy. Soc. Lond.*, 39 (1985) pp.179–89.
69. Reprinted in *Medical Classics*, 5 (1940–1) pp.58–99.
70. Fothergill, J., *Chain of friendship: selected letters of Dr. John Fothergill of London, 1735–1780. With introduction and notes by Betsy C. Corner and Christopher C. Booth* (Cambridge, Mass., 1971). See also Fox, R. H., *Dr. John Fothergill and his friends: chapters in eighteenth century life* (London, 1919); Booth, C. C., 'Dr. John Fothergill and the angina pectoris', *Med. Hist.* 1 (1957) pp.115–22; and Elkinton, J. R., 'Betty

Fothergill and her "Uncle Doctor": an intimate glimpse of Dr. John Fothergill', *Ann. Intern. Med.*, 85 (1976) pp.637–40.

71. Jolley, L., 'Two inquiries about the bibliography of William Cullen', *Bibliotheck*, 1, i (1956) pp.28–9.

72. Crellin J. K., 'William Cullen: his calibre as a teacher, and an unpublished introduction to his *A treatise of the materia medica* (London, 1773)', *Med. Hist.*, 15 (1971) pp.79–87.

73. See Thomson, J., *An account of the life, lectures and writings of William Cullen*, 2 vols (Edinburgh, London, 1859), vol. 2, pp.687–690, which deal with Cullen's published writings; Johnstone, R. W., 'William Cullen', *Med. Hist.*, 3 (1959) pp.33–46; and Stott, R., 'Health and virtue: or, how to keep out of harm's way. Lectures on pathology and therapeutics by William Cullen, *c*.1770', *Med. Hist.*, 31 (1987) pp.123–42.

74. Risse, G. B., 'Dr. William Cullen, physician, Edinburgh: a consultation practice in the eighteenth century', *Bull. Hist. Med.*, 48 (1974) pp.338–51, which refers to his practice of 'consultation by correspondence'.

75. French, R. K., *Robert Whytt, the soul and medicine* (London, 1969). See also Comrie, J. D., 'An eighteenth-century neurologist', *Int. Congr. Hist. Med.*, 5th, Geneva (1925) pp.25–8.

76. Overmier, Judith, A., 'John Brown's *Elementa medicinae*: an introductory bibliographical essay', *Bull. Med. Lib. Assn*, 70 (1982) pp.310–17.

77. O'Malley, C. D., 'A translation of William Withering's *De angina gangraenosa*', *J. Hist. Med.*, 8 (1953) pp.16–45.

78. See Greene, S. W., 'The publication date of William Withering's *A systematic arrangement of British plants* (Ed. 4), London, 1801' *J. Soc. Bib. Nat. Hist.*, 4, i (1962) pp.66–7.

79. Brodman, Estelle, 'Two different plates in Withering's *Account of the foxglove'*, *Bull. Hist. Med.*, 17 (1945) pp.415–17.

80. See, for example, Aronson, J. K., *An account of the foxglove and its medical uses, 1785–1985* (London, 1985) which includes a facsimile of the original monograph; Mann, R. D., *William Withering and the foxglove: a bicentennial selection of letters from the Osler bequest to the Royal Society of Medicine, together with a transcription of 'An account of the foxglove' and an introductory essay. By Ronald D. Mann with the collaboration of Helen Townsend and Joanna Townsend* (Lancaster, 1986) which is a folio volume; Wray, S., D. A. Eisner and D. G. Allen, 'Two hundred years of the foxglove', *Med. Hist.* (Suppl.), (1985) pp.132–50; Whitfield, A. G., 'Bicentenary of "An account of the foxglove", Historical address given at Edgbaston Parish Church, Birmingham', *Br. Heart J.*, 54 (1985) pp.253–5; and McMichael, J., 'William Withering in perspective', *Univ. Birmingham. Hist. J.*, 11 (1967) pp.41–50.

81. 'Among our manuscripts: William Withering' [Autograph letter of 1795], *Acad. Bkman*, 18(2), (1965) pp.7–8.

82. See Hunt, T. (ed.), *The Medical Society of London 1773–1973* (London, 1973).

83. See Price, R., 'Lettsom's letters', *Trans. Med. Soc. Lond.*, 94 (1977–8) pp.1–14; and Newman, C., 'Dr. Lettsom's letters', *Trans. Med. Soc. Lond.*, 90 (1974) pp.31–7. See also Abraham, J. J., *Lettsom, his life, times, friends and descendants* (London, 1933); Pettigrew, T. J., *Memoirs of the life and writings of the late John Coakley Lettsom*, 3 vols (London, 1817); and, for a brief biographical summary, Newman, C., 'John Coakley Lettsom', *Br. Med. J.* (1975) II, pp.382–3.

84. Musto, D. F., 'Benjamin Rush's medical thesis "On the digestion of food in the stomach", Edinburgh, 1768. Translated, and with an historical introduction', *Trans. Stud. Coll. Phycns Philad.*, 33 (1965) pp.121–38.

85. See Rush B., *Medical inquiries and observations upon the diseases of the mind. With an introduction by S. Bernard Wortis* (New York, 1962); this contains a facsimile of the 1812 edition. See also Middleton W. S., 'Gleanings from "Medical Inquiries" and "Observations" of Benjamin Rush', *Trans. Stud. Coll. Phycns Philad.*, 36 (1968) pp.55–60.

86. *The selected writings of Benjamin Rush. Edited by D. D. Runes* (New York, 1947).

87. *The autobiography of Benjamin Rush. His 'Travels through life' together with his*

'Commonplace book' for 1789–1813. Edited with introduction and notes by George W. Corner (Princeton, 1948). See Goodman, N. G., Benjamin Rush, physician and citizen, 1746–1813 (Philadelphia, 1934) with a list of his published writings, pp.382–90; Binger, C. A. L., Revolutionary doctor: Benjamin Rush, 1746–1813 (New York, 1966); Rush, A. R., 'Benjamin Rush MD (1745–1813): his origins and ancestry', Trans. Stud. Coll. Phycns Philad., 44 (1976) pp.9–35; Shryock, R. H., 'The medical reputation of Benjamin Rush: contrasts over two centuries', Bull. Hist. Med., 45 (1971) pp.507–52; Holloway, L. M., 'The many faces of Benjamin Rush: a bibliographic introduction', Trans. Coll. Phycns Philad., 44 (1976) pp.36–8; De Jong, R. N., 'The first American textbook in psychiatry; a review and discussion of Benjamin Rush's "Medical inquiries and observations upon the diseases of the mind"', Ann. Med. Hist, 3rd ser., 2 (1940) pp.195–202; Rush, B., Lectures on the mind. Edited, annotated and introduced by Eric T. Carlson, Jeffrey L Wollock and Patricia S. Noel (Philadelphia, 1981); Woodruff, A. W., 'Benjamin Rush, his work on yellow fever and his British connections', Amer. J. Trop. Med. Hyg., 26 (1977) pp.1055–9; and Holmes, C., 'Benjamin Rush and the yellow fever', Bull. Hist. Med., 40 (1966) pp.246–63.

88.   Baxby, D., 'The genesis of Edward Jenner's "Inquiry" of 1798: a comparison of the two unpublished manuscripts and the published version', Med. Hist., 29 (1985) pp.193–9.

89.   See Ford, E., 'The Sydney reprint of Jenner's "Inquiry"', Med. J. Aust. (1951) II, pp.320–4.

90.   See Blake, J. B., 'An unrecorded Jenner imprint', J. Hist. Med., 9 (1954) pp.233–4.

91.   Razzell P. E., 'Edward Jenner: the history of a medical myth', Med. Hist., 9 (1965) pp.216–29, incorporating a comment by A. W. Downie; a further comment by N. Schuster is contained on pp.381–3. See also Razzell, P., Edward Jenner's cowpox vaccine: the history of a medical myth, 2nd edn (Firle, 1980).

92.   LeFanu, W. R., A bibliography of Edward Jenner, 2nd edn (Winchester, 1985).

93.   Miller, Genevieve (ed.), Letters of Edward Jenner and other documents concerning the early history of vaccination. From the Henry Barton Jacobs collection in the William H. Welch Medical Library (Baltimore, 1983).

94.   See, for example, Letters from the past: from John Hunter to Edward Jenner (London, 1976) which contains 31 letters edited, with some facsimiles, by E. H. Cornelius and A. J. Harding Rains; Colyer, R. J., 'A letter of Edward Jenner (1749–1823)', Med. Hist., 21 (1977) pp.88–9; LeFanu, W. R., 'John Hunter to Edward Jenner: a lost letter discovered', Ann. Roy. Coll. Surg. Engl., 67 (1985) p.266; and LeFanu, W. R., 'Letters from Edward Jenner' [copies of 5 letters to Lady Louisa Brome, 1801–4 given to the College Library] Ann. Roy. Coll. Surg. Engl., 39 (1966) pp.370–2.

95.   See Baron, J., The life of Edward Jenner, 2 vols (1827–38); Underwood, E. A. and A. M. G. Campbell, Edward Jenner: the man and his work. Revised by E. Gethyn-Jones and H. Sanderson (East Grinstead [1981?]); Saunders, P., Edward Jenner: the Cheltenham years, 1795–1823. Being a chronicle of the vaccination campaign (Hanover, N.H., 1982); Baxby, D., Jenner's smallpox vaccine, the riddle of vaccine virus and its origin (London, 1981); LeFanu, W. R, 'Edward Jenner', Proc. Roy. Soc. Med., 66 (1973) pp.664–8; Cameron, Sir Gordon, 'Edward Jenner F.R.S., 1749–1823', Notes Rec. Roy. Soc. Lond., 7 (1949–50) pp.43–53; Palmer, R., 'Illustrations from the Wellcome Institute Library: the Wellcome collection of papers relating to Edward Jenner', Med. Hist., 29 (1985) pp.200–5; also Thornton–Tully, p.191.

96.   See Lewis, Sir Thomas, 'Caleb Hillier Parry, MD, F.R.S. (1755–1822); a great Welsh physician and scientist', Proc. Cardiff Med. Soc., (1940–1) pp.1–19, and Medical Classics, 5 (1940–1) pp.1–20, which contains a chronological biography and bibliography (pp.6–7); Kligfield, P., 'The early pathophysiologic understanding of angina pectoris (Edward Jenner, Caleb Hillier Parry, Allan Burns)', Amer. J. Cardiol., 50 (1982) pp.1433–5.

97.   See [McMichael, W.], The gold-headed cane. Second edition (1828) pp.236–67.

98.   See Crainz, F., 'The editions and translations of Dr. Matthew Baillie's "Morbid anatomy"', Med. Hist., 26 (1982) pp.443–52; and Rodin, A. E., The influence of

Matthew Baillie's Morbid anatomy: biography, evaluation and reprint (Springfield, Ill., 1973), which contains a reprint of the second American edition, 1808.

99. LeFanu, W. R., 'Laënnec and Matthew Baillie', *Ann. Roy. Coll. Surg. Engl.*, 36 (1965) pp.67–8. See also Hill, B., '"Enlightened and honourable" Matthew Baillie, M. D., 1761–1823', *Practitioner*, 220 (1978) pp.490–3.

100. For complete details see Baumgartner, Leona, 'John Howard (1726–1790), hospital and prison reformer; a bibliography', *Bull. Hist. Med.*, 7 (1939) pp.489–534, 595–626; also Durling, R. J., 'John Howard: a bibliographical note', *J. Hist. Med.*, 14 (1959) pp.375–8.

101. See Duveen, D. I. and H. S. Klickstein, 'Note on the French translation of Howard's "State of the prisons"', *J. Hist. Med.*, 10 (1955) pp.114–16.

102. Howard, D. L., *John Howard: prison reformer* (London, 1958).

103. Rendle-Short, M. and J. Rendle-Short, *The father of child care: life of William Cadogan (1711–1797)* (Bristol, 1966); Rendle-Short, J., 'William Cadogan, eighteenth-century physician', *Med. Hist.*, 4 (1960) pp.288–309.

104. Ruhräh, J., *William Cadogan [His Essay on gout]* (New York, 1925); this is a reprint of the tenth edition, and was reprinted with corrections from *Ann. Med. Hist.*, 7 (1925) pp.77–90.

105. Hamilton, D., 'Sir John Pringle', *J. Roy. Army Med. Cps*, 110 (1964) pp.139–47.

106. Selwyn, S., 'Sir John Pringle: hospital reformer, moral philosopher and pioneer of antiseptics', *Med. Hist.*, 10 (1966) pp.266–74.

107. See Lorenz, A. J., 'Some pre-Lind writers on scurvy', *Proc. Nutrition Soc.*, 12 (1953) pp.306–24.

108. Meiklejohn, A. P., 'The curious obscurity of Dr. James Lind', *J. Hist. Med.*, 9 (1954) pp.304–10.

109. Lind, J., 'Nutrition classics, "A treatise of the scurvy" by James Lind, 1753', *Nutr. Rev.*, 41 (1983) pp.155–7.

110. *Lind's treatise on scurvy. A bicentenary volume containing a reprint of the first edition of A treatise of the scurvy ... Edited by C. P. Stewart and Douglas Guthrie* (Edinburgh, 1953).

111. See Wyatt, H. V. and R. E. Hughes, 'James Lind and the prevention of scurvy', *Med. Hist.*, 20 (1976) pp.433–8; Hughes, R. E., 'James Lind and the cure of scurvy: an experimental approach', *Med. Hist.*, 19 (1975) 342–51; Hill, B., 'The father of nautical medicine. James Lind M.D. (1716–1794)', *Practitioner*, 191 (1963) pp.784–8.

112. See Baumgartner, L. and E. M. Ramsey, 'Johann Peter Frank and his "system einer vollständigen medizinischen Polizey"', *Ann. Med. Hist.*, N.S.5 (1933) pp.525–32; N.S.6 (1934) pp.69–90 (bibliography, pp.84–90); and Frank, J. P., *A system of complete medical police. Selections from Johann Peter Frank*, ed. by E. Lesky (Baltimore, 1976).

113. See Frank, J. P., *Johann Peter Frank: Seine Selbstbiographie. Hrsg. eingeleit und mit Erläuterungen versehen von Erna Lesky* (Bern, 1969); Dolan, J. P., 'Johann Peter Frank: father of socialized medicine', *J.S.C. Med. Assn*, 70 (1974) pp.294–6; and the following two articles by C. C. Barnard: 'Bicentenary of J. P. Frank', *Lancet* (1945) I, p.381 (gives details of Frank's writings); and 'The Epistoli Invitatoria (1776) of Johann Peter Frank', *Janus*, 39 (1935) pp.149–64.

114. Doetsch, R. N., 'Lazzaro Spallanzani's "Opusculi" of 1776', *Bact. Rev.*, 40 (1976) pp.270–5.

115. Edited by B. Biagi, the work completed after his death by D. Prandi.

116. See Prandi, D., *Bibliografia della opere di Lazzaro Spallanzani: delle traduzione e degli scritti su di lui* (Florence, 1951); Di Pietro, P., *Lazzaro Spallanzani* (Modena, 1979) written in Italian; Castellani, C., 'Spermatozoan biology from Leeuwenhoek to Spallanzani', *J. Hist. Biol.*, 6 (1973) pp.37–68; and Sandler, I., 'The re-examination of Spallanzani's interpretation of the role of the spermatic animalcules in fertilization', *J. Hist. Biol.*, 6 (1973) pp.193–223; see also Thornton–Tully, pp.187–8.

117. *The letters of Erasmus Darwin. Edited by D. King-Hele* (Cambridge, 1981). See also *The essential writings of Erasmus Darwin, chosen and edited with a linking commentary by Desmond King-Hele* (London, 1968); King-Hele, D., *Doctor of revolution: the*

life and genius of Erasmus Darwin (London, 1977); Moody, J. W. T., 'Erasmus Darwin MD, FRS: a biographical and iconographical note', *J. Soc. Bibliog. Nat. Hist.*, 4 (1964) pp.210–13; Thornton–Tully, pp.188–9.

·118. See Verso, M. L., 'A note on the observations of Hewson and Falconar on the morphology of blood cells, with an account of their theory of blood formation', *Med. J. Australia* (1957) II, pp.431–2; and Dameskek, W., 'William Hewson, thymicologist; father of hematology?' *Blood*, 21 (1963) pp.513–16.

119. See also Bailey, G. H., 'William Hewson, F.R.S. (1739–1774). An account of his life and work', *Ann. Med. Hist.*, 5 (1923) pp.209–24.

120. See Chapter 8.

121. See Thornton–Tully, pp.178–9.

122. A reprint of the two-volume Edinburgh edition of 1786, entitled *First lines of physiology*, was produced in one volume in New York, 1966, with a new introduction by Lester S. King.

123. See Buess, H., 'Albrecht von Haller and his "Elementa physiologiae" as the beginning of pathological physiology', *Med. Hist.*, 3 (1959) pp. 123–31; and Buess, H., 'Zur Enstehung der "Elementa physiologiae" Albrecht Hallers (1708–1777)', *Gesnerus*, 15 (1958) pp.17–35.

124. See also Balmer, H., *Albrecht von Haller* (Berne, 1977) written in German; Roe, S. A. *Matter, life and generation. Eighteenth-century embryology and the Haller-Wolff debate* (Cambridge, 1981); Buess, H., 'William Harvey and the foundation of modern haemodynamics by Albrecht von Haller', *Med. Hist.*, 14 (1970) pp.175–82; Roe, S. A., 'The development of Albrecht von Haller's views on embryology', *J. Hist. Biol.*, 8, (1975) pp.167–90; and Lindskog, G. E., 'Albrecht von Haller. A bicentennial memoir', *Conn. Med.*, 42 (1978) pp.49–57.

125. Bishop, P. J., 'A bibliography of Auenbrugger's "Inventum novum" (1761)', *Tubercle*, 42 (1961) pp.78–90; Rate, R. G., 'Leopold Auenbrugger and the "Inventum novum"', *J. Kans. Med. Soc.*, 67 (1966) pp.30–3.

_6. Bishop, P. J., 'A list of papers, etc. on Leopold Auenbrugger (1722–1809) and the history of percussion', *Med. Hist.*, 5 (1961) pp.192–5. See also Bedford, D. E., 'Auenbrugger's contribution to cardiology. History of percussion of the heart', *Brit. Heart J.*, 33 (1971) pp.817–21.

127. *Phil. Trans. Roy. Soc.*, 85 (1795) pp.177–89. See 'William C. Cruikshank (1745–1800), surgeon of Leicester Square' [Editorial] *J. Amer. Med. Assn*, 214 (1970) 1110–12; and Ochs, S., 'The early history of nerve regeneration, beginning with Cruikshank's observations in 1776', *Med. Hist.*, 21 (1977) pp. 261–74.

128. *Novi Commentarii Academiae Scientiarium Imperialis Petropolitanae*, 12 (1768) pp.403–507; 13 (1769) pp.478–530.

129. See Belloni, L., 'Embryological drawings concerning his "Theorie von Generationen" sent by Caspar Friedrich Wolff to Albrecht Haller in 1764', *J. Hist. Med.*, 26 (1971) pp.205–8.

130. Ostwald's *Klassiker*, Nos.84–5. See Stephens, T. D., 'The Wolffian ridge: history of a misconception', *Isis*, 73 (1982) pp.254–9; Roe, S. A., op. cit. (no. 124 above); and Aulie, R. P., 'Caspar Friedrich Wolff and his "Theoria generationis", 1759', *J. Hist. Med.*, 16 (1961) pp.124–44.

131. See Blezza, F., *Galvani e Volta: la polemica sull' elettricita* (Brescia, 1983) which includes an Italian translation of *De viribus electricitatis*.

132. A translation of Luigi Galvani's *De viribus electricitatis in motu musculari commentarius: commentary on the effect of electricity on muscular motion* (Cambridge, Mass., 1953).

133. *Commentary of the effects of electricity on muscular motion. Translated into English by Margaret Glover Foley with notes and a critical introduction by I. Bernard Cohen, together with a facsimile of Galvani's De viribus electricitatis in motu musculari commentarius (1791) and a bibliography of the editions and translations of Galvani's book prepared by John Farquhar Fulton and Madeline E. Stanton* (Norwalk, Conn., 1953).

134. See Dibner, B., *Luigi Galvani* (Norwalk, Conn., 1971) which comprises an expanded version of a biography prepared for publication in *Encyclopaedia Britannica*, three

of four original drawings illustrating the 1791 edition of 'De viribus electricitatis' being reproduced in a supplement; and Williams, B. I., *The conceptual and empirical basis of Luigi Galvani's work on muscular motion*, PhD Thesis (London, 1975).

135. See Peterkin, G. A. G., 'The birthplace of Robert Willan (Corres.)', *Br. J. Derm.*, 74 (1962) pp.423–4.
136. See Hare, P. J., 'A note on Robert Willan's Edinburgh days', *Br. J. Derm.*, 88 (1973) 615–17.
137. Sutherland, F. M., 'Willan's *Cutaneous diseases*', *J. Hist. Med.*, 13 (1958) pp.92–4; supplements article by Beswick, T. S. L., 'Robert Willan: the solution of a ninety-year-old mystery', *J. Hist. Med.*, 12 (1957) pp.349–65.
138. See Booth, C. C., 'Robert Willan and his kinsmen', *Med. Hist.*, 25 (1981) pp.181–96; Sharma, O. P., 'In memoriam Robert Willan (1757–1812)', *Sarcoidosis*, 2 (1985) pp.158–60; and Sharma, O. P., 'Robert Willan and erythema nodosum', *Int. Congr. Hist. Med.*, 23rd (London, September 1972, 1974) vol.2, pp.1082–6.
139. Pattie, F. A., 'Mesmer's medical dissertation and its debt to Mead's "De imperio solis ac lunae"', *J. Hist. Med.*, 11 (1956) pp.275–87.
140. See also Buranelli, V., *The wizard from Vienna* (New York, [1975]).
141. *Bull. Hist. Med.*, Suppl., N.S. No.3 (Baltimore, 1980).
142. Weiner, D. B., 'The apprenticeship of Philippe Pinel: a new document, "Observations of Citizen Pussin on the insane"', *Amer. J. Psychiat.*, 136 (1979) pp.1128–34; Weiner, D. B., 'The apprenticeship of Philippe Pinel: a new document', *Clio. Med.* 13 (1978) pp.125–33. See also Grange, Kathleen M., 'Pinel and eighteenth-century psychiatry', *Bull. Hist. Med.*, 35 (1961) pp.442–53; Woods, Evelyn A. and E. T. Carlson, 'The psychiatry of Philippe Pinel', *Bull. Hist. Med.*, 35 (1961) pp.14–25; Mackler, B. and E. Bernstein, 'Contributions to the history of psychology. II. Philippe Pinel: the man and his time', *Psychol. Rep.*, 19 (1966) pp.703–20; and Weiner, D. B., 'Philippe Pinel, linguist: his work as translator and editor', *Gesnerus*, 42 (1985) pp.499–509.
143. See Hunter, R. A. and Ida Macalpine, 'William Battie, M.D., F.R.S., pioneer psychiatrist', *Practitioner*, 174 (1955) pp.208–15; and *A treatise on madness. By William Battie, M.D. and Remarks on Dr. Battie's Treatise on madness, by John Monro, M.D. A psychiatric controversy of the eighteenth century. Introduced and annotated by Richard Hunter and Ida Macalpine* (London, 1962).
144. See Leigh, D., 'John Haslam, M.D. – 1764–1844, apothecary to Bethlem', *J. Hist. Med.*, 10 (1955) pp.17–44; and Schiller, F., 'Haslam of "Bedlam", Kitchener of the "Oracles": two doctors under Mad King George III and their friendship', *Med. Hist.*, 28 (1984) pp.189–201.
145. See Graham, J., 'Lavater's *Physiognomy*: a checklist', *Pap. Bib. Soc. Amer.*, 55 (1961) pp.297–308.
146. See Charles, S. T., 'John Jones, American surgeon and conservative patriot', *Bull. Hist. Med.*, 39 (1965) pp.435–49; Peltie, L. T., 'John Jones, an extraordinary American', *Bull. Amer. Coll. Surg.*, 63 (1978) pp.20–5; and Stark, R. B., 'John Jones M.D. 1729–1791, father of American surgery', *N.Y. St. J. Med.*, 76 (1976) pp.1333–8.
147. Austin, R. B., *Early American imprints: a guide to works printed in the United States, 1668–1820* (Washington, 1961); see also Toomey, Thomas Noxon, 'The first general medical treatise published in the western hemisphere', *Ann. Med. Hist.*, N.S.1 (1929) pp.215–28.
148. See also Thornton–Tully, Chapter 7, pp.256–76.
149. Dukes, C. E., 'London medical societies in the eighteenth century', *Proc. Roy. Soc. Med.*, 53 (1960) pp.699–706.
150. Batty Shaw, A., 'The oldest medical societies in Great Britain', *Med. Hist.*, 12 (1968) pp.233–44.
151. See Gray, James, *History of the Royal Medical Society, 1737–1937. Edited by Douglas Guthrie* (Edinburgh, 1952); see also Power, Sir D'Arcy, *British medical societies* (1939) pp.12–19.
152. See Power, Sir D'Arcy, op. cit. (no. 151 above) pp.20–7.
153. Owen, E., 'An oration on the Medical Society of London in the eighteenth century', *Lancet* (1897) I, pp.1388–95.

154. See Dukes, C. E., 'Dr. James Sims (1741–1820); a new appraisal', *Med. Hist.*, 5 (1961) pp.375–83; *Trans. Med. Soc. Lond.*, 78 (1962) pp.178–88.
155. See also Power, Sir D'Arcy, op. cit. (no. 151 above), pp.28–36.
156. See, Pitt, G. N., 'The Hunterian Oration; reflections on John Hunter as a physician and on his relation to the medical societies of the last century. Delivered before the Hunterian Society on Feb. 13th, 1896', *Lancet* (1896) I, pp.1270–4.
157. See Strohl, E. L., 'The Fleece Inn Medical Society', *Surg. Gynec. Obstet.*, 177 (1963) pp.371–4.
158. Bishop, W. J., 'Medical book societies in England in the eighteenth and nineteenth centuries', *Bull. Med. Lib. Assn.*, 45 (1957) pp.337–50.

6 Medical books of the nineteenth century
Geoffrey Davenport

He becomes the true discoverer who establishes the truth, and the sign of the truth is the general acceptance. Whoever, therefore, resumes the investigation of the neglected or repudiated doctrine, elicits its true demonstration, and discovers and explains the nature of the errors which have led to its tacit or declared rejection, may certainly and confidently await the acknowledgements of his right in its discovery.

(Sir Richard Owen)

During the nineteenth century there was an enormous increase in the output of books on all branches of medicine, and it is impossible to record but a fraction of these. Many important advances were made, for research was carried on with increasing vigour. Each important discovery acted as a stepping-stone towards even greater achievements, and where pioneers of previous centuries had hesitatingly put forth new theories, it was now possible to advance at greater speed, owing to improvements in technique, and increased facilities for the research worker. Nevertheless brilliant achievements were also gained despite detrimental circumstances, for it is not necessarily the best equipped laboratory that produces the epoch-making discoveries. It is the man behind the apparatus, and genius has triumphed over conditions that would today be deemed impossible for the encouragement of scientific research.

Research in anatomy, both normal and pathological, and in physiology resulted in many additions to our knowledge of the structure and functions (and dysfunctions) of the human body, particularly of the nervous system. At the same time growing industrialization and the overcrowding of towns led to the need for more efficient systems of sanitation and to the development of public health and preventive medicine.

German anatomists were foremost in the field during the period under consideration. It was considered necessary for all budding anatomists to visit the German schools, for their teaching was renowned throughout the civilized world. The British anatomists were mainly surgeons, for anatomy as a full-time career as yet offered little inducement. France possessed at least two outstanding writers on normal and pathological anatomy, Bichat and Cruveilhier, the former having been described by Garrison as 'the creator of descriptive anatomy'.

Although Bichat's ideas may be regarded as the culmination of eighteenth-century thought on the living body, as Elizabeth Haigh has shown in her recent study,[1] his works, published at the turn of the century, were a great influence, especially on the French school, in the following decades and he may therefore legitimately be taken as beginning the nineteenth century. Marie François Xavier Bichat (1771–1802) served as an army surgeon during the French revolution, and was the author of the following important books: *Traité des membranes en général et de diverses membranes en particulier*, Paris, 1799–1800, of which an American edition was issued at Boston and Cambridge, 1813, and an English edition, London, 1821; *Traité d'anatomie descriptive*, five volumes, Paris 1801–3; *Anatomie générale appliquée à la physiologie et à la médecine* ..., two volumes, Paris, 1802, which was translated into English by George Hayward, Boston, 1822; *Anatomie pathologique* ..., Paris, 1825, an American edition being published at Philadelphia in 1827; *Recherches physiologiques sur la vie et la mort*, An VIII, [1800], representing Bichat's physiological doctrine; his *Oeuvres complètes* appeared in eleven volumes, Paris, 1832, and his manuscript notes are in the Bibliothèque de la Faculté de Médecine, Paris.[2]

Jean Cruveilhier (1791–1873),[3] a native of Limoges, and a pupil of Dupuytren, held the first chair of pathology established in the Paris Faculty. He first described disseminated sclerosis in his *Anatomie pathologique du corps humain* ..., two volumes, Paris, 1829–42, which is one of the most beautifully illustrated books on pathology. Cruveilhier also wrote *Anatomie descriptive*, four volumes, Paris, 1834, which was translated into English, 1841; *Traité d'anatomie pathologique générale* ..., five volumes, Paris, 1849–64; and *Essai sur l'anatomie pathologique en général* ..., two volumes, Paris, 1816. Marie Philibert Constant Sappey (1810–96) was the author of *Anatomie, physiologie, pathologie des vaisseaux lymphatiques*, Paris, 1874–5, which was noted for its excellent illustrations.

Carl von Rokitansky (1804–78), a native of Bohemia who became head of the department of pathological anatomy at the University of Vienna, conducted over 30 000 post-mortems. He was author of the three-volume *Handbuch der pathologischen Anatomie*, Vienna, 1842–46, which was translated into English and published by the New Sydenham Society in four volumes, 1849–54. Rokitansky also contributed a volume on the malformation of the heart, *Die Defekte der Scheidewände des Herzens* ... Vienna, 1875.[4]

Friedrich Gustav Jacob Henle (1809–85) was born at Fürth, near Nuremberg, becoming professor of anatomy successively at Zurich, Heidelberg and Göttingen, after studying at Berlin under Johannes Müller. Henle excelled as an histologist and a lecturer, his microscopical researches covering a very wide field. He illustrated his own works, which include *Symbolae ad anatomiam villorum intestinalium imprimis eorum epithelii et vasorum lacteorum*, Berlin, 1837; *Allgemeine Anatomie* ..., Leipzig, 1841; *Handbuch des systematischen Anatomie des Menschen*, three volumes, Braunschweig, 1856–73; *Pathologische Untersuchungen*, Berlin, 1840; *Handbuch der rationellen Pathologie*, two volumes, Braunschweig,

1846–51, of which an English translation was published at Philadelphia, 1853; and *Beiträge zur Anatomie und Embryologie*, Bonn, 1882. In the first part of *Pathologische Untersuchungen*, entitled *Von den Miasmen und Kontagion, und von den miasmatisch-kontagiösen Krankheiten*, Henle sought to establish that some infectious diseases were caused by a living agent, and this work is now regarded as an important stage in the developing understanding of disease transmission. It was reprinted in the Klassiker der Medizin series, Leipzig, 1910, and translated into English by George Rosen in 1938.[5]

Theodor Schwann (1810–82) was a native of Neuss, near Düsseldorf, and after a period at the University of Louvain, became professor of anatomy and physiology at Liège. He contributed many articles on physiology to journals, and was also the author of the following books: *De necessitate aëris atmosphoerici ad evolutionem pulli in ovo incubato*, Berlin, 1834, his inaugural dissertation; *Mikroskopische Untersuchungen über die Uebereinstimmung in der Struktur und dem Wachtsthum der Thiere und Pflanzen*, Berlin, 1839, of which another edition was published at Leipzig in 1910, and was translated into English by Henry Smith, and published by the Sydenham Society in 1847; and *Anatomie du corps humain*, two parts, Brussels, [1855].[6]

Joseph Hyrtl (1810–94) of Eisenstadt, Hungary, was renowned as a teacher rather than as a research worker, and after being professor of anatomy at Prague, held a similar position at Vienna for thirty years. His *Lehrbuch der Anatomie des Menschen* ..., Prague, 1846, went into 20 editions up to 1889 and was not illustrated until it appeared in two later editions; it was translated into several languages. His *Handbuch der topographischen Anatomie*, Vienna, 1847, was also without illustrations. Hyrtl wrote a manual of dissecting, *Handbuch der praktischen Zergliederungskunst* ..., Vienna, 1860; *Die Corrosions-Anatomie und ihre Ergebnisse*, Vienna, 1873, dealing with his novel method of making anatomical preparations; *Antiquitates anatomicae rariores*, Vienna, 1835; and after his retirement in 1874 Hyrtl wrote several other interesting books, including *Das Arabische und Hebräische in der Anatomie*, Vienna, 1879; *Onomatologia anatomica* ... Vienna, 1880, on medical terminology; and *Die alten deutschen Kunstworte der Anatomie* ..., Vienna, 1884. Hyrtl was a great medical scholar, and the author of numerous other books and papers.[7]

Robert Remak (1815–65) of Posen was an histologist, and the author of many writings on the subject, of which the following are of primary significance: *Observationes anatomicae et microscopicae de systematis nervosi structura*, Berlin, [1838], his inaugural thesis; *Untersuchungen über die Entwickelung des Wirbelthiere*, Berlin, 1851 [1855]; *Diagnostische und pathogenetische Untersuchungen* ..., Berlin, 1845; and *Galvanotherapie der Nerven- und Muskelkrankheiten*, Berlin, 1858, of which a French translation was published at Paris in 1860.[8]

Another brilliant histologist, (Rudolph) Albert von Kölliker, was also the author of about 300 books and papers on physiology and comparative anatomy. Kölliker was born at Zurich on 6 July 1817, and died at Würzburg on 2 November 1905. He studied at Zurich, Bonn, and Heidelberg, and was a pupil of Johannes Müller at Berlin. In 1844 he became professor of physiology and comparative anatomy at Zurich, but three years later went to Würzburg, first teaching physiology, and later adding the chair of anatomy. With Gottfried von Siebold, Kölliker founded and edited the *Zeitschrift für wissenschaftliche Zoologie* in 1849, and in the same year was also prominent in the founding of Die physikalischmedicinische Gesellschaft in Würzburg. Kölliker travelled widely, and was a good linguist, his reminiscences appearing as *Erinnerungen aus meinem Leben*, Leipzig, 1899. Among other volumes he was the author of the following: *Entwicklungsgeschichte des Menschen und die höheren Thiere*, Leipzig, 1861, the first book on comparative embryology, of which a French translation was published at Paris, [1879–] 1882; *Mikroskopische Anatomie*, two volumes, Leipzig, 1850–4; and *Handbuch der Gewebelehre des Menschen*, Leipzig, 1852, of which a sixth edition appeared in three volumes, 1889–1902. The Sydenham Society published the *Manual of human histology*, two volumes, 1853–4, which was translated and edited by George Busk and Thomas Huxley.[9]

Rudolf Ludwig Karl Virchow (1821–1902) was a man of considerable charisma and strong opinions on a wide variety of subjects, who made an enormous number of valuable contributions to the literature of medicine and public health, being the virtual creator of cellular pathology. He also made important contributions to embryology, anthropology, ethnology and history, and was also a politician, supporting the revolution of 1848 and entering the Reichstag in 1880. Virchow was a native of Schavelbein, Pomerania, and graduated at the Friedrich-Wilhelm Institut, Berlin, where he joined the teaching staff in 1847. The following year he left to become a professor at Würzburg, but in 1856 was recalled to Berlin. He founded Virchow's *Archiv für pathologische Anatomie,* of which he was editor from 1847 to 1902, and in 1851 founded Virchow's *Jahresbericht.* Among his more important books the following should be noted: *Gesammelte Abhandlungen zur wissenschaftlichen Medizin*, Frankfort-on-Main, 1856; *Handbuch der speziellen Pathologie und Therapie*, six volumes, Erlangen, 1854; *Die Cellularpathologie in ihrer Begründung auf physiologische und pathologische Gewebelehre* ..., Berlin, 1858, of which there were several editions, including an English translation, London, 1860 (reprinted Birmingham, Ala., 1978) and a French translation, Paris, 1861; *Die krankhaften Geschwülste* ..., three volumes, Berlin, 1863–7; *Die Sektionstechnik in Leichenhause des Charitékrankenhauses*, Berlin, 1875; *Gesammelte Abhandlungen aus dem Gebiet der offentlichen Medizin und der*

Seuchenlehre, two volumes, Berlin, 1879; and *Crania ethnica Americana* ..., Berlin, 1892.[10]

Wilhelm His (1831–1904), a native of Basle, was professor of anatomy at Basle University (1857–72) and then at Leipzig. He conducted research on the histogenesis of tissues, and was a fine artist. In 1876 His founded the *Zeitschrift für Anatomie und Entwicklungsgeschichte*; he was one of the founders of the *Archiv für Anthropologie* (1876) and of the Anatomische Gesellschaft. His more important writings include *Die Häute und Höhlen des Körpers*, Basle, 1865, containing his new classification of tissues; *Untersuchungen über die erste Anlage des Wirbelthierleibes* ..., Leipzig, 1868 on the embryology of the chick; *Anatomie menschlicher Embryonen* ..., three volumes, Leipzig, 1880–5, in which the human embryo is studied as a whole for the first time; *Unsere Körperform und das physiologische Problem ihrer Entstehung. Briefe an einem befreundeten Naturforscher*, Leipzig, 1874; *Beiträge zur normalen und pathologischen Histologie der Cornea*, Basel, 1856; and *Die anatomische Nomenclatur*, Leipzig, 1895, of which an English translation by L. F. Barker was published in 1907.[11] It is not generally appreciated that it was Wilhelm His (1863–1934),[12] a clinician rather than an anatomist like his father, after whom the 'Bundle of His' is named. The younger His discovered the embryonic muscle bundle uniting the right auricle with the ventricles, and described it in an article published in 1893, which was translated into English by T. H. Bast and Weston D. Gardner in 1949.[13]

Julius Friedrich Cohnheim (1839–84) was a native of Demmin, Pomerania, and studied at Berlin and Würzburg. Under Kölliker he became an expert histologist, and later served under Virchow in Berlin for seven years. Cohnheim occupied the chair of pathology at Kiel in 1868, and four years later went to Breslau, where he founded an institute of pathology. In 1878 he became professor of general pathology and pathologic anatomy at Leipzig, and was particularly concerned with the pathology of the circulation. Cohnheim's most important book was the *Vorlesungen über allgemeine Pathologie*, two volumes, Berlin, 1877–80, which was translated by Alexander B. McKee, and published by the New Sydenham Society as *Lectures on general pathology*, three volumes, London, 1889–90. His other writings include *Neue Untersuchungen über die Entzündung*, Berlin, 1873, on inflammation and suppuration; *Die Tuberkulose vom Standpunkte der Infectionslehre*, Leipzig, 1880; *Untersuchungen über die embolischen Processe*, Berlin, 1872; *Ueber die Aufgangen der pathologischen Anatomie*, Leipzig, 1878; and his *Gesammelte Abhandlungen*, Berlin, 1885.[14]

Karl Heinrich von Bardeleben (1849–1918) of Giessen graduated at Berlin in 1871, and was professor at Jena from 1889 to 1918, after having been associated with His at Leipzig. Bardeleben made many anatomical investigations, and with Heinrich Haeckel was the author of *Atlas der topographischen Anatomie des Menschen für Studierende und Aerzte …*, Jena, 1894, of which an English translation appeared in 1906. Bardeleben also wrote *Lehrbuch der systemischen Anatomie des Menschen für Studierende und Aerzte,* Berlin, Vienna, 1906; *Nervensystem und Sinnesorgane,* Leipzig, Berlin, 1913; and edited *Handbuch der Anatomie des Menschen.* Jena, 1896–1915.

British authors are represented by Henry Gray (1827–61), who graduated from St George's Hospital, London, and at the age of twenty-five was elected a Fellow of the Royal Society. He was demonstrator of anatomy, curator of the museum, and later lecturer on anatomy at St George's, but died of smallpox at the early age of thirty-four. He wrote a dissertation in 1853 which was awarded the Astley Cooper Prize of 300 guineas and was published as *On the structure and use of the spleen,* London, 1854, which is very rare, and generally overlooked by those writing of Gray as a 'one-book man'. The volume associated with his name for over a century was first published as *Anatomy, descriptive and surgical* in August 1858 by John W. Parker & Son, and was illustrated by Henry Vankyke Carter (1831–97). The second edition contained several new drawings by John Guise Westmacott (1811–84) and was issued by the same publisher in December 1860, the publishers then selling out to Longman, Green. This was also the last revision by Henry Gray, but it has continued to date under various distinguished editors as the most popular students' textbook of anatomy. The thirty-third edition was published in London in 1962, but the book is also maintained up to date in a separate American edition, the first of which was published in Philadelphia in 1859. The centenary of this event was celebrated by the publication by C. M. Goss of an account of Gray, and a list of the various editions of this remarkable book.[15]

Jones Quain (1796–1865) was the author of *Elements of descriptive and practical anatomy,* London, 1828, of which the eleventh edition was published between 1908 and 1929, and which had several distinguished editors and contributors.[16] With Erasmus Wilson he was the author of *A series of anatomical plates …*, a folio in two volumes published from 1836 to 1842. Jones Quain was professor of general anatomy at University College, London, where his brother Richard Quain (1800–87) became professor of descriptive anatomy, and eventually professor of clinical surgery. Richard Quain edited the 1848 edition of his brother's *Elements*, and was the author of *The anatomy of the arteries of the human body …*, London, 1844; *The diseases of the rectum,* London, 1854, with a second edition in 1855; and *Clinical lectures,* 1884.

Sir Robert Carswell (1793–1857), a native of Paisley, graduated at Aberdeen, and became professor of morbid anatomy at University College, London, in 1828. He has been described as probably the greatest of all illustrators of gross pathology, and he made 2000 water-colour drawings for his *Pathological anatomy. Illustrations of the elementary forms of disease*, London, 1838, a folio of coloured plates drawn upon stone by himself.[17]

Surgery made rapid strides during the nineteenth century, largely at the hands of the following eminent surgeons, and it should be noted that many of these were also prominent anatomists. The introduction of anaesthetics greatly advanced operative surgery, for the insensibility of the patient to pain greatly assisted the operator, who was now able to conduct major operations without haste, while the introduction of antiseptic surgery greatly decreased the risks of surgical intervention. British surgeons predominated during this period, but French and American operators also made important contributions. John Bell (1763–1820) of Edinburgh was a founder of modern vascular surgery, and like his brother, Charles, was also an artist. He wrote *Anatomy of the bones, muscles and joints*, two volumes, Edinburgh, [1793–] 1797, which was reissued in four volumes (1797–1804), with plates drawn by Sir Charles Bell, and was at that time an important book. John Bell was also the author of *Engravings explaining the anatomy of the bones, muscles and joints*, Edinburgh [etc.], three volumes, 1794–1804, the third volume of which was almost entirely by Sir Charles; *Discourse on the nature and cure of wounds*, 1795, of which a German translation was published at Leipzig, 1798, and a French translation, Paris, 1825; and *Principles of surgery*, three volumes in four (Vol. I, Edinburgh, Vols.2–3, London) 1801–8, which is valued for the engravings and historical matter. A second edition by Sir Charles appeared in four volumes, London, 1826. John Bell died in Italy, leaving a posthumously published book entitled *Observations on Italy*, Edinburgh, 1825, one of the best travel books by a medical man.

Sir Charles Bell (1774–1842), also of Edinburgh, excelled his elder brother both as artist and surgeon, and was a leading anatomist, physiologist and neurologist. The plates of his books are mainly from his original drawings, and most of his writings went into several editions and translations. Among these the following are of particular note: *A system of dissections* ..., two volumes, Edinburgh, 1798–1803, written while Bell was still a student, which went into a third edition, London, 1809, and was reprinted in Baltimore, 1814; *Engravings of the arteries* ..., London, 1801, 1806, 1811 and 1824 also went into successive American editions from Philadelphia, 1812, 1816 and 1823, and was translated into German (Leipzig, 1819) and into Latin (Leipzig, 1819); *The anatomy of the brain explained in a series of engravings*, London, 1802, containing twelve coloured plates; *A series of engravings explaining the course of the nerves*, London, 1803 and 1816, with American editions, Philadelphia, 1818 and 1834, and a German translation, Leipzig, 1820; *Essays on the anatomy of expression in painting*, 1806, second edition, 1824, third with the title *The anatomy and philosophy of expression as connected with the fine arts*, 1844, and a seventh edition in 1893;[18] *A system of operative surgery* ..., 2 vols, London, 1807–9, second edition, 1814, with American editions from Hartford, 1812 and 1816, and a translation into German, Berlin, 1815; *Idea of a new anatomy of the brain* ... is undated but was privately printed in London in 1811 in an edition of 100 copies for distribution to friends, and copies of this original edition are rare. It expounds Bell's law based on the discovery of one-way traffic in the nerves, and has been reprinted several times, including English and German texts in 1911, 1936 and 1966.[19] His *Letters concerning the diseases of the urethra*, London, 1810 was published in America in the following year, and appeared in a new edition as *Treatise on the diseases of the urethra, vesica urinaria, prostate and rectum*, London, 1820 and 1822, with a German translation from Weimar, 1821, and a Swedish version from Stockholm in 1824; *A dissertation on gun-shot wounds*, London, 1814; *Illustrations of the great operations of surgery* ..., London, 1821, which was translated into German, Leipzig, 1822–3, and Berlin, 1838; *Observations on injuries of the spine and of the thigh bone*, London, 1824; *The nervous system of the human body* ..., London 1830, incorporating his descriptions of 'Bell's nerve' and 'Bell's palsy', and which was translated into German by H. Romberg, Berlin, 1832; *The hand, its mechanism and vital endowments as evincing design*, 1833, a Bridgewater treatise published by William Pickering, three of the engravings in which are copied without acknowledgement from Cheselden's *Osteographia*, 1733;[20] *Institutes of surgery* ..., two volumes, Edinburgh, 1838, with American printings from Philadelphia in 1840 and 1843; *Practical essays*, two volumes, Edinburgh, 1841–2, with a German translation published in Tübingen, 1842; and many other books and articles in journals. Sir Gordon Gordon-Taylor and E. W. Walls have produced an exhaustive biography of Sir Charles Bell, containing lists of biographical material relating to him, and of his writings.[21]

John Abernethy (1764–1831) eventually became Surgeon to St Bartholomew's Hospital, London, but his fame rests rather upon his reputation as a teacher than as a surgeon. He was the virtual founder of the Medical College at Bart's and attracted numerous pupils who became inspired by his manner of presentation. Abernethy was the author of numerous books and articles in journals, and his lectures were published in several forms and editions. These include *Surgical and physiological essays*, two parts, London, 1793, Part 3, 1797; *Surgical observations, containing a classification of tumours* ..., London, 1804, Part 2, 1806; *Surgical observations on the constitutional origin and treatment of local diseases; and on aneurisms*, London, 1809, called by Abernethy 'My Book',[22] to which he frequently referred his patients, and the eleventh edition of which appeared in 1829; *Surgical observations on diseases resembling syphilis* ..., London, 1810, a fifth edition of which was published in 1826; *Surgical observations on injuries of the head* ..., 1810, with a fourth edition in 1825; *Surgical observations on tumours, and on lumbar abscesses*, London, 1811, the fourth edition of which was published in 1825; *An enquiry into the probability and rationality of Mr. Hunter's theory of life ...*, London, 1814; *Physiological lectures ...*, London, 1817 and 1822; *Lectures on anatomy, surgery, and pathology ...*, 1828, based on lectures printed in the *Lancet* and published without authority by James Bulcock, these were followed two years later by the authorized edition with the title *Lectures on the theory and practice of surgery*, London, 1830; and *Surgical and physiological works ...*, four volumes, London, 1830. Further information on these and other writings by John Abernethy are contained in a biography of him.[23]

France found a successor to the immortal Ambroise Paré in Dominique Jean Larrey (1766–1842), who was described by Napoleon as 'the most virtuous man I have ever known'. Larrey was born at Beaudéan, near Bagnères de Bigorre, Hautes Pyrénées, and rose to become Surgeon-in-Chief to the Imperial armies. Larrey first served in the navy, but excelled on the battlefield, operating in the open in an utterly fearless attempt to save lives. He devised the horse-drawn ambulance, and became surgeon-in-chief of the Hôtel des Invalides. In 1826 he visited England, meeting Astley Cooper, Sir Walter Scott and other eminent men on his visits to Dublin, Edinburgh and Glasgow. He was the author of *Mémoires de chirurgie militaire et campagnes*, four volumes, Paris, 1812–17; *Relation médicale de campagnes et voyages de 1815 à 1840*, Paris, 1841; *Relation historique et chirurgicale de l'expédition de l'Armée d'Orient en Egypte et en Syrie*, Paris, 1803; *Clinique chirurgicale exercée particulièrement dans les camps et les hôpitaux militaires, depuis 1792 jusqu'en 1836*, five volumes, Paris, 1830–6; *Mémoire sur l'ophtalmie régnante en Egypte*, Cairo, An IX [1802], which describes ophthalmia, previously unnoticed since being mentioned in the Papyrus Ebers, but which Larrey recognized as contagious;[24] and *Recueil de mémoires de chirurgie*, Paris, 1821. In these writings Larrey initiated several important advances in surgery. He died at Lyons on his way back to Paris from a visit to the hospitals of Algeria.[25]

Sir Astley Paston Cooper (1768–1841), a native of Brook, Norfolk, was surgeon to Guy's Hospital, and the author of a large number of important works on surgery and anatomy which went into several editions. Chief among these are *The anatomy and surgical treatment of inguinal and congenital hernia*, two parts, London, 1804–7, his first and greatest work; (with Benjamin Travers) *Surgical essays*, two volumes, London, 1818–19; *Treatise on gonorrhoea and syphilis*, London, 1821; *The anatomy of the thymus gland*, London, 1832; *Lectures on the principles and practice of surgery*, three volumes, London, 1824–7; *A treatise on dislocations and on fractures of the joints*, London, 1822;[26] *Observations on the structure and diseases of the testis*, London, 1830; *On the anatomy of the breast*, London, 1840; Sir Astley Cooper also contributed many papers to *Guy's Hospital*

Reports and other periodicals, and Sir Geoffrey Keynes has provided a more complete list of his writings, together with details of his career.[27] Benjamin Travers (1783–1858) who had collaborated with Astley Cooper in *Surgical essays*, was also the author of *An inquiry into the process of nature in repairing injuries of the intestine illustrating the treatment of penetrating wounds and strangulated hernia*, London, 1812; *An inquiry concerning that disturbed state of the vital functions usually denominated constitutional irritation*, London, 1826; *A further inquiry ...*, 1834; *A synopsis of diseases of the eye and their treatment*, London, 1820, with a third edition in 1824, and other writings.[28]

John Lizars (1783–1860) was professor of surgery at the University of London, and later at Edinburgh, being a pupil of John Bell. He was author of *A system of anatomical plates of the human body ...*, two volumes, Edinburgh, 1825, containing 110 coloured illustrations from his own dissections; *Observations on extirpation of diseased ovaria*, 1825; *A system of practical surgery*, two volumes, Edinburgh, London, 1838; and *Elements of anatomy ...*, two volumes, Edinburgh, 1844, and numerous other books.

Sir Benjamin Collins Brodie (1783–1862) was born at Winterslow, Wiltshire, and attended Abernethy's anatomical lectures at Bart's before proceeding to the Great Windmill Street school under James Wilson, after which he became a surgical pupil of Everard Home in 1803, and the following year enrolled at St George's. There he eventually became surgeon in 1822, having been elected FRS in 1810. Brodie served as President of the Royal College of Surgeons (1844) and of the Royal Society, 1858, and was appointed Serjeant Surgeon in 1832. From 1808 to 1830 Brodie lectured on surgery at Great Windmill Street and at St George's Hospital. The latter houses several manuscript volumes of his lectures and case books, as does the Royal College of Surgeons, while one is at the Royal Society of Medicine. Brodie was keenly interested in physiology, and conducted experiments on curare. Many of these were published in the *Philosophical Transactions*, and then in his *Physiological researches*, 1851.[29] Brodie was the author of several significant books, including *Pathological and surgical observations on diseases of the joints*, London, 1818, which went into five editions, the last in 1850, with French (Paris, 1819) and German (Hannover, 1821) translations; *Lectures on the diseases of the urinary organs*, London, 1832, with a fourth edition in 1849; *Lectures illustrative of certain local nervous affections*, London, 1837; *Lectures illustrative of various subjects in pathology and surgery*, London, 1846; *Notes on lithotrity*, London, 1853; and the posthumously published *Works ... Collected and arranged by Charles Hawkins*, three volumes, London, 1865.[30]

George James Guthrie (1785–1856) was an English military surgeon who served in America and Europe, and was also a skilled ophthalmic surgeon. His most important contribution to medical literature was *On gunshot wounds of the extremities requiring the different operations of amputation*, London, 1815, which went into six editions, and a German translation, Berlin, 1821. Guthrie was also the author of *A treatise on the operations for the formation of an artificial pupil ...*, London, 1819; *Lectures on the operative surgery of the eye ...*, London, 1823; *On the diseases and injuries of arteries, with the operations required for their cure*, London, 1830; *On the anatomy and diseases of the neck of the bladder and of the urethra*, London, 1834; *On the anatomy and diseases of the urinary and sexual organs ...*, London, 1836; and *On injuries of the head affecting the brain*, London, 1842. Joseph Hodgson (1788–1869) of Birmingham was a lithotomist, but his most important work was *A treatise on the diseases of the arteries and veins ...*, London, 1815, of which a German translation was published at Hannover, 1817, and a French translation, Paris and Montpellier, 1819.

Robert Liston (1794–1847) was born at Ecclesmachon, Linlithgow-shire, and was educated at Edinburgh University before moving in 1816 to London, where he worked at the London Hospital, and attended Abernethy's lectures. After two years he returned to Edinburgh and taught anatomy. In 1828 he applied for the chair of clinical surgery there but James Syme was appointed. In 1834 University College Hospital was opened, and Liston became the first professor of surgery. He was elected FRS in 1841, and became one of the original Fellows of the RCS Eng. Liston was renowned as an operator, but was rather intolerant and quarrelsome. He was the first surgeon in the British Isles to perform a major operation with the patient under an anaesthetic, this taking place on 21 December 1846. Liston's *Elements of surgery*, London, 1831, and *Practical surgery*, London, 1837, were very popular and went into several editions.[31]

Johann Friedrich Dieffenbach (1792–1847) of Königsberg excelled at operative and plastic surgery, and was the author of *Nonnulla de regeneratione et transplantatione*, Würzburg, 1822, his MD thesis; *Die Transfusion des Blutes und die Infusion der Arzeneien in die Blutgefässe*, Berlin, 1828; *Chirurgische Erfahrungen ...*, three volumes in four, Berlin, 1829–34; *Anleitung zur Krankenwartung*, Berlin, 1832; *Über die Durchschneidung der Sehnen und Muskeln*, Berlin, 1841; *Die Heilung des Stotterns ...*, Berlin, 1841, translated into English by Joseph Travers, London, 1841; *Über das Schielen und die Heilung desselben durch eine Operation*, Berlin, 1842; and *Die operative Chirurgie*, two volumes, Leipzig, 1845–8.[32]

Alfred Armand Louis Marie Velpeau (1795–1867) was surgeon to the Hôpital St Antoine (1828–30), La Pitié (1830–4), the Charité (1834–67), and professor of clinical surgery at the Paris Faculty from 1834 until his death. He was a good teacher and brilliant operator, among his chief works being the *Traité élémentaire de l'art des accouchemens ...*, two volumes, Paris, 1829, of which there are many editions and translations into English, Italian and Spanish; *Nouveaux éléments de médecine opératoire* ..., three volumes, Paris, 1832, with a second edition in four volumes, Paris, 1839, and a printing from Brussels, dated 1835, with a translation into Italian in 1833–[5], and into English in 1847; *Traité complet d'anatomie chirurgicale, générale et topographique* ..., Paris, 1823, with English, German and Italian translations and other later editions; *Dans les plaies de tête* ..., Paris, 1834; *Maladies de l'utérus*, Paris, 1854; and his important volume on diseases of the breast, *Traité des maladies du sein et de la région mammaire*, Paris, 1854, which went into numerous editions, including an English translation in 1856.[33]

James Syme (1799–1870) was a native of Edinburgh and became professor of clinical surgery there in 1833. He succeeded Liston at University College, London, in 1847, but soon returned to his former appointment at Edinburgh. Syme was the first in Scotland to amputate at the hip joint, and was an early exponent of anaesthesia and antiseptic surgery. He wrote several books, of which the following were most popular: *Treatise on the excision of diseased joints*, Edinburgh, 1831; *Contributions to the pathology and practice of surgery*, Edinburgh, 1848; *On diseases of the rectum*, Edinburgh, 1838; and *Observations in clinical surgery*, Edinburgh, 1861.[34]

John Hilton (1805–78) was born at Sible Hedingham, Essex, and went to Guy's in 1824, where he became demonstrator of anatomy in 1828. Elected an original FRCS in 1843, Hilton was President in 1867 and was elected FRS in 1839, becoming surgeon at Guy's Hospital in 1849. His writings include *Notes on some of the developmental and functional relations of certain portions of the cranium. Selected by Frederick William Pavy from the lectures on anatomy delivered at Guy's Hospital by John Hilton*, London, 1855; *On the influence of mechanical and physiological rest in the treatment of accidents and surgical diseases and the diagnostic value of pain*, his Arris and Gale lectures of 1860–2, published in 1863, with a second edition entitled *On rest and pain* ..., London, 1877, and a sixth published in 1950. This is recognized as one of the most significant books in the history of orthopaedic surgery, and is still worthy of study as a timeless classic.[35]

The most prominent surgeon in the United States during the period was Samuel David Gross (1805–84), of Easton, Pennsylvania, who was professor of surgery at Louisville, Kentucky, and then at Jefferson Medical College, Philadelphia, where he had graduated. His writings on pathology and surgery are of special value, but he also wrote biographical studies of Daniel Drake, Valentine Mott, Robley Dunglison, John Hunter, Charles Wilkins Short and Ambroise Paré. He left an autobiography, which was published by his sons (two volumes, Philadelphia, 1887). Gross was the author of the following books: *The anatomy, physiology, and diseases of the bones and joints*, Philadelphia, 1830; *Elements of pathological anatomy*, two volumes, Boston, 1839, of which three editions appeared; *An experimental and critical inquiry into the nature and treatment of wounds of the intestines*, Louisville, 1843; *A practical treatise on the diseases, injuries and malformations of the urinary bladder, and prostate gland, and the urethra*, Philadelphia, 1851, second edition, 1855; and third edition, 1876; *On the results of surgical operations in malignant diseases*, Philadelphia, 1853; *Report on Kentucky surgery ...*, Louisville, 1853; *A system of surgery ...*, two volumes, Philadelphia, 1859, of which a sixth edition appeared in 1882; *Lives of eminent American physicians and surgeons of the nineteenth century*, Philadelphia, 1861; and *History of American medical literature from 1776 to the present time*, Philadelphia, 1876.[36]

Sir William Fergusson (1808–77) was born in Preston Pans, Scotland and became a pupil of Robert Knox (1791–1862), and was later his friend and colleague. Fergusson was a keen advocate of conservative surgery, and was surgeon to the Edinburgh Royal Dispensary and the Royal Infirmary, before moving to London, where he was appointed professor of surgery at King's College, London. Fergusson was President of the Royal College of Surgeons of England (1870), and received a baronetcy in 1866. He invented many surgical instruments and was the author of *A system of practical surgery*, London, 1842, of which a fifth edition was published in 1870; and *Lectures on the progress of anatomy and surgery during the present century*, London, 1867. Fergusson's casebooks are preserved at King's College Hospital, London.[37]

Sir James Paget (1814–99), a native of Great Yarmouth, was one of the first English surgical pathologists. He entered St Bartholomew's Hospital in 1834, and the following year, while still a student, discovered *Trichina spiralis*, reading a paper on the subject before the Abernethian Society. He held several important positions at Bart's becoming the first Warden of the Residential College, and Surgeon in 1861, to become President of the Royal College of Surgeons in 1875. Paget wrote numerous articles for periodicals, including two classic descriptions of diseases, with which his name is associated.[38] His first book was written with his brother Charles, and entitled *Sketch of the natural history of Yarmouth and its neighbourhood*, Yarmouth, 1834. He also wrote *Lectures on tumours*, 1851; *Lectures on surgical pathology delivered at the Royal College of Surgeons of England ...*, two volumes, London, 1853, which went into numerous editions; *Clinical lectures and essays. Edited by Howard Marsh*, London, 1875 and 1879; and *Selected essays and addresses. Edited by Stephen Paget*, London, 1902;[39] and *Studies of old case books*, London, New York, 1891. Seven volumes of his manuscript casebooks are in the Medical College Library, St Bartholomew's Hospital, and there is much material relating to him in the Royal College of Surgeons of England, and elsewhere. Sir James Paget's life presents a model of success, achieved through industrious plodding, without making enemies, yet achieving the position of Serjeant

Surgeon to Queen Victoria, among many other honours. Paget was particularly interested in students, and made a study of their later careers.[40] He catalogued the museum at St Bartholomew's Hospital, and extensive sections of that at the Royal College of Surgeons of England.

Another prominent American surgeon was Henry Jacob Bigelow (1818–90) of Boston, Mass., the son of Jacob Bigelow (1787–1879). H. J. Bigelow was surgeon to the Massachusetts General Hospital, and professor of surgery at Harvard Medical School. He was the first in America to excise the hip-joint, and first described the mechanism of the iliofemoral, or Y-ligament in *The mechanism of dislocation and fracture of the hip* ..., Philadelphia, 1869. Bigelow published many important papers, and was a brilliant operator, inventing many surgical instruments. His Boylston Prize Dissertation of 1844 was published as *A manual of orthopedic surgery* ..., Boston, 1845, and he championed W. T. G. Morton's discovery of the use of ether vapour in *Ether and chloroform: a compendium of their history, surgical use, dangers, and discovery*, Boston, 1848. Bigelow was also the author of *Fragments of medical science and art*, 1846; *Surgical anaesthesia: addresses and other papers*, Boston, 1900; and *Orthopedic surgery and other medical papers*, Boston, 1900.[41]

The immortal Joseph Lister (1827–1912) did not publish a book to announce his discoveries, his writings being found mainly in the *Lancet*. He was born at Upton House, Plaistow, was house-surgeon to Syme at Edinburgh, professor of surgery at Glasgow and Edinburgh, before coming to London as professor at King's College in 1877. The story of his career is full of honour and hard work, and is recounted in the biographies by Sir Rickman Godlee and by Douglas Guthrie.[42] Lister applied to surgery the ideas of Louis Pasteur, and his writings in support of antiseptic surgery were numerous. Some of these were published in his *Collected papers*, two volumes, Oxford, 1909, and a list of his writings as first published has been compiled by William LeFanu,[43] while three of his more important papers have been reprinted, with a further list of his works.[44]

Sir Anthony Alfred Bowlby (1855–1929) was connected with St Bartholomew's Hospital throughout his career, becoming full surgeon in 1903, and was also prominent as a military surgeon during the First World War. He wrote very few books, but a large number of papers.[45] His most important contribution to medical literature was *Surgical pathology and morbid anatomy*, London, 1887, an eighth edition of which, revised by Geoffrey Keynes, was published in 1930. Bowlby also wrote *Injuries and diseases of nerves, and their surgical treatment*, London, 1889, and his Bradshaw Lecture, 1915, Jacksonian Prize Essay, 1882, and Astley Cooper Prize Essay, 1886, were also published in book form.

James Parkinson (1755–1824) lived all his life in Hoxton, London, and was the son of John Parkinson, a surgeon. He was interested in social welfare and became actively engaged in politics, writing several anony-

mous and pseudonymous pamphlets on the subject. Parkinson was also
the author of numerous popular writings on medicine, but he is mainly
remembered for his classic description of paralysis agitans, or 'Parkinson's disease'. This was published as *An essay on the shaking palsy*,
London, 1817 and facsimile editions were printed in 1917 by the American
Medical Association, and in 1959 by Dawsons in London.[46] Parkinson
had been a pupil of John Hunter and of James Macartney and his interest
in geology and evolution was revealed in his *Organic remains of a former
world*, three volumes, London, 1804–11, which went into a second edition
in 1833, and was reprinted in 1850. The following are among Parkinson's
other writings: *Dangerous sports*, London, 1800; *Hints for the improvement
of trusses; intended to render their use less inconvenient, and to prevent the
necessity of an understrap* ..., London, 1802; *The hospital pupil; or an essay
intended to facilitate the study of medicine and surgery* ..., London [etc.],
1800; *Observations on the nature and cure of gout*, London, 1805; *Mad-
houses. Observations on the act for regulating mad-houses*, London, 1811;
and *The villager's friend and physician* ..., London, 1800. James Parkinson
was neglected until L. G. Rowntree investigated his life.[47] A biographical
article by E. Graeme Robertson includes the text of the *Essay on the
shaking palsy*, as do the short biography by Christopher Gardner-
Thorpe[48] and the full-scale biography by A. D. Morris.[49]

Daniel Drake (1785–1852) practised at Cincinnati until 1815, when he
went to Philadelphia, and two years later became professor of materia
medica at Transylvania University. He later occupied other chairs,
founded several medical schools, and was keenly interested in medical
education. Drake wrote several books, including *Natural and statistical
view or picture of Cincinnati*, 1815, which was an extension of his earlier
work, *Notices of Cincinnati, its topography, climate and diseases*, 1810; and
*A systematic treatise, historical, etiological and practical, on the principal
diseases of the interior valley of North America, as they appear in the
Caucasian, African, Indian and Esquimaux varieties of its population*, two
volumes, Cincinnati, 1850–5. This 'masterpiece of medico-geographic
research', as it has been called, contains topography, hydrology, socio-
logy, etc., in the first volume, volume two being devoted to the diseases.
Daniel Drake was one of the foremost physicians of his period, and was
closely connected with several early American medical periodicals.[50]

Born near Angoulême in western France, Jean Baptiste Bouillaud
(1796–1881) was professor of clinical medicine in Paris from 1831 to 1876.
Critical of others of the French school such as G. L. Bayle and Laënnec
for their antipathy to theory, he advocated the use of reasoning together
with observation and experimentation in his *Essai sur la philosophie médicale et sur les généralités de la clinique médicale* ..., Paris, 1836. He
identified the anterior lobes as the speech centre and, refuting Gall, he
showed that the brain controls equilibrium, station and progression.

Bouillaud was also the first to describe rheumatic heart disease as a separate clinical and pathological entity in *Nouvelles recherches sur le rhumatisme articulaire aigu en général, et spécialement sur la loi de coïncidence de la péricardite et de l'endocardite avec cette maladie*, Paris, 1836, and *Traité clinique du rhumatisme articulaire, et la loi de coïncidence des inflammations du coeur avec cette maladie*, Paris, 1840. He also wrote *Traité clinique et physiologique de l'encéphalite …*, Paris, 1825; *Clinique médicale de l'Hôpital de la Charité*, 3 vols, Paris, 1837; and *Traité clinique des maladies du coeur, précédé de recherches nouvelles sur l'anatomie et la physiologie de cet organe*, Paris, 1840.[51]

Pierre Fidèle Bretonneau (1778–1862) of Tours contributed an important book on diphtheria, in which he also described the first successful tracheotomy in croup. This is entitled *Des inflammations spéciales du tissu muqueux et en particulier de la diphthérite, ou inflammation pelliculaire*, Paris, 1826. An English translation was included in the New Sydenham Society's *Memoirs on diphtheria …*, London, 1859.[52]

Jean Nicolas Corvisart (1755–1821) was born in the Ardennes region of France and studied in Paris. Under the 1794 general reform of medical teaching in Revolutionary France, the post of professor of internal clinical medicine was created for him at the Hôpital de la Charité. From 1801 Napoleon was his patient and when the First Consul became Emperor, Corvisart was made Surgeon-General. He was among the first to advocate the replacement of empirical methods of diagnosis with more thorough methods and the use of percussion of the chest as a diagnostic method began to grow following his 1808 translation (mentioned in the previous chapter) of Auenbrugger's *Inventum novum …* under the title *Nouvelle méthode pour reconnaître les maladies internes de la poitrine par la percussion de la cavité* (reprinted Paris, 1968, with an essay pp.109–60 by C. Coury ('Auenbrugger, Corvisart et les origines de la percussion'). His magnum opus, *Essai sur les maladies du coeur et des gros vaisseaux*, Paris, 1806, created cardiac symptomatology and advanced the differentiation between cardiac and pulmonary disorders.[53]

A native of Haute Provence, Gaspard Laurent Bayle (1774–1816) studied medicine first at Montpellier and later became the pupil and successor of Corvisart at La Charité in Paris. He was the friend and teacher of Laënnec and is regarded as the theoretician of the early nineteenth-century Parisian pathologic-anatomical school. *Considérations sur la nosologie, la médecine d'observation, et la médecine pratique; suivies de l'histoire d'une maladie gangréneuse non décrite jusqu'à ce jour* was his MD thesis, Paris, 1802 and was reprinted in *Encyclopédie des sciences médicales*, vol.23, Paris, 1838. He is also known for his work on tuberculosis, *Recherches sur la phthisie pulmonaire*, Paris, 1810 (English translation London and Liverpool, 1815), which combined pathological observations on 900 autopsies with clinical work on tuberculosis patients. He also

wrote (with Jean Bruno Cayol) a 150-page article on cancer in *Dictionnaire des sciences médicales*, vol.3, Paris, 1812, and his nephew A. L. J.
Bayle published two volumes of his writings on cancer, *Traité des maladies
cancéreuses*, Paris, 1839.[54]

François Joseph Victor Broussais (1772–1838) from St Malo in Brittany
spent some time in the Service de Santé Militaire before becoming professor and physician at the Val de Grâce, the Paris military hospital and
medical school, where his courses attracted large and enthusiastic classes.
His first book, *Histoire des phlegmasies ou inflammations chroniques*, Paris,
1808, reported clinical observations and autopsy records collected while
he was a physician in Napoleon's armies. Of several expanded editions,
the last appeared in 1838 and an English translation of the fourth was
published in Philadelphia, 1831. His system of physiological medicine,
first proposed in *Examen de la doctrine médicale généralement adoptée*,
Paris, 1816, was highly influential for about two decades in France and in
several countries abroad, but was eventually almost forgotten. In it, the
phenomena of illness differed from those of health only in intensity and
most illnesses were manifestations of inflammation, requiring copious
bleeding for their treatment. Broussais fought the idea of specificity,
localization of contagion and the third edition of the *Examen de la
doctrine médicale généralement adoptée*, Paris, 1829–34, devoted much
space to attacking the anatomic–pathological school of Laënnec and
Bayle. His fellow Breton Laënnec was among his severest critics. In 1822,
he founded the *Annales de la médecine physiologique*, which ran for 12
years, and published a *Traité de physiologie appliquée à la pathologie*.[55]

Pierre Charles Alexandre Louis (1787–1872) taught in Paris, after studying for six years in Russia, and has been called the founder of medical
statistics.[56] His writings were extremely popular, and include *Recherches
anatomico-pathologiques sur la phthisie ...*, Paris, 1825, which was translated into English by Charles Cowan, Boston, 1836; *Mémoires ou
recherches anatomico-pathologiques sur le ramollissement avec la mem-
brane muqueuse de l'estomac ...*, Paris, 1826, a German translation of this
being published in Berlin in 1827; *Recherches anatomiques, pathologiques
et thérapeutiques sur la maladie connue sous les noms de gastro-entérite ...*,
Paris, 1829, a German version being published at Würzburg, 1830, and an
English translation by H. I. Bowditch, two volumes, Boston, 1836;
Recherches sur les effets de la saignée ..., Paris, 1835, with an English
translation by C. G. Putnam, Boston, 1836; and *Anatomical, pathological
and therapeutic researches on the yellow fever of Gibraltar. Translated from
the manuscript, by G. C. Shattuck*, Boston, 1839.

Diseases of the chest received attention from several noteworthy
physicians, and our knowledge of the subject was greatly increased at their
hands. René Théophile Hyacinthe Laënnec (1781–1826) was born at
Quimper, Brittany, and studied medicine at L'Hôtel Dieu, Nantes, and at

L'Ecole de Médecine, Paris under Jean Nicolas Corvisart, who popularized Auenbrugger's discovery of percussion. In 1812 Laënnec became
physician to the Beaujon Hospital, where he specialized in diseases of the
chest. In 1816 he became chief physician to the Necker Hospital, and it
was here that he invented the stethoscope, first using a roll of paper.
Laënnec became professor of medicine at the Collège de France in 1822,
and the following year was appointed professor of internal medicine in the
Paris Faculty. His book on auscultation was first published in 1819 as *De
l'auscultation médiate* ..., two volumes, Paris, a second revised edition
appearing as *Traité de l'auscultation médiate* ..., two volumes, Paris, 1826,
there being at least three other French editions (1831–1837 and 1879), two
Belgian printings (1828 and 1834), seven English editions (1821, 1827,
1829, 1834, 1838, 1846 and 1923), four American printings (Philadelphia,
1823; New York, 1830, 1835 and 1838); three editions of the German
translation (1822, 1832 and 1839), and an Italian version in four volumes,
Livorno, 1833–6. A reprint of the 1821 English translation was published
in New York, 1962, and a translation of selected passages from *De
l'auscultation médiate (first edition)*; with a biography by W. Hale-White,
London, 1923. H. R. Viets[57] has compiled a bibliography of the various
editions of *De l'auscultation médiate*, based on the Henry Barton Jacobs
Collection in Baltimore, which contains all the editions he lists except one.
There were 19 printings between 1819 and 1839 listed in 1929. A biography covering other aspects of Laënnec's life and writings has been published by Roger Kervran,[58] and some of Laënnec's letters have been
published elsewhere.[59]

The great French clinician Armand Trousseau (1801–67) of Tours, was
professor in the Paris Faculty, physician at the Hôpital St Antoine, and at
the Hôtel-Dieu. He contributed many important books to medical literature, including the following: (with Hermann Pidoux), *Traité de thérapeutique et de matière médicale*, two volumes, Paris, 1836–9, which went into
nine French editions, and was translated into English, Italian and Spanish: (with Hippolyte Belloc) *Traité pratique de la phthisie laryngée, de la
laryngite et des maladies de la voix*, Paris, 1837, also translated into
English and German; *Du tubage de la glotte et de la trachéotomie*, Paris,
1859; and *Clinique médicale de L'Hôtel-Dieu de Paris*, two volumes, Paris,
1861, of which there were several editions, including a German translation, Würzburg, 1866, and an English translation published by the New
Sydenham Society, 1868–72.[60]

Richard Bright (1789–1858), a native of Bristol, graduated at Edinburgh and was prominently associated with Guy's Hospital, contributing
numerous important papers to *Guy's Hospital Reports* as well as to *London
Medical Gazette, The Lancet* and *Medico-Chirurgical Transactions*. Bright
wrote on the cerebral nervous system, chorea, sclerosis, hydrocephalus,
abdominal tumours, jaundice, pancreatic diabetes and pancreatic stea-

torrhea, but he is best remembered for his classic description of chronic nephritis, or 'Bright's disease'. This is described in *Reports of medical cases, selected with a view of illustrating the symptoms and cure of disease, by a reference to morbid anatomy*, two volumes [in three], London, 1827–31.[61] Volume one deals mainly with the kidney, the second volume being concerned with the brain and spinal cord. Both volumes contain beautifully coloured illustrations. Bright's writings have been studied bibliographically by William Hill and by G. A. R. Winston.[62] His Edinburgh MD thesis was published as *Disputatio medica inauguralis de erysipitate contagioso* ..., Edinburgh, 1813, and was reprinted about 1928. With Thomas Addison he commenced to write *Elements of practical medicine*, but only one volume of this, dated 1839, was published. It was actually published in sections, part one appearing in 1836, part two in 1837, and the third part, completing the volume, with a title-page to volume one dated 1839. *Clinical memoirs on abdominal tumours and intumescence* was edited by G. Hilaro Barlow, London, 1860, and was reprinted from *Guy's Hospital Reports* and published by the New Sydenham Society. Another selection of Bright's papers was published as *Original papers of Richard Bright on renal disease. Edited by A. Arnold Osman*, London, 1937. Richard Bright travelled extensively through Holland, Belgium, Germany and Hungary, and himself illustrated the account of his travels published as *Travels from Vienna through Lower Hungary, with some remarks on the state of Vienna during the congress in 1814*, Edinburgh, 1818.[63] A publication attributed to Bright by various sources, entitled *Practical observations on the nature and symptoms of dropsy*, 1839, was written by another person bearing the same name.

Thomas Addison (1795–1860) of Long Benton, Cumberland also graduated in Edinburgh, and went to Guy's Hospital as a colleague of Richard Bright. They collaborated in writing *Elements of the practice of medicine* (see above), and this contains an early accurate account of appendicitis.[64] In 1849 Addison read a paper describing pernicious anaemia and disease of the supra-renal capsules, which was expanded into the classic book *On the constitutional and local effects of disease of the supra-renal capsules*, London, 1855.[65] This contains eleven beautifully coloured plates, and describes the condition generally known as 'Addison's disease'. Addison was also the author of numerous papers in *Guy's Hospital Reports*, including several notable contributions to dermatology,[66] *Medico-Chirurgical Transactions*, *London Medical Gazette*, and *Medical Times*. Many of these were published by the New Sydenham Society as *A collection of the published writings of the late Thomas Addison*, London, 1868. He also wrote *An essay on the operation of poisonous agents upon the living body* (jointly with John Morgan), London, 1829; and *Observations on the disorders of females connected with uterine irritation*, London, 1830. A bibliography of Addison's writings has been compiled by G. A. R.

Winston and William Hill, and several articles and one short book deal with his life and works.[67]

The greatest figure in Irish medicine during his period was Robert James Graves (1796–1853), who was physician to the Meath Hospital, Dublin. He was the author of *A system of clinical medicine*, Dublin, 1843, with a second edition published as *Clinical lectures on the practice of medicine*, Dublin, 1848, which went into several other editions, including a French translation, 1862. His description of exophthalmic goitre, which became known as 'Graves' disease', also 'Parry's disease' and 'Basedow's disease', was first published in 1835, but has been reprinted.[68] *Studies in physiology and medicine*, London, 1863, is a selection from his works edited by William Stokes.

William Stokes (1804–78) was a native of Dublin, finally becoming regius professor of medicine at that University. While still a student he published a small treatise, *An introduction to the use of the stethoscope ...*, Edinburgh, 1825, which was followed by *Two lectures on the application of the stethoscope to the diagnosis and treatment of thoracic disease*, Dublin, 1828. These two books formed the basis for his very important *A treatise on the diagnosis and treatment of diseases of the chest. Part I, Diseases of the lung and windpipe*, Dublin, 1837, of which no more parts were published, but which went into many editions. Stokes wrote *The diseases of the heart and aorta*, Dublin, 1854, which also went into several editions; *Lectures on fever ... Edited by John William Moore*, London, 1874; and *The life and labours in art and archaeology of George Petrie*, London, 1868.[69]

George Bodington (1799–1882) of Sutton Coldfield, anticipated many modern views on the advantages of the open-air treatment of tuberculosis of the lungs, but his work received such unfavourable criticism that he was discouraged from fully developing his ideas. Bodington's little book was entitled *An essay on the treatment and cure of pulmonary consumption*, 1840 and was reprinted at Lichfield and London in 1906, with a portrait and obituary notice. The *Essay* was also published by the New Sydenham Society in a volume of *Selected essays*, 1901.[70]

Austin Flint, Senior (1812–86) of Petersham, Massachusetts, was a pioneer in cardiology, and in auscultation and percussion. His books include *Clinical reports on continued fever ...*, Buffalo, 1852, and Philadelphia, 1855; *Physical exploration and diagnosis of diseases affecting the respiratory organs*, Philadelphia, 1856, which went into several editions; *A practical treatise on the diagnosis, pathology, and treatment of diseases of the heart*, Philadelphia, 1859; *A treatise on the principles and practice of medicine ...*, Philadelphia, 1866, of which several editions were published; and *Phthisis ...*, Philadelphia, 1875. His paper 'On cardiac murmurs', published in *American Journal of Medical Science*, 44, 1862, was reprinted by the same journal in vol.265, 1973, pp.236–55.[71]

Thomas Hodgkin (1798–1866) was born at Tottenham and graduated at Edinburgh in 1823. He lectured on pathology at Guy's Hospital, and in 1832 contributed the classic description of lymphadenoma, later known as 'Hodgkin's disease'.[72] He also contributed an excellent account of aortic insufficiency. ('On the retroversion of the valves of the aorta', *London Medical Gazette*, 3 (1828–9) pp.433–43). Hodgkin was the author of *Hints relating to cholera in London* ..., London, 1832; *Lectures on the morbid anatomy of the serous and mucous membranes*, two volumes, London, 1836–40, which was translated into German, Leipzig, 1843–4; and *Narrative of a journey to Morocco in 1863 and 1864*, London, 1866. Hodgkin was a Quaker, and died in Jaffa in 1866 while engaged on philanthropic work.[73]

John Conolly (1794–1866), who was born at Market Rasen, Lincolnshire, graduated MD Edinburgh with an inaugural dissertation entitled *De statu mentis in insania et melancholia*, 1821. He became professor of medicine at University College, then newly founded as the University of London, in 1828, and in 1839 took charge of the Middlesex Asylum at Hanwell. Conolly was a pioneer in the humane treatment of the mentally sick, and was the author of *An inquiry concerning the indications of insanity, with suggestions for the better protection and care of the insane*, London, 1830, which was reprinted in facsimile in 1964, with annotations and an introduction by Richard Hunter and Ida Macalpine, who have similarly reproduced Conolly's *The construction and government of lunatic asylums and hospitals*, London, 1847 (London, 1968) and *The treatment of the insane without mechanical restraint*, London, 1856 (Folkestone, 1973). His Croonian lectures ('On some of the forms of insanity') at the Royal College of Physicians, 1849, printed in *The Lancet* and then reprinted in book form, London, 1849, were reprinted by St Bernard's Hospital, Southall, in 1960.[74] He was the author of several other writings, including the anonymous *An address to parents, on the present state of vaccination in this country ... By a Candid Observer*, London, 1822, a clue to the authorship of which is contained in his *Observations on vaccination, and on the practice of inoculating for the small-pox* ..., Stratford-Upon-Avon, 1824.[75]

Franz Joseph Gall (1758–1828) was born near Pforzheim in Baden, Germany, began his medical studies in Strasbourg and graduated MD in Vienna in 1785. His first work *Philosophischmedizinische Untersuchungen über Natur and Kunst im kranken und gesunden Zustand des Menschen*, Vol.1, Vienna, 1791 (vol.2 never published), deals mainly with practical medicine. With his co-worker Johann Christoph Spurzheim (1776–1832), he founded 'organology', generally known as phrenology, to establish an anatomy and physiology of the brain and a new psychology. Prevented by the Austrian Emperor from lecturing at the university, Gall and Spurzheim left Vienna and eventually settled in Paris, where Gall spent the remainder of his life. Although their ideas on the functions of the separate parts of the brain were controversial and are often regarded as misconceived nowadays, their investigations gave considerable impetus to the study of neuroanatomy. They published *Anatomie et physiologie du système nerveux ...*, 4 vols, Paris, 1810–19, and *Sur les fonctions du cerveau et sur celles de chacune de ses parties*, 6 vols, Paris, 1822–5 (English translation by W. Lewis, Boston, 1835). George Combe translated selections from Gall and others in *On the functions of the cerebellum by Drs Gall, Vimont and Broussais*, Edinburgh, 1838. J. L. Choulant, *Vorlesungen über die Cranioscopie*, Dresden, Leipzig, 1844, contains a nearly complete bibliography of publications for and against Gall before 1840.[76]

Marshall Hall (1790–1857) was born at Basford near Nottingham in the English midlands and received his MD from the University of Edinburgh in 1812. While practising medicine in Nottingham, 1816–24, he published *On diagnosis*, London, 1817, a revised version of part 1, 1822 (2nd edn with the title *The principles of diagnosis*, 2 vols in 1, London, 1833–4) and *On the mimoses ...*, London, 1818, 2nd edn with the title *A descriptive, diagnostic and practical essay on disorders of the digestive organs and general health*, London, 1820. He moved to London in 1826, but held no hospital appointment there, and his work on the physiology of the vascular and nervous systems, particularly the reflex function was more accepted abroad than in Britain. He introduced the term 'reflex' in his paper in *Phil. Trans. Roy. Soc.*, 123 (1833) pp.635–65, 'On the reflex function of the medulla oblongata and the medulla spinalis'. His other works included *Memoirs on the nervous system*, London, 1837; *New memoir on the nervous system*, London, 1843; *On the diseases and derangements of the nervous system, in their primary forms and in their modifications by age, sex, constitution, hereditary predisposition, excesses, general disorder, and organic disease*, London, 1841; *Synopsis of cerebral and spinal seizures of inorganic origin and of paroxysmal form as a class; and of their pathology as involved in the structures and actions of the neck*, London, [1851]; *Principles and theory of the practice of medicine, including a third edition of the author's work on diagnosis*, London, 1837; *Commentaries on some of the more important diseases of females*, London, 1827, 2nd edn 1830; *Prone and postural respiration in drowning and other forms of apnoea or suspended respiration*, edited by his son Marshall Hall, London, 1857.[77]

Marie Jean Pierre Flourens (1794–1867) was born near Béziers in southern France and studied medicine in Montpellier and Paris. Eventually he left clinical medicine to devote himself to physiological research, notably on the nervous system and brain function. He introduced the idea of coordination and the importance of its role in nervous physiology. His conclusions were often expressed in an authoritarian manner, however, with insufficient caution or comparison of his experimental results with those of others. His books reveal the range of his interests: *Recherches expérimentales sur les propriétés et fonctions du système nerveux dans les animaux vertébrés*, Paris, 1824 (2nd edn, 1842); *Expériences sur le système nerveux ... faisant suite aux Recherches expérimentales ...*, Paris, 1825; *Cours sur la génération, l'ovologie et l'embryologie*, Paris, 1836; *Histoire de la découverte de la circulation du sang*, Paris, 1854 (2nd edn, 1857), which was translated into English; *Cours de physiologie comparée*, Paris, 1856; *De l'instinct et de l'intelligence des animaux. De la vie de l'intelligence*, Paris, 1858. In *Examen de la phrénologie*, Paris, 1842, he opposed Gall's ideas, and he repudiated every idea of localization in the brain. *Examen du livre de M. Darwin sur l'origine des espèces*, Paris, 1864, revealed him an opponent of Darwin's theory of evolution.[78]

Pierre Paul Broca (1824–80) was born near Bordeaux and became surgeon to the Necker Hospital and, in 1868, professor of clinical surgery in the Paris Faculty of Medicine. He made important contributions to anatomy, pathology, surgery, cerebral function and anthropology, but is probably best known for his role in the discovery of cerebral localization, a concept that began with the phrenologists but was denied by Flourens and those who were influenced by his ideas. From 1850 to his death Paul Broca produced 223 papers and monographs. Among the monographs are *De l'étranglement dans les hernies abdominales et des affections qui peuvent le simuler*, Paris, 1853 (2nd edn, 1856); *Des anévrismes et de leur traitement*, Paris, 1856; and *Traité des tumeurs*, 2 vols, Paris, 1866–9. *Atlas d'anatomie descriptive du corps humain*, edited by Broca, C. Bonamy and E. Beau, Paris, 1844–66, includes vol.3, *La splanchnologie* by Broca. A selection of his papers, *Mémoires sur le cerveau de l'homme et des primates*, ed. S. Pozzi, was published Paris, 1888, and a translation into English of his 1865 report, 'Localization of speech in the third left frontal convolution' appeared in 1986.[79]

The eminent French neurologist Jean Martin Charcot (1825–93) was also a pioneer in psychotherapy. A native of Paris, he was associated with the Salpêtrière from 1862, and became professor of pathological anatomy, and later professor of clinical neurology at the Faculty of Medicine. He was the author of a number of significant writings, including *Leçons sur les maladies des vieillards et les maladies chroniques*, Paris, 1867, which was translated into English by William S. Tuke, and published by the New Sydenham Society in 1881; *Leçons sur les maladies du système nerveux faites à La Salpêtrière*, five volumes, Paris, also published by the New Sydenham Society in English, three volumes, 1877–89; *Leçons sur les localisations des maladies du cerveau*, Paris, 1876, translated into English by Edward P. Fowler, New York, 1878, and by William Baugh Hadden, New Sydenham Society, 1883; *Leçons sur les maladies du foie, des voies biliaires et des reins*, Paris, 1877; (with Paul Marie Louis Pierre Richer), *Les démoniaques dans l'art*, Paris, 1887; *Oeuvres complètes*, nine volumes, Paris, 1888–94; *Les difformés et les malades dans l'art*, Paris, 1889; and (with Jean Albert Pitres), *Les centres moteurs corticaux chez l'homme*, Paris, 1895. Georges Guillain has contributed an authoritative biography of Charcot, which contains a list of his writings available in English translations.[80]

Friedrich Theodor von Frerichs (1819–85) of Aurich was a graduate of Göttingen, where he became professor, before proceeding to Kiel, Breslau and Berlin successively. He contributed numerous articles to periodicals, and was the author of a book on Bright's disease, *Die Bright'sche Nierenkrankheit und deren Behandlung*, Braunschweig, 1851; on diseases of the liver, *Klinik der Leberkrankheiten*, two volumes and atlas, Braunschweig, 1858–61, which was translated into English by Charles Murchison, and published by the New Sydenham Society, two volumes, 1860–1, with an American edition in three volumes, New York, 1879; and *Ueber der Diabetes*, Berlin, 1884, of which a French translation was published at Paris in 1885.

A native of Hythe, Charles Hilton Fagge (1838–83) became physician to Guy's Hospital, and was distinguished in pathology, dermatology and cardiology. His textbook, *The principles and practice of medicine*, two volumes, London, 1886, was completed after his death by Philip Henry Pye-Smith (1840–1914) and Sir Samuel Wilks (1824–1911). A fourth edition was published in 1901. Fagge translated Hebra's *On diseases of the skin*, two volumes, 1866–8 for the Sydenham Society. Ferdinand von Hebra (1816–80) was born in Moravia, studied medicine in Vienna, and became assistant to Josef Skoda (1805–81). Hebra contributed original descriptions of several conditions, and he devised a classification of skin diseases based on their pathological anatomy. His *Atlas der Hautkrankheiten* was published in ten parts, Vienna, 1856–76.[81]

Another eminent dermatologist, Sir William James Erasmus Wilson (1809–84), lectured on anatomy and physiology at Middlesex Hospital, and endowed a chair of dermatology at the Royal College of Surgeons of England, to which he was appointed. He was a keen philanthropist, and was responsible for the transport of Cleopatra's Needle to this country. Erasmus Wilson was the author of numerous books and papers, and a list of these is included in a biographical study by R. M. Hadley.[82] They include *Practical and surgical anatomy*, London, 1838; *The anatomist's vade mecum ...*, London, 1839, which went into an eighth edition in 1861; *A practical and theoretical treatise on the diagnosis, pathology and treatment of diseases of the skin ...*, London, 1842, which went into several editions; *Lectures on dermatology delivered at the Royal College of Surgeons of England, 1876–1878 ...*, 1878; *A history of the Middlesex Hospital during the first century of its existence*, 1845; *Healthy skin: a popular treatise on the skin and hair ...*, 1845, seventh edition, 1866, and an Italian translation published in 1855; *On ringworm ...*, 1847; and *Portraits of diseases of the skin*, 1855.

Puerperal fever was greatly to be feared in midwifery, and several authors wrote on the subject without effectively proving its nature and cause. John Burton (1697–1771) in his book *An essay towards a complete new system of midwifery* ..., London, 1751; John Leake (1729–92) in his *Practical observations on the child-bed fever*, London, [1772]; Charles White (1728–1813) in *A treatise on the management of pregnant and lying-in-women*, London, 1773; and particularly Alexander Gordon (1752–99) in *A treatise on the epidemic puerperal fever of Aberdeen*, London, 1795 all contributed to the solution of the problem of puerperal fever without convincing the world. This was left to Ignaz Semmelweis and Oliver Wendell Holmes (1809–94). The latter is more generally known as a poet, but he was also a physician and anatomist of repute. Born at Cambridge, Mass., Holmes graduated from Harvard in 1829; he taught anatomy and physiology there for many years, and was also attached to Massachusetts General Hospital. In 1843 Holmes lectured to the Boston Society for Medical Improvement on *The contagiousness of puerperal fever*, a lecture which was afterwards published in a periodical.[83] This was enlarged and published in book form as *Puerperal fever, as a private pestilence*, Boston, 1855.[84] Ignaz Philipp Semmelweis (1818–65) was a native of Budapest, and spent his life studying the causes of child-bed fever. In 1855 he became the professor of midwifery at Pesth University, and first proclaimed his doctrine of the cause of puerperal fever while in Vienna in 1847. But he wrote nothing to advance his claims until 1857, when he decided to prepare a book on the subject. This was published as *Die Aetiologie, der Begriff und die Prophylaxis des Kindbettfiebers*, Budapest, Vienna and Leipzig, 1861.[85] Unfortunately Semmelweis was ridiculed for his efforts, and became insane as the result of persecution. He died in an asylum in Vienna following a dissection wound. Yet his work on puerperal fever was perhaps more thorough and convincing than any previously attempted, as is conveyed by the biography by Sir William J. Sinclair.[86] The writings of Semmelweis were issued as *Gesammelte Werke* ..., Jena, 1905, and a bibliography of his writings, and of literature on puerperal fever up to 1949, has been compiled by Frank P. Murphy.[87]

Sir James Young Simpson (1811–70) was a native of Bathgate, Scotland, and became professor of obstetrics at Edinburgh in 1840. He invented several new instruments, introduced iron wire sutures, the long obstetric forceps, the uterine sound, the sponge tent, and made valuable contributions to archaeology and the history of medicine. But, above all, Simpson is remembered as the first to use chloroform in midwifery, and he wrote many papers on the subject. Most of his scattered writings were collected together in *Obstetric memoirs and contributions ... Edited by W. O. Priestley and Horatio R. Storer*, two volumes, Edinburgh, 1855–6; *Selected obstetrical and gynaecological works ... Edited by J. Watt Black*, Edinburgh, 1871; *Anaesthesia, hospitalism, hermaphroditism, and a propo-*

sal to stamp out small-pox and other contagious diseases ... *Edited by Sir W. G. Simpson,* Edinburgh, 1871; and *Clinical lectures on the diseases of women ... Edited by Alexander R. Simpson*, Edinburgh, 1872. Sir James Simpson was also the author of *Archaeological essays ...*, two volumes, 1872, and *Acupressure ...*, Edinburgh, 1864.[88]

James Marion Sims (1813–83) was born at Lancaster, South Carolina, and graduated at Jefferson Medical College in 1835. In 1849 he operated successfully for vesico-vaginal fistula, and three years later published the results of his cases in the *American Journal of the Medical Sciences*.[89] Sims became chief of the Women's Hospital of the State of New York when it was opened in 1855, and later visited Europe. He wrote *Clinical notes on uterine surgery ...*, London, and also New York, 1866, while residing in England, the book going into several editions, including a German translation. Sims also wrote *The story of my life ... Edited by his son, H. Marion Sims*, New York, 1884, and 1888.[90]

Sir Thomas Spencer Wells (1818–97) of St Albans, served in the Navy following qualification, but left the service in 1848. He practised as an ophthalmic surgeon, and then became surgeon to the Samaritan Hospital. Spencer Wells is recognized as a pioneer of abdominal surgery, and he perfected the operation of ovariotomy. Among his numerous writings, a list of which has been compiled,[91] the following books are of special interest: *Practical observations on gout ...*, London, 1854; *Diseases of the ovaries ...*, two volumes, London, 1865–72, which went into several editions, including a German translation, Leipzig, 1874; *Notebook for cases of ovarian and other abdominal tumours*, London, 1865; *On ovarian and uterine tumours ...*, London, 1882; and *Diagnosis and surgical treatment of abdominal tumours*, London, 1885, which also appeared in several editions. John A. Shepherd has written an invaluable biography of Spencer Wells.[92]

Another eminent gynaecologist, Robert Lawson Tait (1845–99) was born in Edinburgh but settled in Birmingham in 1871. He possessed wonderful skill as an operator and, although an opponent of Lister, had remarkably good results from his operations. Lawson Tait wrote several books, in addition to numerous articles in periodicals, the more important being his *Diseases of women ...*, London, 1877; *General summary of conclusions from one thousand cases of abdominal section*, Birmingham, 1884; and *Lectures on ectopic pregnancy and pelvic haematocele*, Birmingham, 1888.[93]

Ophthalmology progressed at the hands of Frans Cornelis Donders (1818–89) of Tilburg, Holland, who commenced his professional career as an army surgeon, but from 1862 confined his attention to physiology and ophthalmology. His greatest work was first published by the New Sydenham Society as *On the anomalies of accommodation and refraction of the eye*, London, 1864, the English version being that of William Daniel

Moore. Donders was the author of a large number of publications, mostly in Dutch, but the more important have appeared in English, French and German translations, and include a volume on the physiology of stuttering, *De physiologie der spraakklanken* ..., Utrecht, 1870.[94]

Sir William Paget Bowman (1816–92) made important contributions to anatomy and physiology, before confining himself entirely to ophthalmology. He made useful improvements in operative technique and was the author of *Lectures on the parts concerned in the operations on the eye, and on the structure of the retina* ..., London, 1849. Bowman's *Collected papers* ..., London, 1892, were published in two volumes.[95]

Friedrich Wilhelm Ernst Albrecht von Graefe (1828–70) of Berlin, has been described as the 'greatest of all eye surgeons'. He was a professor at Berlin University, and in 1854 founded the *Archiv für Ophthalmologie*, which contains most of his writings. Von Graefe also wrote, among others, *Symptomenlehre der Augenmuskellähmungen*, Berlin, 1867; and *Klinische Vorträge über Augenheilkunde* ..., Berlin, 1871.[96]

The inventor of the ophthalmoscope, Hermann Ludwig Ferdinand von Helmholtz (1821–94) was a native of Potsdam, and served for a time as an army surgeon. He held chairs of anatomy, physiology and pathology at various universities, finally taking the chair of physics at Berlin, and from 1871 Helmholtz devoted himself entirely to physics. He invented several optic instruments, and his writings on physiological optics include *Beschreibung eines Augen-spiegels zur Untersuchung der Netzhaut in lebenden Auge*, Berlin, 1851, which was translated into English by Thomas Hall Shastid, Chicago, 1916; *Ueber die Erhaltung der Kraft* ..., Berlin, 1847; *Die Lehre von den Tonempfindungen als physiologische Grundlage für die Theorie der Musik*, Braunschweig, 1863, which went into several editions, including a French translation, and an English translation by A. J. Ellis, 1875, with a second edition in 1885, and a reprint, New York, 1954; *Handbuch der physiologischen Optik*, Leipzig, 1867; and *Wissenschaftliche Abhandlungen*, Leipzig, 1882–95.[97]

Physiology attracted the attention of several eminent French scientists during the nineteenth century,[98] and it also made progress in certain other countries, but Magendie and Claude Bernard were supreme at the heights of their careers. François Magendie (1783–1855) was born at Bordeaux, but graduated and lived most of his life in Paris. His early interest was in pharmacology, upon which subject he presented several memoirs to the Academy of Sciences, but he also dabbled in anatomy and surgery before renouncing these to take up medicine and experimental physiology. In 1826 Magendie went to the Salpêtrière, until 1830, when he removed to the Hôtel-Dieu. In 1831 he occupied the chair of medicine at the Collège de France. Magendie wrote a large number of articles, and he founded and edited the *Journal de Physiologie expérimentale*, 1821–31. His more important books include the following: *Précis élémentaire de physiologie*, two volumes, Paris, 1816–17 (second edition, 1823, third edition 1834, and fourth edition 1836, this latter being a reprint of the third, which was destroyed by fire) translated into English by John Revere (Baltimore, 1822), by E. Milligan (Philadelphia, 1824), into German, two volumes, Tübingen, 1826, while a French edition published in Brussels contains some plates from Jules Cloquet's atlas instead of Magendie's illustrations; *Recherches physiologiques et médicales sur les causes, les symptômes et le traitement de la gravelle*, Paris, 1818, translated into German, Leipzig, 1820 and 1830, and into Dutch, Rotterdam, [n.d.]; *Leçons sur le choléra morbus ...*, Paris, 1832; *Leçons sur les fonctions et les maladies du système nerveux, professées au Collège de France*, Paris, 1839–41; *Phénomènes physiques de la vie ...*, Paris, 1842; and *Recherches physiologiques et cliniques sur le liquide céphalo-rachidien ou cérébro-spinal*, Paris, 1842.[99]

Claude Bernard (1813–78) was a pupil of Magendie, and is considered to be the founder of experimental medicine. He became 'interne' to Magendie in 1839, and subsequently held the position of physician to the Hôtel-Dieu, later becoming professor of medicine at the Collège de France. Bernard gave private lectures and conducted research, the results of his experiments being communicated to scientific societies, and many of his articles appeared in the *Comptes rendus de la Société de Biologie*. His work on the digestive and vasomotor systems was of particular importance, for he discovered glycogen,[100] investigated the vasomotor nerves, and the action of the pancreatic juice. Bernard wrote extensively in journals, and the following books represent his more important items: *Nouvelle fonction du foie considéré comme organe producteur de matière sucrée chez l'homme et les animaux*, Paris, 1853, which was translated into German, Würzburg, 1853; *Leçons de physiologie expérimentale appliquée à la médecine ...*, two volumes, Paris, 1855–6; *Mémoire sur le pancréas et sur le rôle du suc pancréatique dans les phénomènes digestifs, particulièrement dans la digestion des matières grasses neutres*, Paris, 1856; *Leçons sur les effets des substances toxiques et medicamenteuses*, Paris, 1857; *Leçons sur la physiologie et la pathologie du système nerveux*, two volumes, Paris, 1858; *Leçons sur les propriétés physiologiques et les altérations pathologiques des liquides de l'organisme*, two volumes, Paris, 1859; *Introduction à l'étude de la médecine expérimentale*, Paris, 1865, translated into English by Henry Copley Greene, New York, 1927, and reprinted in facsimile in 1949, and which was intended to be an introduction to a larger 'Principles' which never appeared; *Leçons sur les propriétés des tissus vivants. Recueillies, rédigées et publiées par Émile Alglave*, Paris, 1866; *Leçons de pathologie expérimentale*, Paris, 1872; *Leçons sur les anesthétiques et sur l'asphyxie*, Paris, 1875; *Leçons sur la chaleur animale, sur les effets de la chaleur et sur la fièvre*, Paris, 1876;[101] *Leçons sur le diabète et la glycogénèse animale*, Paris, 1877; *La science expérimentale*, Paris, 1878; *Leçons sur les phénomènes de la vie communs aux animaux et aux végétaux*, two volumes, Paris, 1878–9; and *Leçons de physiologie opératoire*, Paris, 1879.[102]

Charles Édouard Brown-Séquard (1817–94) was a native of the Isle of Mauritius, and studied in Paris under Claude Bernard, before occupying the chair of physiology at Harvard in 1864. He later became professor of pathology at L'École de Médecine, Paris, practised as a physician in New York and London, and finally succeeded Bernard at L'École de Médecine. Brown-Séquard was a neurologist who became interested in endocrinology in his later years, and was the author of *Experimental researches applied to physiology and pathology*, New York, 1853; *Courses of lectures on the physiology and pathology of the central nervous system* ..., Philadelphia, 1860; and *Lectures on the diagnosis and treatment of the principal forms of paralysis of the lower extremities*, London, 1861.[103]

Although he was not trained as a laboratory physiologist, William Beaumont's experiments on gastric juice through a gastric fistula in the half-breed Alexis St Martin, rank him as a pioneer in the physiology of digestion. William Beaumont (1785–1853) of Connecticut, was a United States Army Surgeon, and in 1822 attended St Martin, who had been wounded by the accidental discharge of a rifle. The wound healed, leaving a fistula through into the stomach, and Beaumont conducted his experiments by this means. In 1824 he sent a complete report on the case to Surgeon General Lovell, who sent it to the *Medical Recorder*, and it was printed in 1825 under the name of Joseph Lovell by mistake. Lovell stimulated and advised Beaumont throughout his work, and their correspondence has been investigated by Estelle Brodman.[104] Beaumont later published his observations in book-form as *Experiments and observations on the gastric juice, and the physiology of digestion*, 1833, which was printed on thin paper by S. P. Allen of Plattsburgh, the sale of the edition being placed in the hands of Lilly, Wait & Co., of Boston. In 1838, Andrew Combe published a British edition at Edinburgh, while a second edition of the American imprint was published by Chauncey Goodrich at Burlington, Vermont, 1847. This second edition bears on the title-page the words 'Corrected by S. Beaumont, M.D.' Samuel Beaumont, cousin of William, endeavoured in vain to suppress this, as he had certainly not made any corrections, but had merely looked through the script. A facsimile of the first edition, with a biography of Beaumont by Sir William Osler, was issued in 1929, and a German translation was published in Leipzig in 1834. Jesse S. Myer wrote a reliable memoir of William Beaumont, which gives full details of his life, experiments and writings.[105] Beaumont's pioneer work soon received recognition in England,[106] Germany, France and Russia, and in the United States was eventually followed up by Walter B. Cannon, Walter C. Alvarez, Anton J. Carlson, and Arno B. Luckhardt, who persuaded Beaumont's heirs to give certain mementoes to the University of Chicago. The bulk of Beaumont's notes and records had previously been deposited in Washington University School of Medicine Library, St Louis, Missouri.[107]

Jan Evangelista Purkyně (Johann Purkinje) (1787–1869), eminent Czech scientist, physiologist and pioneer in the use of the microscope held successively several chairs of physiology. In 1842 the Prussian Government erected for him a Physiology Institute at Breslau, but eight years later he returned to Prague. Purkinje contributed many important papers to periodicals, and the results of much of his research are contained in the dissertations by his students. His inaugural dissertation on subjective visual phenomena was published as *Beiträge zur Kenntniss des Sehens in subjectiver Hinsicht*, Prague, 1819, and Purkinje was also the author of *Beobachtungen und Versuche zur Physiologie der Sinne ...*, Prague, 1823; *Commentatio de examine physiologico organi visus et systematis cutanei ...*, Breslau [1823], the first study of finger-prints; *Subjectae sunt symbolae ad ovi historiam ante incubationem ...*, Breslau [1825], containing the first description of the germinal vesicle in the embryo; and his works were collected together and printed as *Opera omnia*, volumes one to five, Prague, 1918–51, and *Opera selecta*, Prague, 1948.[108]

Johannes Peter Müller (1801–58) of Coblenz has been called the founder of scientific medicine in Germany and the greatest German physiologist of his period, while he was also keenly interested in biology, comparative morphology, and pathology. He founded the *Archiv für Anatomie, Physiologie, und wissenschaftliche Medicin* in 1834, and contributed numerous papers to this and other periodicals. His books include *De respiratione foetus ...*, Leipzig, 1823; *Zur vergleichenden Physiologie des Gesichtssinnes ...* Leipzig, 1826; *Über die phantastischen Gesichtserscheinungen ...*, Coblenz, 1826; *Bildungsgeschichte der Genitalien ...*, Düsseldorf, 1830; *De glandularum secernentium structura penitiori ...*, Leipzig, 1830; *Handbuch der Physiologie des Menschen für Vorlesungen*, two volumes, Coblenz, 1834–40, which was translated into French and English; *Über den feinern Bau und die Formen der krankhaften Geschwülste*, Berlin, 1838; and *Untersuchungen über die Eingeweide der Fische*, Berlin, 1845.[109]

Eduard Friedrich Wilhelm Pflüger (1829–1910) was professor of physiology at Bonn, and in 1868 founded the *Archiv für die gesamte Physiologie*, which is still published as *Pflügers Archiv*. To this journal Pflüger contributed most of his important articles, and he also introduced many new physiological instruments. His books include *Die sensorischen Funktionen des Rückenmarks der Wirbelthiere ...*, Berlin, 1853; *Untersuchungen über die Physiologie der Electrotonus*, Berlin, 1859; and *Über die Eierstöcke der Saügethiere und des Menschen*, Leipzig, 1863.

Sir Michael Foster (1836–1907) was one of the pioneers of British physiology, and was professor of physiology at Cambridge. His more important writings include *The elements of embryology*, London, 1874, written with Francis M. Balfour, a second edition appearing in 1883, and of which a French translation by E. Rochefort was published in Paris in 1877; *A course of elementary practical physiology*, London, 1878, written with John Newport, with a French translation by F. Prieur, Paris, 1886; *A textbook of physiology*, London, 1876, of which seven editions were printed, with translations into German, Italian and Russian; *Claude Bernard*, London, 1899, in the Masters of Medicine series; and *Lectures on the history of physiology during the sixteenth, seventeenth and eighteenth centuries*, Cambridge, 1901, reprinted New York, 1970.[110]

The leading figure in German physiology in the second half of the century was Carl Ludwig (1816–95). He was born at Witzenhausen in central Germany and studied at more than one German university before graduating in medicine at Marburg. He taught at Zurich and Giessen and in 1865 accepted the new chair of physiology at Leipzig. His chemical laboratory and physiological institute were regarded as models, and among his friends and companions in the creation of modern physiology were Helmholtz and Du Bois-Reymond. Where instruments were lacking he developed them, for example the kymograph for recording variations in fluid pressure. It is said that at the time of his death almost every physiologist who was active had at some juncture studied with him. Among his more important publications were *Lehrbuch der Physiologie des Menschen*, 2 vols, Heidelberg, 1852–6 (2nd edn 1858–61), the first modern textbook of physiology, and *Die physiologischen Leistungen des Blutdrucks*, Leipzig, 1865.[111].

Emil Heinrich Du Bois-Reymond (1818–96) was born in Berlin into a family which came from Neuchâtel in Switzerland. He studied under Schwann, Schleiden and Johannes Müller and was a friend of Ludwig and Helmholtz. In 1858, on the death of Müller, he became professor of physiology in Berlin. His principal research interest was in the electrical phenomena thought to be involved in various life processes and his first paper on the subject was published in 1843. *Untersuchungen über thierische Elektricität*, 2 vols in 3, Berlin, 1848–84, collected his writings on this theme. Extracts from it were translated into English by his friend Henry Bence Jones and published under the title *On animal electricity, being an abstract of the discoveries of Emil Du Bois-Reymond*, London, 1852, and the American Charles E. Morgan's *Electrophysiology and therapeutics*, New York, 1868, contained most of it, translated and rearranged with additional material of later date. Du Bois-Reymond's *Abhandlungen zur allgemeinen Muskel- und Nervenphysik*, 2 vols, Leipzig, 1875–7, consisted mainly of papers published previously in journals. He edited the physiological section of *Archiv für Anatomie, Physiologie und wissenschaftliche Medizin*.[112]

In France the most eminent student of electricity in physiology and medicine was Guillaume Benjamin Amand Duchenne de Boulogne (1806–

75). His examination of the electrophysiology of the muscular system and the application of his results to pathological conditions made him the founder of electrotherapy. His ideas and experiments were published in *De l'électrisation localisée et de son application à la physiologie, à la pathologie et à la thérapeutique*, Paris, 1855 (atlas 1862) (2nd edn 1861, 3rd edn 1872); *Mécanisme de la physionomie humaine, ou analyse électro-physiologique de l'expression des passions*, Paris, 1862; and *Physiologie des mouvements démontrée à l'aide de l'expérimentation électrique et de l'observation clinique, et applicable à l'étude des paralysies et des déformations*, Paris, 1867. The New Sydenham Society published *Selections from the clinical works of Dr Duchenne (de Boulogne)*; translated, edited and condensed by G. V. Poore, London, 1883.[113]

Étienne-Jules Marey (1830–1904) is notable for his adoption and advocacy of the two techniques in experimental physiology of graphic recording and cinematography. Born at Beaune, he studied medicine in Paris, at the Hôpital Côchin, and wrote his dissertation on the circulation of the blood using recording instruments which were modified versions of those developed by Carl Ludwig. In his early work he sought to apply his methods and results to pathology and clinical diagnosis and aimed to simplify instruments so that they could be used by the clinical diagnostician. After 1868, when he accepted the chair of 'natural history of organized bodies' at the Collège de France, in succession to Flourens, he concentrated on the study of human and animal locomotion. He wrote over 150 scientific papers and among his monographs were *Recherches sur le pouls au moyen d'un nouvel appareil enregistreur, le sphygmographe*, Paris, 1860; *Physiologie médicale de la circulation du sang, basée sur l'étude graphique des mouvements du cœur et du pouls artériel avec application aux maladies de l'appareil circulatoire*, Paris, 1863; *Du mouvement dans les fonctions de la vie*, Paris, 1868; *La machine animale: locomotion terrestre et aërienne*, Paris, 1873 (2nd edn 1878); *La circulation du sang à l'état physiologique et dans les maladies*, Paris, 1881 (see Plate 8); *Le mouvement*, Paris, 1894.[114]

The work of Ivan Petrovitch Pavlov (1849–1936) on the nervous mechanism of gastric secretion, and on conditioned reflexes, won for him the Nobel Prize in 1904. Pavlov was director of the Institute for Experimental Medicine, Leningrad, and his most important books are *Lectures on the work of the principal digestive glands* [in Russian], St Petersburg, 1897, with a French version, Paris, 1901, and an English translation by W. H. Thompson, London, 1902 and 1910; and *Conditioned reflexes ... Translated by G. V. Anrep*, London, 1927, and of which an American edition by W. Horsley Gantt was published as *Lectures on conditioned reflexes*, two volumes, New York, 1928–41, and reprinted in London, 1964. Pavlov's *Selected works*, edited by K. J. Koshtoyants, were published in Moscow in 1955.[115]

Medical botany was the subject of an important work written by Jacob Bigelow (1787–1879) of Massachusetts, who has been described as 'one of the greatest American botanists'. He was professor of materia medica at Harvard, and his three-volume *American medical botany*, Boston, 1817–20 contains 60 plates and 6000 coloured engravings. Bigelow was also the author of *Florula Bostoniensis ...*, Boston, 1814; *A treatise of the materia medica ...*, Boston, 1822; *A discourse on self-limited diseases*, Boston, 1835; *Nature in disease illustrated in various discourses and essays ...*, Boston, 1854; and *Modern inquiries: classical, professional and miscellaneous*, Boston, 1867. Matthias Jakob Schleiden (1804–81) was also interested in medical botany, among other subjects, and wrote *Grundzüge der wissenschaftlichen Botanik ...*, two parts, Leipzig, 1842–43, which was translated into English by Edwin Lankester, London, 1849; *Handbuch der medicinisch-pharmaceutischen Botanik ...*, two volumes, Leipzig, 1852–9; *Zur Theorie des Erkennens durch den Gesichtssinn*, Leipzig, 1863, and *Das Salz ... Leipzig*, 1875.[116]

Johann Ludwig Wilhelm Thudichum (1829–1901) was neglected until recent years, but is now acknowledged for his early suggestion of cholecystostomy,[117] his pioneer work on the chemistry of the brain, and his experiments on haemoglobin, urinary pigments, and on the chemistry of wine and beer. Born on 27 August 1829 at Bugingen, Thudichum studied under Liebig at Giessen, and under Bunsen at Heidelberg, but in 1853 he emigrated to London, later becoming naturalized and known also by the Anglicized form of his forenames, John Louis William. He was the first director of the Laboratory of Chemistry and Pathology at St Thomas's Hospital, but resigned after six years and became a leading otolaryngologist. Thudichum published over 200 scientific papers, and his notebooks and chemical preparations were discovered in the stable of his former home by Otto Rosenheim (1871–1955). They are preserved in the National Institute for Medical Research at Mill Hill. Thudichum was the author of *A treatise on the pathology of the urine ...*, London, 1858, with a second edition in 1877; *A treatise on gall-stones: their chemistry, pathology and treatment*, London, 1863; *A treatise on the origin, nature and varieties of wine ...*, London, New York, 1872; *A manual of chemical physiology, including its point of contact with pathology*, London, 1872; *A treatise on the chemical constitution of the brain ...*, London, 1884,[118] of which a Russian translation was published, 1885–6, and a greatly enlarged German edition was printed with the title *Die chemische Konstitution des Gehirns des Menschen und der Tiere ...*, Tübingen, 1901; *Grundzüge der anatomischen und klinischen Chemie ...*, Berlin, 1886; and *Briefe über offentliche Gesundheitspflege ihre bisherigen Leistungen und heutigen Aufgaben*, Tübingen, 1898.[119]

Sir Thomas Lauder Brunton (1844–1916), a native of Roxburghshire, was eminently concerned with pharmacology and therapeutics. He was connected with St Bartholomew's Hospital as lecturer on materia medica and pharmacology, and as a physician. Lauder Brunton wrote many books and papers, several collections of the latter being reproduced in book form, and his work on the action of drugs on the heart, and on the use of amyl nitrite was of special importance. His books include *On digitalis* ..., London, Edinburgh, 1868, which was his graduation dissertation; *Pharmacology and therapeutics* ..., London, 1880, being the Goulstonian Lectures for 1877; *The Bible and science*, London, 1881; *Textbook of pharmacology, therapeutics and materia medica*, London, 1885, which was translated into French, German, Italian and Russian; *On disorders of digestion, their consequences and treatment*, London, 1886; *An introduction to modern therapeutics* ..., London, New York, 1892, being the Croonian Lectures for 1889; *Lectures on the actions of medicines* ..., London, New York, 1897; *Therapeutics of the circulation* ..., London, 1908; *On disorders of assimilation, digestion* ..., London, New York, 1901; *Collected papers on physical and military training*, London, 1887–1915; *Collected papers on circulation and respiration*, two volumes, London, New York, 1906–16.[120]

Louis Pasteur (1822–95) has been called the founder of the science of bacteriology, although he was a professor of chemistry at Strasbourg, Lille, and Paris, where he spent the last years of his life at the Institut Pasteur, built in his honour. The story of his career is well known,[121] and Pasteur's more important writings include *Études sur le vin* ..., Paris, 1866; *Études sur les maladies des vers à soie* ..., two volumes, Paris, 1870; *Études sur le vinaigre* ..., Paris, 1868; *Études sur la bière* ..., Paris, 1876, which was translated into English as *Studies on fermentation* ..., London, 1879; and *La théorie des germes et ses applications à la médecine et à la chirurgie*, 1878. His works were collected together and published as *Oeuvres*, two volumes, Paris, 1922, and as *Oeuvres de Pasteur, réunies par Pasteur Vallery-Radot*, Paris, 1933–9. Pasteur influenced many research workers to continue the study of bacteria, and Lord Lister was greatly indebted to Pasteur, as his theories were based on the findings of the latter.

Robert Koch (1843–1910) has been named the 'Father of preventive medicine' and he conducted research on the aetiology of anthrax, demonstrating the bacillus; on wound infections; on tuberculosis, his greatest discovery being the tuberculosis bacillus, while he did important work on tuberculosis vaccine; on cholera in Egypt and India; on rinderpest in South Africa; plague in India; and on malaria in Italy. Koch was awarded the Nobel Prize in 1905. His writings include *Untersuchungen über die Aetiologie der Wundinfektionskrankheiten*, Leipzig, 1878, which was translated into English by W. Watson Cheyne, and published by the New Sydenham Society in 1880; *Reise-Berichte über Rinderpest, Bubonenpest in Indien und Africa, Tsetse- oder Surrakrankheit, Texasfieber, tropische Malaria, Schwarzwasserfieber*, Berlin, 1898; and *Gesammelte Werke* ..., two volumes [in three], Leipzig, 1912. In 1899, with Flügge, Koch founded the *Zeitschrift für Hygiene*.[122]

Physiological chemistry, later to become known as biochemistry, made important advances at the hands of Liebig and Hoppe-Seyler. Justus von Liebig (1803–73) of Darmstadt, has been called the founder of agricultural chemistry, and he was a pioneer in physiological chemistry. He first introduced the word 'metabolism'. Liebig founded the *Annalen der Pharmacie*, which later became *Annalen der Chemie*, and is familiarly known as Liebig's *Annalen*. His numerous writings include *Die organische Chemie in ihrer Anwendung auf Physiologie und Pathologie*, Braunschweig, 1842, which was translated into English (New York, 1842 and London, 1846); *Chemische Untersuchung über das Fleisch und seine Zubereitung zum Nahrungsmittel*, Heidelberg, 1847, translated into English as *Research on the chemistry of food*, London, 1847; and *Die Chemie in ihrer Anwendung auf Agricultur und Physiologie*, two volumes, Braunschweig, 1865.[123] Ernst Felix Immanuel Hoppe-Seyler (1825–95) of Freiburg, was professor of applied chemistry at Tübingen, and professor of physiological chemistry at Strasbourg. He founded the *Zeitschrift für physiologische Chemie*, which contains many of his papers, and was the author of *Anleitung zur pathologisch-chemischen Analyse für Aerzte und Studirende*, Berlin, 1858; *Allgemeine Biologie*, Berlin, 1877; and *Physiologische Chemie*, two volumes, Berlin, 1877–9.[124]

Thomas Southwood Smith (1788–1861) has been called 'the intellectual father of our modern public health system'. Brought up near Yeovil in Somerset and educated in Bristol as a Calvinist, he became a Unitarian minister and studied medicine in Edinburgh. For many years he was both a doctor and a minister, 'physician to body and soul' as he put it, and his first book, *Illustrations of divine government*, Glasgow, 1816, with four more editions to 1866, contains the germ of his ideas on sanitary reform, his belief that the disease attendant upon poverty is preventable and therefore should be prevented. On moving to London in 1820, as well as furthering his medical education in the London hospitals, he joined the circle around the Utilitarian philosopher Jeremy Bentham, so influential on many aspects of social reform in Britain. He wrote on sanitary topics for the *Westminster Review* and consolidated this work in his important monograph *A treatise on fever*, London, 1830. He also wrote *The philosophy of health*, 2 vols, London, 1835–7 and various later editions, the first work published in England to give an account of William Beaumont's studies on the physiology of digestion; *Epidemics considered with relation to their common nature and to climate and civilization*, Edinburgh, 1856; and after his death a collection of his writings and official reports appeared under the title *The common nature of epidemics and their relation to climate and civilization. Also remarks on contagion and quarantine*, London, 1866.[125]

Not all important writers on public health matters in the nineteenth century were doctors. Sir Edwin Chadwick (1800–1890), as Secretary to the British Poor Law Board and later Commissioner to the short-lived General Board of Health, was a most vigorous promoter of sanitary reform, although many of his ideas were derived from Southwood Smith. George Rosen has called his *Report on an Inquiry into the sanitary condition of the labouring population of Great Britain*, London, 1842, written for the Poor Law Commissioners, 'the fundamental document of modern public health'. He also wrote *A supplementary report on ... the practice of interment in towns*, London, 1843. The 1842 report was reprinted with an introduction by M. W. Flinn, Edinburgh, 1965 (2nd edn 1987). Chadwick organized and substantially drafted the *First report of the Commissioners for inquiry into the state of large towns and populous districts*, 2 vols, London, 1844, and with T. Southwood Smith and Lord Ashley he wrote the *Report of the General Board of Health on the epidemic cholera of 1848 and 1849*, London, 1850.[126]

Although William Farr (1807–83) began his career as a medical practitioner, he is remembered as the pioneer of vital statistics who applied rigorous mathematical methods to the study of health and disease. Born in Shropshire, England, he first studied medicine locally in Shrewsbury and later in Paris, where he came under the influence of Pierre Louis among others. The annual reports of the General Register Office of England and Wales, of which he, the 'examiner and compiler of abstracts', not the Registrar-General, was the author from its establishment in 1839 to his retirement in 1880, hold a significant place in the literature of epidemiology. For the Registrar-General he wrote the *Report on the mortality of cholera 1848–49*, London, 1852. A large selection of his writings was published in a volume, *Vital statistics*, London, 1885 (reprinted Metuchen, NJ, 1975).[127]

Sanitary reform was championed by one of the most prominent medical men of the nineteenth century, Sir John Simon (1816–1904) who became surgeon to St Thomas's Hospital, and in 1848 was appointed the first Medical Officer of Health for the City of London. Afterwards he was Medical Officer to the Privy Council and the Local Government Board. He was the author of: *Observations regarding medical education*, London, 1842; *A physiological essay on the thymus gland*, London, 1845; *On the aims and philosophic method of pathological research*, London, 1847–48; *General pathology as conducive to the establishment of rational principles for the diagnosis and treatment of diseases*, London, 1850; *Reports relating to the sanitary condition of the City of London*, London, 1854; and of *Personal recollections*, which was privately printed in 1894 and 1903. Probably his most significant books, however, were *English sanitary institutions ...*, London, 1890, and *Public health reports ...*, 2 vols, London, 1887, the latter a compilation of his writings, some from his annual reports as the government's chief medical officer.[128] These reports, with their appendixes on a variety of public health matters, like William Farr's annotations to the Registrar-General's reports, form an important part of the literature on the growing understanding of public health and epidemic disease, even though government reports are not normally regarded nowadays as 'literature' in the narrower sense.

Max von Pettenkofer (1818–1901) organized sanitary reform in Munich, where he taught at the university. He founded the discipline of experimental hygiene and despite Louis Pasteur's discoveries was reluctant for many years to believe that bacteria were the prime cause of many infectious diseases. He wrote over 20 monographs and 200 separate articles in German medical and scientific journals between 1842 and 1898 and founded and co-edited *Archiv für Hygiene*, 1883–. His view that cholera was transmitted through soil, not water, was opposed to that of John Snow and William Budd in England and was expressed in such works as *Untersuchungen und Beobachten über die Verbreitungsart der Cholera ...*, Munich 1855; *Boden und Grundwasser in ihren Beziehung zu Cholera und Typhus*, Munich, 1869; and *Zum gegenwärtigen Stand der Cholerafrage*, Munich, 1887.[129]

Charles Creighton (1847–1927) was another British pioneer of epidemiology, but his popularity suffered on account of his anti-Jenner writings and his heterodox views on various subjects. Among his numerous writings, the following are of special interest: *Contributions to the physiology and pathology of the breast and its lymphatic glands*, London, 1878; *Bovine tuberculosis in man ...*, London, 1881; *A history of epidemics in Britain ...*, two volumes, Cambridge, 1891–4, his most important work, which was reissued with much new material in 1965; *Microscopic researches on the formative property of glycogen*, two parts, London, 1896–9; and *Contributions to the physiological theory of tuberculosis*, London, 1908. Creighton also translated for the New Sydenham Society August Hirsch's *Handbook of geographical and historical pathology*, three volumes, 1883–6.

Biology has received attention in Thornton–Tully, but brief mention is necessary of certain authorities whose writings influenced medical science. Sir Richard Owen (1804–92) was the author of many books and articles on comparative anatomy and physiology, including *Odontography ...*, two volumes, London, 1840–5; *On the classification and geographical distribution of the mammalia ...*, London, 1859; and *On the anatomy of the vertebrates*, three volumes, London, 1866–8. Charles (Robert) Darwin (1809–82), the brilliant naturalist, most of whose writings, based on painstaking experiments, are still worthy of careful study, wrote a book on natural selection which is of primary significance in the history of science. Among many published books, the following three of Darwin's works are possibly of particular significance: *On the origin of species by means of natural selection*, London, 1859; *The descent of man, and selection in relation to sex*, two volumes, London, 1871; and *The expression of the emotions in man and animals*, London, 1873. Thomas Henry Huxley (1825–95), a staunch supporter of Darwin, also wrote many volumes on comparative anatomy, including *Evidence as to man's place in nature*, London, 1863; *Lessons in elementary physiology*, London, 1866, which went into thirty editions; *Lectures on the elements of comparative anatomy ...*, London, 1864; *A manual of the anatomy of vertebrated animals*, London, 1864; *A manual of the anatomy of invertebrated animals*, London, 1877; *On the physical basis of life*, London, 1868; his *Scientific memoirs ... Edited by Sir Michael Foster and E. Ray Lankester*, were published in four volumes, with a supplementary volume, London, 1898–1903. Ernst Heinrich Philipp August Haeckel (1834–1919), while differing on certain points from Darwin, championed the latter's cause in Germany, and was the author of several important books, including *Generelle Morphologie der Organismen*, two volumes, Berlin, 1866; *Natürliche Schöpfungsgeschichte ...*, Berlin, 1868, translated into French (Paris, 1874), and into English by E. Ray Lankester, two volumes, London, 1876; and *Anthropogenie, oder Entwicklungsgeschichte des Menschen ...*, Leipzig, 1874, which went into several editions, including a French version (Paris, 1877) and an English translation in two volumes, London, 1883.

It is impossible to write on nineteenth-century medical literature without referring to the writings on anaesthesia. Many of these consist of articles in periodicals, or pamphlets, and some are extremely rare. During 1946 the centenary of the introduction of anaesthetics was celebrated, and much was written upon the subject, while a book by Thomas E. Keys provides a valuable summary of the history of surgical anaesthesia.[130] This includes an extensive chronology and numerous references, in an attempt to evolve order from a chaotic series of claims and counter-claims for priority. Without delving too far back into history for the earliest use of anaesthesia, we would mention certain pioneers, most of whom published something on the subject: Henry Hill Hickman (1800–30), Crawford Williamson Long (1815–78), Horace Wells (1815–48), William Thomas Green Morton (1819–68), Sir James Young Simpson (1811–70) and John Snow (1813–58), who wrote a book on ether entitled *On the inhalation of the vapour of ether in surgical operations ...*, London, 1847, followed by the posthumously published volume *On chloroform and other anaesthetics; their action and administration. Edited with a memoir of the author by Benjamin W. Richardson*, London, 1858.[131] Snow was born at Heworth, near York on 15 March 1813, coming to London in 1836 to study at the Great Windmill St School and Westminster Hospital. He went into practice, and first gave anaesthetics in St George's Hospital in the Dental Out-patients' Department. He demonstrated his methods at University College Hospital, and became anaesthetist to several hospitals. Snow is also eminent for his work on cholera, which he described in his book *On the mode of communication of cholera*, London, 1849, which went into a second edition in 1855, and was reprinted in 1936 and 1949.[132]

Following medical studies in London, Edinburgh and Paris, William Budd (1811–80) was appointed physician to the Dreadnought Seaman's Hospital ship at Greenwich, but resigned after he nearly died from typhoid fever. For a time he assisted his father in general practice in North Tawton, Devon, the place of his birth, but from 1842 settled in Bristol where he was physician to two hospitals and lecturer in medicine in the Bristol Medical College. He was a pioneer epidemiologist whose doctrine that specific infective agents determine the epidemic phenomena of communicable diseases made him a forerunner of the Pasteurian germ theory of disease. His first contribution to the literature, not published at the time, was his essay submitted (unsuccessfully) in 1839 for the 1840 Thackeray prize of the Provincial Medical and Surgical Association, *An essay on the causes and mode of propagation of the common continued fevers of Great Britain and Ireland*, now edited from the manuscript with a foreword and afterword by Dale C. Smith, Baltimore, 1984. His short book, *Malignant cholera: its mode of propagation and its prevention*, London, 1849, appeared about a month after Snow's work on the same subject. Like Snow he concluded that the disease is waterborne. Budd published papers on other communicable diseases of man and animals and his major work was *Typhoid fever: its nature, mode of spreading and prevention*, London, 1873, consolidating studies published in journals over a number of years.[133]

The careers of certain figure-heads of nineteenth-century medicine extended well into the twentieth century, and some of their more significant writings were published in that period. They are briefly mentioned here for the importance of their writings printed before 1900. Sir Jonathan Hutchinson (1828–1913), who wrote extensively on syphilis and leprosy, including *Syphilis*, London, 1887; *On leprosy and fish-eating*, London, 1906; *Archives of Surgery*, eleven volumes, 1889–99, written entirely by Hutchinson: and *Illustrations of clinical surgery*, two volumes, London, 1878–88.[134] Silas Weir Mitchell (1829–1914), a pioneer in neurology and a great teacher, who was physician to the Philadelphia Orthopedic Hospital and Infirmary for Nervous Diseases, wrote *Fat and blood ...*, Philadelphia, 1877, which went into many editions; and was translated into French, German, Italian, Spanish and Russian; *Wear and tear ...*, Philadelphia, 1871; *The early history of instrumental precision in medicine*, New Haven, 1892; *Injuries of nerves and their consequences*, Philadelphia, 1872, which was translated into French, Paris, 1874; *Lectures on diseases of the nervous system, especially in women*, Philadelphia, 1881; *Characteristics*, New York, 1892, and many other books, including novels and poems.

John Hughlings Jackson (1835–1911) was born in Yorkshire, and studied at the York Hospital and St Bartholomew's Hospital, London. His first appointment was to the dispensary of the York Hospital and from 1859 he held posts at the London Hospital as lecturer on pathology and physician. From 1862 to 1906 he was on the staff of the National Hospital for the Paralysed and Epileptic, where a colleague for a few years and an influence on his thinking was Brown-Séquard. He himself profoundly influenced the neurological sciences by applying the data of abnormal functioning to the elucidation of the normal action of the nervous system in approximately 320 papers published between 1861 and 1909. These included 'Unilateral epileptiform seizures, attended by temporary defect of sight', in *Medical Times and Gazette*, 1 (1863) pp.588–9, the condition known from his excellent description as 'Jacksonian epilepsy'; and his 1884 Croonian lectures to the Royal College of Physicians, 'On the evolution and dissolution of the nervous system', printed in both *British Medical Journal* and *Lancet*, 1 (1884). Two selections of his writings have appeared: *Neurological fragments of John Hughlings Jackson*, London, 1925; and *Selected writings* ..., edited for the guarantors of *Brain* by J. Taylor, 2 vols, London, 1931–2.[135]

Sir David Ferrier (1843–1928) from Aberdeen, studied medicine in Edinburgh and from 1872 to 1889 held the chair of forensic medicine in King's College Hospital Medical School, London, in succession to W. A. Guy of whose *Principles of forensic medicine* he co-authored the 4th to 6th editions, 1875–88. He was physician to King's College Hospital and to the National Hospital for the Paralysed and Epileptic, where he was a colleague of Hughlings Jackson. He is best known as an experimental (rather than clinical) neurologist and *The functions of the brain*, London, 1876 (2nd edn 1886) is one of the most significant contributions to the knowledge of cerebral localization. Ferrier's Goulstonian lectures to the Royal College of Physicians, *The localization of cerebral diseases*, London, 1878, were translated into French as *De la localisation des maladies cérébrales*, with an additional 'mémoire' by J. M. Charcot and A. Pitres, Paris, 1879.[136]

Among important English writers on clinical neurology at the end of the century was Sir William Richard Gowers (1845–1915). Born in London, he trained at University College Hospital, London, where he later held several posts, eventually becoming professor of clinical medicine. From 1870 he was also on the staff of the National Hospital for the Paralysed and Epileptic. He wrote *A manual and atlas of medical ophthalmoscopy*, London, 1879 (2nd edn 1882; 3rd edn 1890); *The diagnosis of diseases of the spinal cord*, London, 1880 (2nd edn 1881; 3rd edn 1884); *Epilepsy and other chronic convulsive diseases*, London, 1881 (2nd edn

1901); *Lectures on the diagnosis of diseases of the brain*, London, 1885 (2nd edn 1887); *A manual of diseases of the nervous system*, 2 vols, London, 1886–8 (2nd edn 1892–3); *The border-land of epilepsy: faints, vagal attacks, vertigo, migraine, sleep symptoms, and their treatment*, London, 1907.[137]

Pierre Marie (1853–1940) was born in Paris and studied medicine there. He was an outstanding student of Charcot at the Salpêtrière and the Bicêtre and is best known for his work in neurology. His publications include *L'acromégalie*, Paris, 1890; the New Sydenham Society published *Essays on acromegaly* by Pierre Marie and J. D. Souza-Leite, London, 1891; *Leçons sur les maladies de la moëlle*, Paris, 1892, issued in English by the New Sydenham Society as *Lectures on diseases of the spinal cord*, London, 1895. A collection of his writings appeared as *Travaux et mémoires*, 2 vols, Paris, 1926–8.[138]

Theodor Albrecht Edwin Klebs (1834–1913), discoverer of the diphtheria bacillus, and an eminent pathologist, was the author of *Beiträge zur pathologischen Anatomie der Schusswunden*, Leipzig, 1872; *Handbuch der pathologischen Anatomie*, two volumes, Berlin, 1868–80; *Die allgemeine Pathologie ...*, two volumes, Jena, 1887–9; and *Die causale Behandlung der Tuberculose ...*, Hamburg and Leipzig, 1894.[139] Sir Thomas Clifford Allbutt (1836–1925) edited *A system of medicine*, eight volumes, London, 1896–8, of which a second edition (with Sir Humphry Davy Rolleston) was published from 1906 to 1911; and with W. S. Playfair and others, *A system of gynaecology*, London, 1896 and 1906. Allbutt was the author of several other books, mostly published after 1900.[140]

Bernard Naunyn (1839–1925) studied metabolism in diabetes, and diseases of the liver and pancreas, and was one of the founders of the *Archiv für experimentelle Pathologie und Pharmakologie*. He wrote *Klinik der Cholelithiasis*, Leipzig, 1892, which was translated into English by Archibald E. Garrod, London, 1896; *Der Diabetes mellitus*, Vienna, 1898, with a second edition in 1898; a volume of his memoirs appeared in 1925 as *Erinnerungen, Gedanken und Meinungen*, Berlin. Sir William Osler (1849–1919) was the author of *The cerebral palsies of children*, London, 1889; *On chorea and choreiform affections*, London, 1894; and *The principles and practice of medicine*, New York, 1892, of which Osler revised nine editions, and which went into a sixteenth edition, 1947. It was translated into French (1908), German (1909), Spanish (1915) and Chinese (1915, 1921, 1925).[141]

Sir Patrick Manson (1844–1922), the father of tropical medicine, was born at Old Meldrum, near Aberdeen, at which University he was educated. He wrote *The Filaria sanguinis hominis and certain new forms of parasitic disease in India, China, and warm countries*, London, 1883; and *Tropical diseases ...*, London, 1898, of which a sixteenth edition appeared in 1965 and a French translation, Paris, 1904.[142]

Wilhelm Conrad Röntgen (1845–1932) was professor of physics at Strasbourg, Giessen, Würzburg and Munich, and received the Nobel Prize in 1901. His discovery of X-rays, also known as Roentgen rays, was first described in 'Eine neue Art von Strahlen' (*Sitzungsber. d. phys. med. Gessellsch. zu Würzburg*, 1895, pp.132–41). This was printed at the end of the proceedings for 1895, and reprints with yellow wrappers were published with the date 'Ende 1895', but without a separate title-page. Four more editions of this were printed during 1896. A facsimile was published in 1938.[143]

Elie Metchnikoff (1845–1916) was born near Kharkoff, and gave up a promising career to work with Pasteur in Paris. Metchnikoff was awarded the Nobel Prize in 1908, and the following books are the more important of his numerous writings: *Lektsii o sravnitelnoi patologii vospaleniy*, St Petersburg, 1892, on the pathology of inflammation, translated into French in 1892, and into English the following year; *L'immunité dans les maladies infectieuses*, Paris, 1901, which was translated into English in 1905; and *Quelques remarques sur le lait aigri*, Paris, 1906.[144]

Santiago Ramón y Cajal (1852–1934), a native of Aragon, was a prominent histologist, and conducted invaluable research on the anatomy of the nervous system. His writings include *Die Retina der Wirbelthiere*, Wiesbaden, 1894; *Manual de histología normal y de técnica micrográfica* ..., Valencia, 1889; *Elementos de histología normal y técnica micrográfica* ..., Madrid, 1895; *Textura del sistema nervioso*, two volumes, Madrid, 1899–1904; *Degeneration and regeneration of the nervous system* ..., two volumes, London, 1928. *Studies on the cerebral cortex* was published in 1955, and *Studies on vertebrate neurogenesis* in 1960.[145]

Camillo Golgi (1843–1926) was born at Corteno in the province of Brescia, Italy. He became a lecturer on histology at the University of Pavia in 1875 and after a short spell at Siena university, he was made professor of histology at Pavia, later becoming professor of general pathology. His original techniques of colouration of nerve cells enabled great progress to be made in the study of the microscopic anatomy of the nervous system. He published many papers in journals from 1873 onwards and his *Opera omnia* appeared in 4 vols, Milan, 1903–29. He shared the Nobel Prize with Ramón y Cajal in 1906.[146]

Christian Albert Theodor Billroth (1829–94), born on the island of Rügen in north Germany, was professor of surgery in Zurich and, from 1867, at the university of Vienna. A brilliant surgeon and teacher, he is regarded as the founder of modern gastric surgery. Among his publications are *Die allgemeine chirurgische Pathologie und Therapie in fünfzig Vorlesungen*, Berlin, 1863 (16th edn 1906), translated into English from the 4th edition as *General surgical pathology and therapy*, New York, 1871, and again from the 8th German edition and published by the New

Sydenham Society, 2 vols, London, 1877–8; *Chirurgische Klinik*, 4 vols, Berlin, 1869–79, with an English translation published by the New Sydenham Society under the title *Clinical surgery: extracts from the reports of surgical practice between the years 1860–1876*, London, 1881; *Ueber das Lehren und Lernen der medizinischen Wissenschaften*, Vienna, 1876; and *Die Krankheiten der Brustdrüsen*, Stuttgart, 1880. A collection of his letters has appeared in English translation: *The intimate Billroth: letters to his confidante, the Billroth–Seegen letters*; edited by K. B. Absolon, 2nd edn, Rockville, Md, 1986.[147]

Sir Frederick Treves (1853–1923) of Dorchester was one of the foremost abdominal surgeons of his period, and among numerous other books was the author of *Intestinal obstruction ...*, London, 1884; *A manual of operative surgery*, two volumes, London, 1891; *Surgical applied anatomy*, London, 1892, of which a fourteenth edition appeared in 1962, and *The student's handbook of surgical operations*, London, 1892, published in a tenth edition in 1957.[148]

Théodore Martin Tuffier (1857–1929) was one of the most prominent French surgeons of his day, and was the first surgeon to transport patients from the field of battle by aeroplane. He popularized spinal anaesthesia in France, and was a pioneer in the surgical treatment of phthisis. Tuffier was the author of *Chirurgie du poumon ...*, Paris, 1897; (with P. Desfosses), *Petite chirurgie pratique*, Paris, 1903, the seventh edition of which appeared in 1926; *Semeiological importance of the examination of the blood in surgery* (in Russian, translated from an unpublished manuscript), Moscow, 1905; *Chirurgie de l'estomac ...*, Paris, 1907; and (with J. Martin) *Traitement chirurgical de la tuberculose pulmonaire ...*, Paris, [1909].

Paul Ehrlich (1854–1915) of Strehlen, Silesia, has been described as the founder of haematology, and was prominent in research on infectious diseases, experimental pharmacology and therapeutics, on dyestuffs and tissue staining. Ehrlich introduced salvarsan ('606') and neosalvarsan ('914') in the treatment of syphilis, and was the author of numerous articles and books, including the following during the nineteenth century: *Das Sauerstoffbedürfniss des Organismus. Eine farbenanalytische Studie*, Berlin, 1885; and *Farbenanalytische Untersuchungen zur Histologie und Klinik des Blutes*, Berlin, 1891. *Die Anaemie* (with A. Lazarus), 2 vols, Vienna, 1898–1900, was translated, with some additional sections, as *Diseases of the blood*, Philadelphia, 1905. Ehrlich's *Collected papers. Collected and edited by F. Himmelweit*, were published in four volumes, 1956–65, and he has also been the subject of a definitive biography by Martha Marquardt.[149]

It is rare for a country general practitioner to become renowned for his contributions to scholarship, but Francis Adams (1796–1861) of Banchory was outstanding for his remarkable translations of Greek medical classics. Adams was born on 13 March 1796 at Lumphanan, on Deeside, and entered King's College, Aberdeen, where he qualified MA in 1813. He then came to London and qualified as MRCS, but settled down to general practice in Banchory for the remainder of his life. He later received honorary degrees from Aberdeen, Glasgow and Oxford, and was offered the chair of Greek at Aberdeen, but declined. Adams began his translation of Paul of Aegina in November 1827 and completed it on 28 April 1829. Volume one was published in 1834, but the printer failed, and the whole work was later issued by the Sydenham Society as *The seven books of Paulus Aegineta*, three volumes, 1844–7. He completed his English version of Hippocrates in about four months, and it was published by the Sydenham Society as *The genuine works of Hippocrates*, two volumes, London, 1849. Later editions were published in New York in 1886 and 1891, and even as recently as 1950, and despite more modern translations, Adam's version was republished by an American publisher. His translation of *The Extant works of Aretaeus the Cappadocian* was published by the Sydenham Society in 1856. Adams was also the author of *On the construction of the placenta*, 1858, which had previously appeared in the *Medical Times and Gazette*.[150]

A general survey of medical items published in the United States of America during the nineteenth century was published by Thomas E. Keys, who groups the items by subjects, and a wider conspectus covering the development of medical literature in America, with references to medical societies, journals, and medical schools has been prepared by Gertrude L. Annan.[151]

The nineteenth century saw the foundation of numerous British medical societies, many of which are still active, and the tendency towards specialization became noticeable.[152] The following short list illustrates this trend, and it should be noted that certain societies also formed sections for special branches of medicine. The Edinburgh Obstetrical Society and the Royal Microscopical Society were founded in 1839; the Pathological Society of London, 1846; the Epidemiological Society, London, 1850; the Odontological Society of Great Britain, 1856; the Obstetrical Society of London, 1858; the Physiological Society of England, 1876;[153] the Glasgow Obstetrical and Gynaecological Society, 1885; and the North of England Obstetrical and Gynaecological Society, 1890.

In 1841 the Reading Pathological Society was formed, the oldest society in Great Britain devoted to pathology. At one time the Society issued annual reports, but the proceedings were later incorporated in the *Royal Berkshire Hospital Reports*. Annual addresses are delivered at meetings of the Society, among prominent orators being Sir Jonathan Hutchinson, Sir Frederick Treves, Sir Thomas Lauder Brunton, Sir John Bland-Sutton, and Sir Humphry Rolleston.[154]

In 1830 the Ophthalmological Society of the United Kingdom was founded by Sir William Bowman, who became its first President. A library was commenced four years later with about 100 volumes, and the collection is now housed at the Royal Society of Medicine, where the meetings of the Society are also held. The *Transactions* of the Society are issued periodically. Two years later than the Ophthalmological Society appeared the West London Medico-Chirurgical Society, which published proceedings until 1896, and then issued the *West London Medical Journal*.

Several societies were formed in Birmingham, and in 1824 the Birmingham Medical Library was founded in Mr. Belcher's bookshop in New Street, where a room was kept for members. It was succeeded there by the Medical Circulating Book Society (1831–81). The Social Medical Society (1849) and the Midland Medical Society (1854) were also formed in the city, and in 1875 the Birmingham Medical Institute was registered. Its library had books from the General Hospital, the old Birmingham Medical Library, and the Midland Medical Society. The Institute moved to a new building in 1880, and was again rehoused in 1957.[155]

Also in 1882 appeared the Royal Academy of Medicine in Ireland, which was formed by the amalgamation of four societies, the Association of Fellows and Licentiates of the King and Queen's College of Physicians in Ireland (1816), later the Medical Society of the College of Physicians, which published *Transactions* from 1817 to 1830, and from 1832 the *Dublin Journal of Medical and Chemical Science*; the Surgical Society of Ireland (1831);[156] the Pathological Society (1838); and the Obstetrical Society, each of which published *Proceedings*. These were amalgamated in 1882 as the Academy of Medicine in Ireland, the title 'Royal' being added in 1887. The Academy published *Transactions* from 1893 to 1920, followed by the *Dublin Journal of Medical Science*, which since 1922 has been known as the *Irish Journal of Medical Science*.

Yet another example of a specialized medical society exists in the Anatomical Society of Great Britain and Ireland, which was founded in 1887 by Charles Barrett Lockwood. The official organ of the Society is the *Journal of Anatomy*, formerly the *Journal of Anatomy and Physiology*, which was taken over by the Society in 1916.

Several Canadian medical societies were founded in the nineteenth century, but many of them were short-lived. The Quebec Medical Society was started in November, 1826 but it lapsed after a period, until it was revived in 1844. The Medico-Chirurgical Society of Upper Canada was formed in 1833, but probably disappeared before 1844, when the Toronto and Home District Medico-Chirurgical Society was established. The Medico-Chirurgical Society of Montreal was founded in 1843, and in the following year the Medical Society of Halifax, Nova Scotia was formed, which in 1854 became the Medical Society of Nova Scotia. Following several abortive attempts to establish a national medical association, the Canadian Medical Association was formed in 1869, but was not incorporated until 1909. Its official organ, the *Canadian Medical Association Journal* was first issued in January, 1911.[157] A resolution suggesting the formation of the Royal College of Physicians and Surgeons of Canada was advanced in 1920, but it was not incorporated until 1929.[158]

The United States of America saw great activity in the formation of medical societies during the nineteenth and twentieth centuries, and they would require a separate volume just to name them. Several medical societies were formed in New York, and a Medical Society of the State of New York existed from 1794 to 1806; its minute books are preserved in the New York Academy of Medicine Library. Membership was confined to New York City, and the present Medical Society of the State of New York was established in 1807, the first meeting being held in February of that year. A comprehensive history of this Society has been contributed in a series of papers by Norman Shaftel, Emerson Crosby Kelly and John F. Rogers.[159]

The Medical Society of the County of Queens was founded in 1806, and in 1899 the title was changed to the Queens-Nassau Medical Society. It became the Nassau County Medical Society in 1921.[160]

The oldest student medical society in the States, the Boylston Medical Society of Harvard University, was founded by Ward Nicholas Boylston in 1811.[161]

The Medical Society of Virginia was formed by 17 Richmond and Manchester physicians in December, 1820, monthly meetings were held, and a library was established. In 1826 it became inactive until 1841, when meetings were resumed, and in 1852 it became a State organization. In the same year the Medico-Chirurgical Society of Richmond City was founded, sharing office accommodation with the Medical Society. The former became inactive about 1855, but was reorganized in January, 1866 as the Richmond Academy of Medicine. A rival Richmond Medical and Surgical Society functioned for ten years, but in 1890 they merged as the Richmond Academy of Medicine and Surgery, the last two words being dropped from the title at the beginning of this century. The Academy was housed in a new building in 1932, and contains the valuable library donated by Joseph L. Miller.[162]

The first meeting of the American Medical Association, the United States counterpart of the British Medical Association, was held in Philadelphia on 5 May 1847. Founded for the advancement of medical education, the Association published volumes of *Transactions* until in 1883 the *Journal of the American Medical Association* was established, which has continued its useful career weekly since that date, and is the most widely circulated medical journal in the world. The American Medical Association publishes several specialist journals, among numerous other activities, and its centenary was celebrated by the publication of a very full *History* by Morris Fishbein.[163]

In 1843 was founded a society, the sole object of which was the publication of important works not readily accessible. This was the Sydenham Society, which continued to publish medical classics, and also translations from French and German, until 1858, when 29 publications had been issued. A declining membership decided its decease, and at the winding-up meeting, Jonathan Hutchinson, who voted for the continuance of the Society, was challenged to form a new one. This he proceeded to do, assisted by Sedgwick Saunders and Bevill Peacock, and the New Sydenham Society was formed to continue the policy of the old Sydenham Society. Many prominent men held official positions in the New Sydenham Society, its presidents including Sir Thomas Watson, Sir James Paget, John Hilton, Sir George Burrows, Sir Prescott Hewitt, Hughlings Jackson, Sir Thomas Spencer Wells and Sir Watson Cheyne. The Society had many important publications to its credit, including Trousseau's *Clinical medicine*, Hirsch's *Handbook of geographical and historical pathology*, Hebra's *Diseases of the skin*, Casper's *Forensic medicine*, Frerichs' *Diseases of the liver*, Cohnheim's *Lectures on pathology*, and many others. It published an annual *Year-book* from 1860 for six years, and then biennially until 1875; also collected editions of the works of British authors, including Addison, Gull, Warburton Begbie, and Abraham Colles. A medical lexicon and several volumes of collected essays were also issued, but in 1907 the work of the Society was discontinued, after the issue of 195 publications, not including periodicals.[164]

Notes

1. Haigh, E. S., *Xavier Bichat and the medical theory of the eighteenth century* (London, 1984).
2. Binet, Léon, 'M. F. Xavier Bichat', *Sem. Hôp. Paris*, 32 (1956) pp.3985–9; Maulitz, R. C., *A treatise on membranes: concepts of tissue structure, function and dysfunction, from Xavier Bichat to Julius Cohnheim* (PhD thesis, Duke University, 1973), (Ann Arbor, MI, 1979); Canguilhem, G., *DSB*, 2 (1970) pp.122–3; Albury, W. R., 'Experiment and explanation in the physiology of Bichat and Magendie', *Stud. Hist. Biol.*, 1 (1977) pp.47–131. This includes a transcription of manuscripts by Bichat; Pickstone, J. V. 'Bureaucracy, liberalism and the body in post-revolutionary France; Bichat's physiology and the Paris school of medicine', *Hist. Sci.*, 19 (1981) pp.115–42.
3. Huard, P., and M. J. Imbault-Huard, 'La vie et l'oeuvre de Jean Cruveilhier, anatomiste et clinicien', *Episteme*, 8 (1974) pp.46–57; Genty, M., 'Jean Cruveilhier (1791–1874)', *Biographies médicales*, 3 (1932–4) pp.293–308; Huard, P., *DSB*, 3 (1971) pp.489–91.
4. Rokitansky, Carl von, *Selbstbiographie und Antrittsrede*, ed. by E. Lesky (Wien, 1968); Miciotto, R. J., *Carl Rotikansky: nineteenth-century pathologist and leader of the New Vienna School* (PhD thesis, Johns Hopkins University, 1979), (Ann Arbor, MI, 1981).
5. Rosen, G., 'Jacob Henle and William Farr', *Bull. Hist. Med.*, 9 (1941) pp.585–9; Robinson, V., *The life of Jacob Henle* (New York, 1921); Carter, K. C., 'Koch's postulates in relation to the work of Jacob Henle and Edwin Klebs', *Med. Hist.*, 29 (1985) pp.353–74; Evans, A. S., 'Causation and disease: the Henle–Koch postulates

revisited', *Yale J. Biol. Med.*, 49 (1976) pp.175–95; Hintzsche, E., *DSB*, 6 (1972) pp.268–70.

6. Florkin, M., *Naissance et déviation de la théorie cellulaire dans l'oeuvre de Theodore Schwann*, Paris, 1960; Watermann, R., *Theodor Schwann: Leben und Werk* (Dusseldorf, 1960); Maulitz, R. C., 'Schwann's way: cells and crystals', *J. Hist. Med.*, 26 (1971) pp.422–37; Florkin, M., *DSB*, 12 (1975) pp.240–45; Causey, Gilbert, *The cell of Schwann* ... (Edinburgh, London, 1960); see also Thornton–Tully.

7. Steyer, G. E., 'Joseph Hyrtl als komparativer Anatomist', *Anat. Anz.*, 48 (1980) pp.462–73; Steudel, J., *DSB*, 6 (1972) pp.618–19; Patzelt, Viktor, 'Josef Hyrtl. Sein Werk nach 100 Jahren', *Anat. Anz.*, 103 (1956) pp.160–75.

8. Kisch, B., *Forgotten leaders in modern medicine: Valentin, Gruby, Remak, Auerbach* (Philadelphia, 1954); Anderson, C. T., 'Robert Remak and the multinucleated cell: eliminating a barrier to the acceptance of cell division', *Bull. Hist. Med.*, 60 (1986) pp.523–43; Hintzsche, E., *DSB*, 11 (1975) pp.367–70.

9. Zuppinger, H., *Albert Kölliker (1817–1905) und die mikroskopische Anatomie* (Zurich, 1974); Hildebrand, R., 'Rudolf Albert von Koelliker und sein Kreis', *Würzburg. med.-hist. Mitt.*, 3 (1985) pp.127–57; Hintzsche, E., *DSB*, 7 (1973) pp.437–40; Cameron, Sir Roy, 'Rudolf Albert v. Koelliker (1817–1905)', *Ann. Sci.*, 11 (1955) pp.166–72; Ehler, E., 'Albert von Kölliker. Zum Gedächtnis. *Zeitschrift für Wissenschaftliche Zoologie*', 84 (1906) pp.1–26.

10. Virchow, R. L. C., *Collected essays on public health and epidemiology*, ed. by L. J. Rather, 2 vols (Canton, Mass., 1985); Maulitz, R. C., 'Rudolf Virchow, Julius Cohnheim and the program of pathology', *Bull. Hist. Med.*, 52 (1978) pp.162–82; Simon, H. and P. Krietsch, *Rudolf Virchow und Berlin* (Berlin, 1985); Winter, K., *Rudolf Virchow* (Leipzig, 1976); Humboldt-Universität zu Berlin, Universitätsbibliothek, *Rudolf Virchow (1821–1902): Auswahlbibliographie* (Berlin, 1983); Unger, H., *Virchow, ein Leben für die Forschung* (Hamburg, 1953); Boenhum, F. (ed.), *Virchow: Werk und Wirkung* (Berlin, 1957); Virchow, R. L. C., *Disease, life and man: selected essays*, trans. and intro. by L. Rather (Stanford, Calif., 1959); Risse, G. B., *DSB*, 14 (1976) pp.39–44; Ackerknecht, Erwin H., *Rudolf Virchow, doctor, statesman, anthropologist* (Madison, Wisconsin, 1953) (with list of his writings, pp.290–92); Cameron, Sir Roy, 1858 [Symposium in honour of the centenary of Virchow's 'Cellular pathology', 1858–1958] *J. Clin. Path*, 11 (1958) pp.463–72.

11. Ludwig, E. (ed.), *Wilhelm His der Ältere: Lebenserinnerungen und ausgewählte Schriften* (Berne, 1965); Querner, H., *DSB*, 6 (1972) pp.434–6; Picken, Laurence, 'The fate of Wilhelm His', *Nature*, 178 (1956) pp.1162–5.

12. *Wilhelm His der Anatomen: ein Lebensbild* (Berlin, 1931); Bast, T. H., and Weston D. Gardner, 'Wilhelm His, Jr., and the Bundle of His', *J. Hist. Med.*, 4 (1949) pp.170–87.

13. *Arbeiten aus der Medizinische Klinik zu Leipzig* (1893) pp.14–49; *J. Hist. Med.*, 4 (1949) pp.298–318.

14. Thom, A. *et al.*, 'Julius Cohnheim (20.7.1839–15.8.1884) und sein Werk. Beiträge einer Festveranstaltung', *Zbl. Allg. Path.*, 130 (1985) pp.281–347; Maulitz, R. C., 'Rudolf Virchow, Julius Cohnheim and the program of pathology', *Bull. Hist. Med.*, 52 (1978) pp.162–82; Maulitz, R. C., *A treatise on membranes: concepts of tissue structure, function and dysfunction, from Xavier Bichat to Julius Cohneim* (PhD thesis, Duke University, 1973), (Ann Arbor, MI, 1979).

15. Goss, Charles Mayo, *A brief account of Henry Gray and his Anatomy, descriptive and surgical. During a century of its publication in America* (Philadelphia, 1959); Poynter, F. N. L., 'Gray's Anatomy: the first hundred years', *Br. Med. J.*, (1958) ii, pp.610–11; Edwards, George, 'Henry Gray, F.R.S., 1827–1861', *St George's Hosp. Gaz.*, 43 (1958) pp.87–8; Brockbank, William, 'The centenary of a false prophecy: a warning to reviewers', *Med. Hist.*, 2 (1958) pp.67–8; Williams, W. C., *DSB*, 5 (1972) pp.514–15.

16. O'Rahilly, R., 'Quain's "Elements of anatomy"', *Irish J. Med. Sci.*, No.290 (1950) pp.34–8.

17. Reckert, H., *Das unbekannte Werk des Pathologen Robert Carswell (1793–1857)*, (Cologne, 1982).

18. Knecht, K., *Charles Bell, the anatomy of expression (1806): die Ausdruckstheorie des Anatomen und Chirurgen Sir Charles Bell (1774–1842) und ihre Beziehung zur Asthetik des 19. Jahrhunderts* (Cologne, 1978).
19. Cole, F. J., 'Bell's law', *Notes Rec. Roy. Soc. Lond.*, 11 (1955) pp.222–7.
20. Spector, Benjamin, 'Sir Charles Bell and the Bridgewater treatises', *Bull. Hist. Med.*, 12 (1943) pp.314–22; see also *Medical Classics*, 1 (1936–7) pp.81–190 (chronological biography; bibliography, pp.84–96); LeFanu, W. R., 'Charles Bell and Cheselden', *Med. Hist.*, 5 (1961) p.196.
21. Gordon-Taylor, Sir Gordon and E. W. Walls, *Sir Charles Bell, his life and times* (Edinburgh, London, 1958); Gordon-Taylor, Sir Gordon, 'The life and times of Sir Charles Bell. Thomas Vicary Lecture delivered at the Royal College of Surgeons of England on 28th October 1954', *Ann. Roy. Coll. Surg. Engl.*, 18 (1956) pp.1–24; Bell, John W., 'The Bells of Edinburgh', *Surgery*, 38 (1955) pp.794–805; *Letters of Sir Charles Bell, selected from his correspondence with his brother George Joseph Bell* (1870); Cranefield, Paul F., *The way in and the way out: Francois Magendie, Charles Bell and the roots of the spinal nerves* (New York, 1974), (this includes a facsimile of Bell's annotated copy of his *Idea of a new anatomy of the brain*, priv. print., 1811. A facsimile of the *Idea*, with a bio-bibliography, was also published London, 1966); Amacher, P., *DSB*, 1 (1970) pp.583–4.
22. Power, Sir D'Arcy, 'Epoch-making books in British surgery. XI. "My Book", by John Abernethy', *Br. J. Surg.*, 17 (1929–30), pp.369–72.
23. Thornton, John L., *John Abernethy: a biography* (1953), (list of writings, pp.164–8); Thornton, John L., 'John Abernethy, 1764–1831', *St Bart's Hosp. J.*, 68 (1964) pp.287–93; Franklin, Alfred White, 'The tribulations of John Abernethy ...', ibid., pp.283–7, 335–40.
24. Roberts, A.E.S., 'Dominique Jean Larrey, 1766–1842', *Med. J. Southw.*, 71 (1956) pp.134–5.
25. Bechet, Paul E., 'Jean Dominique Larrey, a great military surgeon', *Ann. Med. Hist.*, N.S.9 (1937) pp.428–36; Soubiran, A., *Le baron Larrey, chirurgien de Napoléon* (Paris, 1967); Dible, J. H., *Napoleon's surgeon* (London, 1970); Richardson, R. G., *Larrey: surgeon to Napoleon's imperial guard* (London, 1974).
26. Power, Sir D'Arcy, 'Epoch-making books in British surgery. XII. Sir Astley Cooper's "Treatise on dislocations and fractures"', *Br. J. Surg.*, 17 (1929–30) pp.573–7.
27. Keynes, Sir Geoffrey, 'The life and works of Sir Astley Cooper, Bart.', *St Bart's Hosp. Rep.*, 55 (1922) pp.9–36 (bibliography, pp.35–6); Hill, W., 'Sir Astley Cooper: a bibliography', *Guy's Hosp. Rep.*, 117 (1968) pp.235–55; Cooper, Bransby Blake, *The life of Sir Astley Cooper ...*, 2 vols (1843); Symonds, Sir Charters J., 'Astley Paston Cooper', *Guy's Hosp. Rep.*, 90, Nos 2–4 (1940–1) pp.73–103 (special issue dedicated to Sir Astley Paston Cooper in commemoration of the centenary of his death); Brock, R. C., *The life and work of Astley Cooper* (Edinburgh, 1952).
28. Monafo, William, 'Benjamin Travers, scientific surgeon', *Surg. Gynec. Obstet.*, 120 (1965) pp.587–90.
29. Thomas, K. Bryn, 'Benjamin Brodie: physiologist', *Med. Hist.*, 8 (1964) pp.286–91.
30. Brodie, Sir Benjamin Collins, *Autobiography*, 2nd edn (1865); Acland, Sir Henry W., *Biographical sketch of Sir Benjamin Brodie* (1864); Holmes, Timothy, *Sir Benjamin Collins Brodie* (1898), (Masters of Medicine); *Medical Classics*, 2 (1937–8) pp.883–954 (chronological biography, eponyms, bibliography, pp.885–93); LeFanu, W. R., 'Sir Benjamin Brodie, F.R.S. (1783–1862)', *Notes Rec. Roy. Soc. Lond.*, 19 (1964) pp.42–52; Jones, Arthur Rocyn, 'Sir Benjamin Collins Brodie', *J. Bone Jt Surg.*, 36B (1954) pp.496–501; Riches, Sir Eric, 'A manuscript of Benjamin Collins Brodie's surgical lectures, 1822: with some notes on the history of stricture and stone', *Proc. Roy. Soc. Med.*, 51 (1958) pp.1049–54; Goodfield, G. J., *DSB*, 2 (1970) pp.482–4.
31. Fleming, Percy, 'Robert Liston, the first professor of clinical surgery at U.C.H', *Univ. Coll. Hosp. Mag.*, 11 (1926) pp.176–85; Patterson, M. J. L., 'Robert Liston', *St Bart's Hosp. J.*, 62 (1958) pp.135–41; Littlewood, A. H. M., 'Robert Liston (1794–1847)', *Br. J. Plast. Surg.*, 13 (1960–1) pp.97–101.

32. Lampe, R., *Dieffenbach* (Leipzig, 1934); Genschorek, W., *Wegbereiter der Chirurgie: Johann Friedrich Dieffenbach, Theodor Billroth* (Leipzig, 1982).

33. *Bretonneau et ses correspondants: ouvrage comprenant la correspondence de Trousseau et de Velpeau avec Bretonneau, publié avec une biographie et des notes, par P. Triaire*, 2 vols (Paris, 1892); Genty, M., *Biographies médicales*, 2 (1929–31) pp.297–328.

34. Shepherd, J. A., *Simpson and Syme of Edinburgh* (Edinburgh, 1969); Graham, James M., 'James Syme (1799–1870)', *Br. J. plast. Surg.*, 7 (1954–5) pp.1–12.

35. 'Classic articles in colonic and rectal surgery. John Hilton 1805–78. On the influence of mechanical and physiological rest in the treatment of accidents and surgical diseases, and the diagnostic value of pain', *Dis. Colon Rect.*, 30 (1987) pp.304–13.

36. Wagner, F. B., Jr, 'Revisit of S. D. Gross, M.D.', *Surg. Gynec. Obstet.*, 152 (1981) pp.663–74; Gross, Samuel D., *Autobiography ... with sketches of his contemporaries* (New York, 1972), (facsimile reprint of Philadelphia 1887 edn).

37. Bennett, J. P., 'Sir William Fergusson, Bart., 1808–1877', *Ann. Roy. Coll. Surg. Engl.*, 59 (1977) pp.484–7; Ewing, M., 'Sir William Fergusson (1808–1877)', *J. Roy. Coll. Surg. Edin.*, 22 (1977) pp.127–35; Gordon-Taylor, Sir Gordon, 'Sir William Fergusson, Bt., F.R.C.S., F.R.S. (1808–1877)', *Med. Hist.*, 5 (1961) pp.1–14 (a list of his papers is given on p.13).

38. On disease of the mammary areola preceding cancer of the mammary gland', *St Bart's Hosp. Rep.*, 10 (1874) pp.87–9; 'On a form of chronic inflammation of bones (osteitis deformans)', *Med. Chir. Trans.*, 60 (1877) pp.37–64; and 65 (1882) pp.225–36 (both of these are included in *Medical Classics*, 1 (1936–7) pp.5–78; bibliography, pp.7–21). See also Power, Sir D'Arcy, 'Eponyms. V. Sir James Paget', *Br. J. Surg.*, 10 (1922–3) pp.1–3, 161–4.

39. See also *Memoirs and letters of Sir James Paget. Edited by Stephen Paget* (London, 1901); Bett, W. R., 'Life and works of Sir James Paget', *St Bart's Hosp. J.*, 33 (1925–6) pp.21–6; Paget, Stephen, 'Sir James Paget ...', ibid., 9 (1901–2) pp.17–21; Shenoy, B. V. and B. W. Scheitauer, 'Paget's perspectives on pathology', *Mayo Clin. Proc.*, 63 (1988) pp.184–92; Whitfield, A. G. W., Beloved Sir James: the life of Sir James Clark, Bart, physician to Queen Victoria, 1788–1870 ([Sutton Coldfield, 1982]).

40. Thornton, John L., 'Sir James Paget's notes on his students', *Ann. Roy. Coll. Surg. Engl.*, 21 (1957) pp.199–201.

41. *A memoir of Henry Jacob Bigelow* (Boston, 1900).

42. Godlee, Sir Rickman John, *Lord Lister* (1917); Leeson, John Rudd, *Lister as I knew him* (1927); Guthrie, Douglas, *Lord Lister, his life and doctrine* (Edinburgh, 1949); the *Scottish Medical Journal*, 10, ix, Sept. 1965, is a Lister centenary issue; Wangensteen, O.H. 'Nineteenth-century wound management of the parturient uterus and compound fracture: the Semmelweis–Lister priority controversy', *Bull. N.Y. Acad. Med.*, 46 (1970) pp.565–96; Fisher, R. B., *Joseph Lister, 1827–1912* (London, 1977); Fox, N. J., 'Scientific theory choice and social structure: the case of Joseph Lister's antisepsis, humoral theory and asepsis', *Hist. Sci.*, 26 (1988) pp.367–97; Dolman, C. E., *DSB*, 8 (1973) pp.399–413.

43. LeFanu, William, *A list of the original writings of Joseph, Lord Lister, O. M.* (Edinburgh, London, 1965); *Lister Centenary Exhibition at the Wellcome Historical Medical Museum. Handbook, 1927* (1927), (chronological list of Lister's writings, pp.155–66; biographies etc., pp.167–75; Johnson and Johnson, *Lister and the ligature: a landmark in the history of modern surgery ...* (New Brunswick, N. J., 1925), (bibliography of his writings, pp.83–9);

44. *Medical Classics*, 2 (1937–8) pp.5–101 (chronological biography; bibliography, pp.9–15); 'Classics in infectious diseases. On the antiseptic principles of the practice. Reprinted from *The Lancet*, 1867, 2, pp.353–56', *Dis. Colon Rect.*, 25 (1982) pp.173–8 (also in *Rev. Infect. Dis.*, 9 (1987) pp.421–6).

45. Obituary notice in *St Bart's Hosp. Rep.*, 63 (1930) pp.1–17 (list of books and papers, pp.11–17).

46. It was also published in 1922 in *Arch. Neurol. Psych.*, 7, pp.681–710; and in *Medical Classics*, 2 (1937–8) pp.957–97, with chronological biography and bibliography; a German translation was published in 1912 in Sudhoff's *Med. Klass.* See also *James*

Parkinson (1755–1824). A bicentenary volume of papers dealing with Parkinson's disease, incorporating the original 'Essay on the shaking palsy'. Edited by Macdonald Critchley. With the collaboration of William H. McMenemey, Francis M. R. Walshe, J. Godwin Greenfield (London, New York, 1955), (biographical essay by W. H. McMenemey, pp.1–143).

47. Rowntree, L. G., 'James Parkinson', *Bull. Johns Hopkins Hosp.*, 23 (1912) pp.33–45.

48. Robertson, E. Graeme, 'James Parkinson and his Essay on the shaking palsy', *Roy. Melbourne Hosp. Clin. Rep.* (25 Dec. 1955) pp.1–14; Gardner-Thorpe, C., *James Parkinson 1755–1824*, 2nd edn (Exeter, 1988).

49. Morris, A. D., *James Parkinson: his life and times [published posthumously], edited with a new chapter on progress in treating 'Parkinson's disease' since Parkinson's time by F. Clifford Rose* (Basle, 1989). A copy of A. D. Morris's full typescript has been deposited in the Library of the Royal College of Physicians of London (MS.820).

50. Horine, E. F. H., *Daniel Drake (1785–1852), pioneer physician of the midwest* (Philadelphia, 1961); Mansfield, E. D., *Memoirs of the life and services of Daniel Drake, M.D.* (New York, 1975), (reprint of 1855 Cincinnati edn); Drake, Daniel, *Malaria in the interior valley of North America: a selection by N. D. Levine from A systematic treatise* ... (Urbana, Ill., 1964); Drake, Daniel, *Physician to the West: selected writings on science and society, ed. by H. D. Shapiro* (Lexington, Ky, 1970).

51. Stookey, B., 'Jean-Baptiste Bouillaud and Ernest Aubertin. Early studies on cerebral localization and the speech center', *JAMA*, 184 (1963) pp.1024–9; Rolleston, J. D., 'Jean-Baptiste Bouillaud, 1796–1881, a pioneer in cardiology and neurology', *Proc. Roy. Soc. Med.*, 24 (1931) pp.1253–62; Busquet, P., *Biographies médicales*, 1 (1927–8) pp.251–64.

52. Aron, E., *Bretonneau: le médecin de Tours* (Paris, 1979); Mutzner-Scharplatz, U., *Pierre Bretonneau (1778–1862) der Entdecker der Diphtherie* (Zurich, 1965); *Bretonneau et ses correspondants: ouvrage comprenant la correspondance de Trousseau et de Velpeau avec Bretonneau, publié avec une biographie et des notes, par P. Triaire*, 2 vols (Paris, 1892); Rousseau, A., *DSB*, 2 (1970) pp.444–5; Apert, E., *Biographies médicales*, 6 (1937–9) pp.209–54.

53. See Ganière, Paul, *Corvisart, médecin de Napoléon* (Paris, 1951); Touche, Marcel, *Jean Nicolas Corvisart, praticien célèbre, grand maître de la médecine* (Paris, 1968); Coury, Charles, 'La méthode anatomo-clinique et ses promoteurs en France: Corvisart, Bayle et Laënnec', *Méd. de France*, 224 (1971) pp.13–22; Ganière, P., *DSB*, 3 (1971) pp.426–8.

54. Rousseau, A., 'Gaspard Laurent Bayle (1774–1816): le théoricien de l'École de Paris', *Clio Med.*, 6 (1971) pp.205–11; Coury, Charles, op. cit. in note no.53 above; Huard, P. and M. J. Imbault-Huard, 'Gaspard Laurent Bayle: ou la méthodologie de la médecine anatomo-clinique ...', *Gaz. Méd. de France*, 81 (1974) pp.4943, 4946, 4949; Bayle, A. L. J. and A. J. Thillaye (eds), *Biographie médicale*, Paris (1855) vol.2, pp.884–99.

55. Braunstein, J. F., *Broussais et le matérialisme: médecine et philosophie au XIXe siècle* (Paris, 1986); Ackerknecht, E. H., 'Broussais or a forgotten medical revolution', *Bull. Hist. Med.*, 27 (1953) pp.320–43; Bonnette, P., *Broussais: sa vie, son oeuvre, son centenaire, 1772–1838* (Paris, 1939); Huard, P., *DSB*, 2 (1970) pp.507–9.

56. Greenwood, M., 'Louis and the numerical method' in *The medical dictator and other essays* (London, 1936), (reprinted London, 1986) pp.75–87; Muellener, E. R., 'Pierre Charles Alexandre Louis (1787–1872). Genfer Schuler und die "méthode numérique"', *Gesnerus*, 24 (1967) pp.46–74; Bariety, M., 'Louis et la méthode numérique', *Clio Med.*, 7 (1972) pp.177–83; Bollet, A. J., 'Pierre Louis: the numerical method and the foundation of quantitative medicine', *Amer. J. Med. Sci.*, 266 (1973) pp.92–101; Piquemal, J., 'Succès et décadence de la méthode numérique en France à l'époque de Pierre Charles Alexandre Louis', *Méd. de France*, 250 (1974) pp.11–22, 59–60.

57. Viets, Henry R., '"*De l'auscultation médiate*" of Laënnec', *Arch. Surg.*, 18 (1929) pp.1280–97.

58. Kervran, Roger, *Laënnec, his life and times ... Translated from the French by D. C. Abrahams-Curiel* (Oxford, 1960).

59. LeFanu, W. R., 'Laënnec and Matthew Baillie', *Ann. Roy. Coll. Surg. Engl.*, 36

(1965) pp.67–8; Thayer, W. S., 'On some unpublished letters of Laënnec', *Bull. Johns Hopkins Hosp.*, 31 (1920) pp.425–35; Huard, P. and M. D. Grmek, 'Les élèves étrangers de Laënnec', *Rev. Hist. Sci. (Paris)*, 26 (1973) pp.315–37; Duffin, J., *Laënnec: entre la pathologie et la clinique* (Paris, doct. thesis Sorbonne, 1985); Duffin, J., 'The medical philosophy of R. T. H. Laënnec (1781–1826)', *Hist. Philos. Life Sci.*, 8 (1986) pp.195–219; Duffin, J. M., 'The cardiology of R. T. H. Laënnec', *Med. Hist.*, 33 (1989) pp.42–71; Heaf, F., *DSB*, 7 (1973) pp.556–7; Coury, Charles, op. cit. in note no.53 above.

60. Gomez, Domingo M., *Trousseau (1801–1867)* (Paris, 1929); *Bretonneau et ses correspondants: ouvrage comprenant la correspondance de Trousseau et de Velpeau avec Bretonneau*, op. cit. in note no. 52 above. Genty, M., *Biographies médicales*, 2 (1929–31) pp.265–96.

61. Hale-White, Sir William, 'Richard Bright and his discovery of the disease bearing his name', *Guy's Hosp. Rep.*, 107 (1958) pp.294–307 (reprinted from ibid., 71 (1921) pp.1–20); Keith, Norman M. and Thomas E. Keys, 'Contributions of Richard Bright and his associates to renal disease', *Arch. Intern. Med.*, 94 (1954) pp.5–21; Cameron, S. J. and L. E. Becker, 'Richard Bright and observations in renal histology', *Guy's Hosp. Rep.*, 113 (1964) pp.159–71; Hale-White, Sir William, 'Bright's observations other than those on renal disease', *Guy's Hosp. Rep.*, 107 (1958) pp.308–22; Kark, R. M. and D. T. Moore, 'The life, work, and geological collections of Richard Bright, M.D. (1789–1858) ...', *Arch. Nat. Hist.*, 10 (1981) pp.119–51; Kark, R. M., *Physician extraordinary: Dr. Richard Bright (1789–1858)* (Montpelier, Vermont, 1986); Bright, P., *Dr. Richard Bright (1789–1858)* (London, 1983); King, L. S., *DSB*, 2 (1970) pp.463–5.

62. Hill, William, 'Richard Bright: a bibliography', *Guy's Hosp. Rep.*, 107 (1958) pp.531–42 (reprinted from *Guy's Hosp. Gaz.*, 64 (1950) pp.373–9, 393–7, 439–42, 454–7, 472–83); Winston, G. A. R., 'Richard Bright and his published writings: a review', *Guy's Hosp. Gaz.*, 72 (1958) pp.483–8.

63. Garrison, Fielding H., 'Richard Bright's travels in Lower Hungary: a physician's holiday', *Johns Hopkins Hosp. Bull.*, 23 (1912) pp.173–82; Oliver, Jean, 'Materials for a portrait of Richard Bright as a young man', *J. Mount Sinai Hosp.*, 24 (1957) pp.1057–65.

64. Brock, Sir Russell Claude, 'Addison and appendicitis', *Guy's Hosp. Rep.*, 109 (1960) pp.273–9.

65. This was published in *Lond. Med. Gaz.*, N.S.8 (1849) pp.517–18, and was later reprinted in *A collection of the published writings of the late Thomas Addison* (1868) pp.211–39, as well as in *Klassiker der Medizin*, no.20 (1912) and in *Medical Classics*, 2 (1937–8) pp.233–80 (which also contains a chronological biography and a bibliography). A facsimile edition was published in London, 1968, and the text plus selected illustrations were included in *Great men of Guy's*, ed. by W. Ober (Metuchen, N. J., 1973). See also Long, Esmond R., 'Thomas Addison and his discovery of idiopathic anaemia', *Ann. Med. Hist.*, N.S.7 (1935) pp.130–2.

66. Moynahan, E. J., 'Addison's place in dermatology', *Guy's Hosp. Rep.*, 109 (1960) pp.262–8.

67. Winston, G. A. R. and William Hill, 'Bibliography of the published writings of Thomas Addison, M.D.' ibid., pp.280–3 (included in a special issue of the journal, with Dodds, Sir E. C., 'Thomas Addison and after', and the Brock and Moynahan papers cited in notes 64 and 66 above). See also Brooks, Charles M., 'Thomas Addison, M.D., F.R.C.P., 1794–1860', *Newcastle Med. J.*, 27 (1962–3) pp.255–72; Bishop, P. M. F., 'Dr. Addison and his work', *Guy's Hosp. Rep.*, 104 (1955) pp.275–94 (and *Proc. Roy. Soc. Med.*, 48 (1955) pp.1032–8); Benjamin, J. A., *DSB*, 1 (1970) pp.59–60; Pallister, G., *Thomas Addison, M.D., F.R.C.P. (1795–1860)*, [Newcastle-upon-Tyne, 1975]; Rather, L. J., *Addison and the white corpuscles: an aspect of nineteenth-century biology* (London, 1972).

68. *Lond. Med. Surg. J. (Renshaw)*, 7 (1835) pp.516–17 (reprinted in *Medical Classics*, 5 (1940–1) pp.21–43; contains chronological biography; bibliography, pp.23, 24; and reprints his description of exophthalmic goitre).

69. Mulcahy, Ristéard, '"Diseases of the heart and aorta", by William Stokes (1854). A

modern clinical review', *Irish J. Med. Sci.*, No.350 (1955) pp.53–66; Stokes, Sir William, *William Stokes, his life and work (1804–1878)*, (1898; bibliography of his writings, pp.243–7).

70. Cyriax, R. J., 'George Bodington (1799–1882), pioneer of open air treatment of pulmonary tuberculosis. With bibliography', *Brit. J. Tuberc.*, 35 (1941) pp.58–68.

71. See *Medical Classics*, 4 (1939–40) pp.843–920 (contains chronological biography; bibliography, pp.845–59; and list of biographies).

72. 'On some morbid appearances of the absorbent glands and spleen', *Medico-chirurgical Trans.*, 17 (1832) pp.68–114 (reprinted in *Medical Classics*, 1, no.7 (1937) pp.741–70).

73. Kass, E. H., 'Thomas Hodgkin MD (1798–1866): an annotated bibliography', *Bull. Hist. Med.*, 43 (1969) pp.138–75; Rose, M., *Curator of the dead: Thomas Hodgkin (1798–1866)* (London, 1981); Rosenfeld, L., 'Thomas Hodgkin (1798–1866): morbid anatomist and social activist', *Bull. N.Y. Acad. Med.*, 62 (1986) pp.193–205; Kass, A. M. and E. H. Kass *Perfecting the world: the life and times of Dr Thomas Hodgkin (1798–1866)* (Boston, 1988).

74. Clark, Sir James, *A memoir of John Conolly; comprising a sketch of the treatment of the insane in Europe and America* (1869); Scull, A., 'John Conolly: a reconsideration', *J. Roy. Soc. Med.*, 81 (1988) pp.67–70; Scull, A., 'A brilliant career? John Conolly and Victorian psychiatry', *Vict. Stud.*, 27 (1984) pp.203–35; Scull, A., 'A Victorian alienist: John Conolly, FRCP, DCL (1794–1866)', in W. F. Bynum, R. Porter and M. Shepherd (eds), *The anatomy of madness* .. vol. 1 (London, 1985) pp.103–50.

75. Hunter, Richard A. and Ida Macalpine, 'An anonymous publication on vaccination by John Conolly (1794–1866)', *J. Hist. Med.*, 14 (1959) pp.311–19.

76. Temkin, O., 'Gall and the phrenological movement', *Bull. Hist. Med.*, 21 (1947) pp.275–321; Ackerknecht, E. H. and H. V. Vallois, *François Joseph Gall et sa collection* (Paris, 1955), (English translation, Madison, WI, 1956); Critchley, M., 'Neurology's debt to F. J. Gall (1758–1828)', *Br. Med. J.*, 2 (1965) pp.775–81; Lantéri-Laura G., *Histoire de la phrénologie: l'homme et son cerveau selon F. J. Gall* (Paris, 1970); Lesky, Erna (ed.), *Franz Joseph Gall, 1758–1828, Naturforscher und Anthropologe: ausgewählte Texte* (Berne, 1979); Heintel, Helmuth and Brigitte Heintel, *Franz Joseph Gall Bibliographie* (Stuttgart, 1985); Heintel, H., *Leben und Werk von Franz Joseph Gall, eine Chronik* (Würzburg, 1986); Young, R. M., *DSB*, 5 (1972) pp.250–6.

77. Hall, Charlotte, *Memoirs of Marshall Hall, by his widow* (London, 1961); Erez-Federbusch, R., *Marshall Hall, 1790–1857. Physiologe und Praktiker* (Zurich, 1983); Manuel, D. F., 'Marshall Hall, F.R.S. (1790–1857): a conspectus of his life and work', *Notes Rec. Roy. Soc.*, 35 (1980) pp.135–66; Jefferson, Sir Geoffrey, 'Marshall Hall, the grasp reflex and the diastaltic spinal cord', in E. A. Underwood (ed.), *Science, medicine and history*, vol.2 (Oxford, 1953) pp.303–20 (reprinted in Jefferson, Sir Geoffrey, *Selected papers* (London, 1960) pp.73–93).

78. Bernard, Claude, *Discours de réception [à l'Académie Française] de M. Claude Bernard: réponse de M. Patin ... 1869* (Paris, 1869), (the 'Discours' is a biographical sketch of Flourens); Legée, Georgette, 'Physiologie et phrénologie au temps du physiologiste Pierre Flourens', *Int. Congr. Hist. Med.*, (27th, 1980, Barcelona), Actas (1981) vol.1, pp.91–7; Legée, Georgette, 'Les résultats de Pierre Flourens sur les fonctions du cerveau jugés par F. J. Gall, J. Bouillaud et D. Ferrier', *Hist. et Nat.*, No.11 (1977) pp.45–58; Legée, Georgette, 'Les découvertes de Marie-Jean-Pierre Flourens sur l'action des substances toxiques et des anesthétiques', *Hist. Sci. Med.*, 8 (1974) pp.757–71; Kruta, V., *DSB*, 5 (1972) pp.44–5.

79. Schiller, F., *Paul Broca: founder of French anthropology, explorer of the brain* (Berkeley, Calif., 1979); Huard, P., 'Paul Broca (1824–1880)', *Rev. Hist. Sci. (Paris)*, 14 (1961) pp.47–86 (includes a bibliography); Huard, P., 'Vingt ans de réflexions sur Paul Broca', *Hist. Sci. Méd.*, 15 (1981) pp.23–8; Berker, E. A. et al., 'Translation of Broca's 1865 report. Localization of speech in the third left frontal convolution', *Arch. Neurol.*, 43 (1986) pp.1065–72; Clarke, E., *DSB*, 2 (1970) pp.477–8.

80. Guillain, Georges, *J-M. Charcot, 1825–1893: his life, his work ... Edited and trans-*

lated by Pearce Bailey (1959), (English translation of Charcot's writings, pp.192–93; French version, Paris, 1955); Owen, A. R. G., *Hysteria, hypnosis and healing: the work of Jean-Martin Charcot* (London, 1971); Didi-Huberman, G., *Invention de l'hystérie: Charcot et l'iconographie photographique de la Salpêtrière* (Paris, 1982); Nicale, M. S., 'The Salpêtrière in the age of Charcot: an institutional perspective on medical history in the late nineteenth century', *J. Contemporary Hist.*, 20 (1985) pp.703–31; Tetry, A., *DSB*, 3 (1971) p.205.

81. Stillians, Arthur W., 'Ferdinand von Hebra', *Quart. Bull. Northw. Univ. Med. Sch.*, 33 (1959) pp.141–5.

82. Hadley, R. M., 'The life and works of Sir William James Erasmus Wilson, 1809–1884', *Med. Hist.*, 3 (1959) pp.215–47 (writings, pp.243–5); Everett, M. A., 'Erasmus Wilson and the birth of the specialty of dermatology', *Int. J. Derm.*, 17 (1978) pp.345–52.

83. In *New Engl. Quart. J. Med. Surg.*, Boston, 1 (1842–3) pp.503–30.

84. Both reprinted in *Medical Classics*, 1 (1936–7), pp.195–268 (contains chronological biography, and bibliography, pp.196–201); Busby, M. J. and A. E.Rodin, 'Relative contributions of Holmes and Semmelweis to the understanding of the etiology of puerperal fever', *Texas Rep. Biol. Med.*, 34 (1976) pp.221–37; Hoyt, E. P., *The improper Bostonian: Dr Oliver Wendell Holmes* (New York, 1979).

85. See *Medical Classics*, 5 (1940–1) pp.339–773 (contains chronological biography; bibliography, and translation of this classic, pp.350–773). New English translation, ed. with an introduction by K. Codell Carter, published as *The etiology, concept and prophylaxis of childbed fevers* (Madison, Wisc., 1983).

86. Sinclair, Sir William J., *Semmelweis, his life and doctrine: a chapter in the history of medicine* (Manchester, 1909), (Publications of the University of Manchester, Medical Series, No. XI); Slaughter, Frank G., *Immortal Magyar. Semmelweis, conquerer of childbed fever*, (New York, 1950); Lesky, Erna, *Ignaz Philipp Semmelweis und die Wiener medizinische Schule* (Vienna, 1964); Wangensteen, O. H., 'Nineteenth-century wound management of the parturient uterus and compound fracture: the Semmelweis–Lister priority controversy', *Bull. N.Y. Acad. Med.*, 46 (1970) pp.565–96; Gortvay, G. and I. Zoltan, *Semmelweis: his life and work* (Budapest, 1968); Benedek, I., *Ignaz Philipp Semmelweis 1818–1865* (Vienna, 1983); Carter, K. C., 'Semmelweis and his predecessors', *Med. Hist.*, 25 (1981) pp.57–72; Carter, K. C., 'Ignaz Semmelweis, Carl Mayrhofer and the rise of germ theory', *Med. Hist.*, 29 (1985) pp.331–53; Risse, G. B., *DSB*, 12 (1975) pp.294–9.

87. Murphy, Frank P., 'Ignaz Philipp Semmelweiss (1818–1865). An annotated bibliography', *Bull. Hist. Med.*, 20 (1946) pp.653–707; see also Colebrook, Leonard, 'The story of puerperal fever, 1800–1950', *Br. Med. J.*, (1956) I, pp.247–52.

88. Duns, John, *Memoir of Sir James Y. Simpson* (Edinburgh, 1873); Gordon, Henry Laing, *Sir James Young Simpson and chloroform (1811–1870)*, (1897) (Masters of Medicine); Selwyn, S., 'Sir James Simpson and hospital cross-infection', *Med. Hist.*, 9 (1965) pp.241–8; Thornton, John L., 'The relationship between James Matthew Duncan and Sir James Simpson', *Med. Illustrated*, 3 (1949) pp.261–5; Simpson, M., *Simpson, the obstetrician: a biography* (London, 1972); Russell, K. F. and F. M. C. Forster, *A list of the works of Sir James Young Simpson 1811–1870: a centenary tribute* (Melbourne, 1971); Shepherd, J. A., *Simpson and Syme of Edinburgh* (Edinburgh, 1969).

89. Reprinted in *Medical Classics*, 2 (1937–8) pp.663–712 (contains chronological biography; bibliography, pp.665–70).

90. Harris, Seale and Francis Williams Browin, *Woman's surgeon: the life story of J. Marion Sims* (New York, 1950); and Carmichael, Emmett B. J., 'Marion Sims, inventor, physician, surgeon', *J. Internat. Coll. Surg.*, 33 (1960) pp.757–62.

91. Collingworth, C. J., 'List of Sir Thomas Spencer Wells' published writings, arranged chronologically', *Trans. Obstet. Soc. Lond.*, 40 (1898) pp.91–101.

92. Shepherd, John A., *Spencer Wells: the life and work of a Victorian surgeon* (Edinburgh, London, 1965); Power, Sir D'Arcy, 'Eponyms XXIII. Spencer Wells' forceps', *Br. J. Surg.*, 14 (1926–7) pp.385–9.

93. Flack, Isaac Harvey, *Lawson Tait, 1845–1899* (1949); McKay, William John Stew-

art, *Lawson Tait, his life and work: a contribution to the history of abdominal surgery and gynaecology* (1922); Risdon, W., *Robert Lawson Tait* (London, 1967); Shepherd, J. A., *Lawson Tait, the rebellious surgeon (1845–1899)* (Lawrence, Kansas, 1890); Shepherd, J. A., 'The contribution of Robert Lawson Tait to the development of abdominal surgery', *Surg. Annu.*, 18 (1986) pp.339–49.

94.   Laage, R. J. Ch. V. ter, *DSB*, 4 (1971) pp.162–4.
95.   *Medical Classics*, 5 (1940–1) pp.249–336 (contains chronological biography; bibliography, pp.251–4); Thomas, K. B., 'The manuscripts of Sir William Bowman', *Med. Hist.*, 10 (1966) pp.245–56; Grondana, F., 'Structure et fonction du rein selon William Bowman', *Clio Med.*, 6 (1971) pp.195–204; Thomas, K. B., *DSB*, 2 (1970) pp.375–7.
96.   Muenchow, W., *Albrecht von Graefe* (Leipzig, 1978).
97.   M'Kendrick, John Gray, *Hermann Ludwig Ferdinand von Helmholtz* (1899); Crombie, A. C., 'Helmholtz', *Sci. Amer.*, 198 (1958) pp.94–102; Helmholtz number of *Proc. Staff Mtgs Mayo Clinic*, 26, xii, 6 June 1951 (includes Keys, Thomas E., 'Contributions leading to the invention of the ophthalmoscope', pp.209–16; and Rucker, C. Wilbur, 'The development of the ophthalmoscope and of knowledge of the interior of the eye', pp.271–21); *Selected writings*, ed. with an introduction by R. Kahl (Middletown, Conn., 1971); Turner, R. S., *DSB*, 6 (1972) pp.241–53. See also Thornton–Tully.
98.   Olmsted, J. M. D., 'French contributions to physiology in the XIX century', *Texas Rep. Biol. Med.*, 13 (1955) pp.306–16.
99.   Olmsted, J. M. D., *François Magendie, pioneer in experimental physiology and scientific medicine in XIX century France ... With a preface by John F. Fulton* (New York, 1944), (list of Magendie's writings, pp.271–7); Deloyers, L., *François Magendie: précurseur de la médecine expérimentale* (Brussels, 1970); Albury, W. R., 'Experiment and explanation in the physiology of Bichat and Magendie', *Stud. Hist. Biol.*, 1 (1977) pp.47–131; Theodorides, J. *et al.*, 'Présence et actualité de François Magendie (1783–1855)', *Hist. Sci. Méd.*, 17 (1983) pp.321–80: Grmek, M. D., *DSB*, 9 (1974) pp.6–11; Cranefield, Paul F., *The way in and the way out: François Magendie, Charles Bell and the roots of the spinal nerves* (New York, 1974).
100.   Young, Frank G., 'Claude Bernard and the discovery of glycogen. A century of retrospect', *Br. Med. J.*, (1957) I, pp.1431–7; Young, Frank G., 'Claude Bernard and the theory of the glycogenic function of the liver', *Ann. Sci.*, 2 (1937) pp.47–83.
101.   Siegel, Rudoph E., 'Vascular catheterization during the 19th century: Claude Bernard's studies on animal heat', *Surgery*, 55 (1964) pp.595–601; Olmsted, J. M. D., *Claude Bernard, physiologist* (New York, 1938), (contains list of more important writings, pp.257–62); Foster, Sir Michael, *Claude Bernard* (1899) (Masters of Medicine); Virtanen, Reino, *Claude Bernard and his place in the history of ideas* (Lincoln, Nebraska, 1960); *Medical Classics*, 3 (1938–9, pp.513–617), (contains chronological biography; bibliography of 221 items, pp.518–40; list of biographies; reprints of papers on sugar in animal body, pp.552–80; and on digestion, pp.581–617).
102.   Holmes, F. L., *Claude Bernard and animal chemistry: the emergence of a scientist* (Cambridge, Mass., 1974); Grmek, M. D., *Raisonnement expérimental et recherches toxicologiques chez Claude Bernard* (Geneva, 1973); Schiller, J., *Claude Bernard et les problèmes scientifiques de son temps* (Paris, 1967); Schiller, J., 'Claude Bernard et la médecine', *Hôp. à Paris*, 11 (1970) pp.447–67; Grmek, M. D. (comp.), *Catalogue des manuscrits de Claude Bernard; avec la bibliographie de ses travaux imprimés et des études sur son oeuvre* (Paris, 1967); Grmek, M. D., *DSB*, 2 (1970) pp.24–34; Bernard, Claude, *Lectures on the phenomena of life common to plants and animals (vol.1)*, translated by H. H. Hoff *et al.* (Springfield, Ill., 1974); Cranefield, P. F. (ed.), *Claude Bernard's revised edition of his Introduction à l'étude de la médecine expérimentale* (New York, 1976).
103.   Olmsted, J. M. D., *Charles-Édouard Brown-Séquard: a nineteenth-century neurologist and endocrinologist* (Baltimore, 1946); Goody, William, 'Some aspects of the life of Dr. C. E. Brown-Séquard', *Proc. Roy. Soc. Med.*, 57 (1964) pp.189–92; Role, André, *La vie étrange d'un grand savant: le professeur Brown-Séquard, 1817–1894* (Paris, 1977); Grmek, M. D., *DSB*, 2 (1970) pp.524–6.

104. Leake, Chauncey D., 'Beaumont's belly', *J. Internat. Coll. Surg.*, 36 (1961) pp.252–60; Brodman, Estelle, 'Scientific and editorial relationships between Joseph Lovell and William Beaumont', *Bull. Hist. Med.*, 38 (1964) pp.127–32.
105. Myer, Jesse S., *Life and letters of Dr. William Beaumont, including hitherto unpublished data concerning the case of Alexis St. Martin ... With an introduction by Sir William Osler* (St Louis, 1912); new edn with a reprint of the 1st edn of *Experiments and observations on the gastric juice ...* (St Louis, 1981); see also Miller, William Snow, 'William Beaumont, M.D. (1785–1853)', *Ann. Med. Hist.*, N.S.5 (1933) pp.28–51; Cohen, J. B. (ed.), *The career of William Beaumont and the reception of his discovery* (New York, 1980); Rosen, G., *DSB*, 1 (1970) pp.542–5.
106. Poynter, F. N. L., 'The reception of William Beaumont's discovery in England. Two additional early references', *J. Hist. Med.*, 12 (1957) pp.511–12; Rosen, G., 'The reception of William Beaumont's discovery. Some comments on Dr. Poynter's note', ibid., 13 (1958) pp.404–6; Poynter, F. N. L., 'New light on the reception of William Beaumont's discovery in England', ibid., pp.406–9.
107. Pizer, Irwin H., 'Source materials and the library: the dispersion of the Beaumont papers', *Bull. Med. Lib. Assn*, 52 (1964) pp.328–36.
108. John, H. J., 'Jan Evangelista Purkyně, Czech scientist and patriot (1787–1869)', *Proc. Roy. Soc. Med.*, 46 (1953) pp.933–40; John, H. J., *Jan Evangelista Purkyně: Czech scientist and patriot, 1787–1869* (Philadelphia, 1959); Kruta, V., *J. E. Purkyně (1787–1869) physiologist: a short account of his contribution to the progress of physiology, with a bibliography of his works* (Prague, 1969); Kruta, V., 'J. E. Purkyně's contribution to the cell theory', *Clio Med.*, 6 (1971) pp.109–20; *Jan Evangelista Purkyně 1787–1869. Centenary symposium ... Prague ... 1969* (Brno, 1971); Kruta, V., *DSB*, 11 (1975) pp.213–17.
109. Ebbecke, Ulrich, *Johannes Müller, der grosse rheinische Physiologe. Mit einem Neudruck von Johannes Müllers Schrift Über die phantastischen Gesichtserscheinungen* (Hannover, 1951); Koller, Gottfried, *Das Leben des Biologen Johannes Müller, 1801–1858* (Stuttgart, 1958); Lohff, Brigitte R., *Johannes Müller (1801–1858) als akademischer Lehrer* (Hamburg University thesis, 1977); Steudel, J., *DSB*, 9 (1974) pp.567–74.
110. Geison, G. L., *Sir Michael Foster and the Cambridge school of physiology: the scientific enterprise in late Victorian society* (Princeton, N.J., 1978); Geison, G. L., *DSB*, 5 (1972) pp.79–84.
111. Schroeer, H., *Carl Ludwig: Begründer der messenden Experimentalphysiologie 1816–1895* (Stuttgart, 1967); *Zwei grosse Naturforscher des 19. Jahrhunderts: ein Briefswechsel zwischen Emil du Bois-Reymond und Karl Ludwig*, ed. by Estelle du Bois-Reymond and P. Diepgen (Leipzig, 1927); English translation, *Two great scientists of the nineteenth century: correspondence of Emil du Bois-Reymond and Carl Ludwig*, ed. by P. F. Cranefield (Baltimore, 1982); Rosen, G., *DSB*, 8 (1973) pp.540–2.
112. *Zwei grosse Naturforscher des 19. Jahrhunderts*, op. cit. in note 111 above; Cranefield, P. F., 'Charles E. Morgan's *Electrophysiology and therapeutics*: an unknown English version of Du Bois-Reymond's *Thierische Elektricität*', *Bull. Hist. Med.*, 31 (1957) pp.172–81; Marseille, J., *Das physiologische Lebenswerk von E. du Bois-Reymond, mit besonderer Berücksichtigung seiner Schuler*, MD dissertation, Münster, 1967 (includes a complete bibliography of his writings); Rothschuh, K. E. and E. Tutte, 'Emil du Bois-Reymond (1818–1896): Bibliographie, Originalien und Sekundärliteratur', in *Beiträge zur Geschichte der Naturwissenschaften und der Medizin: Festschrift für Georg Uschmann zum 60. Geburtstag* (Halle/Saale, 1975) pp.113–36; *Naturwissen und Erkenntnis im 19. Jahrhundert: Emil du Bois-Reymond*, ed. by G. Mann (Hildesheim, 1981); Ruff, P. W., *Emil du Bois-Reymond* (Leipzig, 1981); Rothschuh, K. E., *DSB*, 4 (1971) pp.200–5.
113. Guilly, P. J. L., *Duchenne de Boulogne* (Paris, 1936); Jokl, E., 'Guillaume Benjamin Amand Duchenne de Boulogne et la physiologie des mouvements', *Episteme*, 1 (1967) pp.273–83.
114. *E. J. Marey and cardiology: physiologist and pioneer of technology, 1830–1904. Selected writings in facsimile with comments and summaries, a brief history of the life and work and a bibliography by H. A. Snellen* (Rotterdam, 1980); Espinosa, R. E. *et*

al., 'J. B. A. Chauveau, E. J. Marey and their resolution of the apex beat controversy through intracardiac pressure recordings', *Mayo Clin. Proc.*, 58 (1983) pp.197–202; Gross, M., *DSB*, 9 (1974) pp.101–3.
115. Gray, J. A., *Pavlov* (Douglas, Isle of Man, 1979); Frolov, Y. P., *Pavlov and his school: the theory of conditioned reflexes* (London, 1938); Babkin, B. P., *Pavlov: a biography* (Chicago, 1949); Grigorian, N. A., *DSB*, 10 (1974) pp.431–6.
116. Klein, M., *DSB*, 12 (1975) pp.173–6.
117. Sparkman, Robert S., 'The early development of gall-bladder surgery. Centennial of the proposed cholecystostomy of J. L. W. Thudichum', *Br. Med. J.* (1959) ii, pp.753–4.
118. Reprinted, with a new historical introduction, by David L. Drabkin, Hamden, Conn., 1962 (Archon Books).
119. Drabkin, David L., *Thudichum: chemist of the brain* (Philadelphia, 1958), (contains an annotated bibliography of his writings, pp.209–34); Hunter, Richard A. and Ida Macalpine, 'Dr. Thudichum on the contents of perspiration as discharging the matter of disease, 1860', *J. Hist. Med.*, 17 (1962) pp.190–1; McIlwain, Henry, 'Thudichum and the medical chemistry of the 1860s to 1880s', *Proc. Roy. Soc. Med.*, 51 (1958) pp.127–32.
120. Bynum, W. F., *DSB*, 2 (1970) pp.547–8.
121. The most authoritative source of information is the biography by René Vallery-Radot, *The life of Pasteur ... Translated from the French by Mrs. R. L. Devonshire. With a foreword by Sir William Osler*, 2 vols (1911); see also Dubos, René J., *Louis Pasteur, freelance of science* (1951); Nicolle, Jacques, *Louis Pasteur: a master of scientific enquiry* (1961), (French edn, Paris, 1953; German edn, Berlin, 1959); James, D. E., 'Louis Pasteur's final judgment: host reactions, soil or terrain', *Hunterian Soc. Trans.*, 42 (1983–4) pp.69–90; Wrotnowska, D., *Pasteur, professeur et doyen de la Faculté des Sciences de Lille (1854–1857)* (Paris, 1975); Hume, E. D., *Béchamp or Pasteur? a lost chapter in the history of biology; founded upon a manuscript by M. R. Leverson*, 2nd edn (London, 1932); Geison, G. L., *DSB*, 10 (1974) pp.350–416.
122. *Medical Classics*, 2 (1937–8) pp.175–880 (contains chronological biography; bibliography of 81 items, pp.720–31); obituaries in *Br. Med. J.* (1910) i, pp.1384–9, and *Lancet* (1910) i, pp.1583–8; Schadewaldt, H., *Robert Koch et la bactériologie de son temps* (Paris, 1969); Barlow, C. and P. Barlow, *Robert Koch*, Geneva (1971); Genschorek, W., *Robert Koch: Leben, Werk, Zeit* (Leipzig, 1975), (title of 5th edn: *Robert Koch: selbstloser Kampf gegen Seuchen und Infektionskrankheiten*, Leipzig, 1982); Dolman, C. E., *DSB*, 7 (1973) 420–35; Evans, A. S., 'Causation and disease: the Henle–Koch postulates revisited', *Yale J. Biol. Med.*, 49 (1976) pp.175–95; Carter, K. C., 'Koch's postulates in relation to the work of Jacob Henle and Edwin Klebs', *Med. Hist.*, 29 (1985) pp.353–74.
123. Hofmann, A. W. von, *The life work of Liebig in experimental and philosophic chemistry ...* (Faraday lecture 1875), (London, 1876); Paoloni, C., *Justus von Liebig. Eine Bibliographie sämtlicher Veröffentlichungen mit biographischen Anmerkungen* (Heidelberg, 1968); Strube, I., *Justus von Liebig* (Leipzig, 1973); Hall, V. M. D., 'The role of force or power in Liebig's physiological biochemistry', *Med. Hist.*, 24 (1980) pp.20–59; Brock, W. H., 'Liebigiana: old and new perspectives', *Hist. Sci.*, 19 (1981) pp.201–18; *Justus von Liebig und August Wilhelm Hofmann in ihren Briefen (1841–1873)*, ed. by W. H. Brock (Weinheim, 1984); Holmes, F. L., *DSB*, 8 (1973) pp.329–50; Liebig, J. von, *Animal chemistry*, introduction by F. L. Holmes (New York, 1964); Pelling, M., 'Morbid poisons and process: Justus Liebig', in her *Cholera, fever and English medicine, 1825–1865* (Oxford, 1978) pp.113–45.
124. Fruton, J. S., *DSB*, 6 (1972) pp.504–6.
125. Lewes, Mrs C. L., *Dr Southwood Smith: a retrospect* (Edinburgh, 1898); Poynter, F. N. L., 'Thomas Southwood Smith – the man (1788–1861)', *Proc. Roy. Soc. Med.*, 55 (1962) pp.381–92; Pelling, M., 'The origins of official doctrine: Chadwick and Southwood Smith', in her *Cholera, fever and English medicine, 1825–1865* (Oxford, 1978) pp.1–33.
126. Richardson, Sir B. W., *The health of nations: a review of the works of Edwin Chadwick, with a biographical dissertation*, 2 vols (London, 1887); Greenwood, M.,

Some British pioneers of social medicine (London 1948) pp.47–58; Finer, S. E., *The life and times of Sir Edwin Chadwick* (London, 1952); Lewis, R. A., *Edwin Chadwick and the public health movement, 1832–1854* (London, 1952); Watson, R., *Edwin Chadwick, poor law and public health* (London, 1970); Pelling, M., op. cit. in note no.125 above.

127. Greenwood, M., *The medical dictator and other biographical studies* (London, 1986) pp.53–71 (reprint of London, 1936 edn); Greenwood, M., *Some British pioneers of social medicine* (London, 1948) pp. 61–80; Eyler, J. M., *Victorian social medicine: the ideas and methods of William Farr* (Baltimore, 1979); Pelling, M., 'Epidemiology as medical science: William Farr', in her *Cholera, fever and English medicine, 1825–1865* (Oxford, 1978) pp.82–112.

128. Lambert, Royston, *Sir John Simon, 1816–1904, and English social administration* (1963), (contains a list of his writings, pp.628–31); Greenwood, M., *Some British pioneers of social medicine* (London, 1948) pp.83–94.

129. Hume, E. E., *Max von Pettenkofer, his theory of the etiology of cholera, typhoid fever and other intestinal diseases: a review of his arguments and evidence* (New York, 1927); Pettenkofer, Max Joseph von, 'The value of health to a city. Two lectures, delivered in 1873 ...; translated with an introduction by Henry E. Sigerist', *Bull. Hist. Med.*, 10 (1941) pp.473–503, 593–613; Kissalt, K., *Max von Pettenkofer* (Stuttgart, 1948); Evans, A. S., 'Pettenkoffer revisited: the life and contributions of Max von Pettenkofer (1818–1901)', *Yale J. Biol. Med.*, 46 (1973) pp.161–76; Goerke, H., 'Die Bedeutung der Chemie für die hygienischen Arbeiten Max von Pettenkofers', *Int. Congr. Hist. Med. (24th, 1974, Budapest) Acta* (1976) vol.2, pp.779–83; Dolman, C. E. *DSB*, 10 (1974) pp.556–63.

130. See centenary numbers of the *Br. Med. J.*, 12 Oct. 1946, *Br. Med. Bull.*, 4, ii (1946) and *Post. Grad. Med. J.*, (Oct. 1946); Keys, Thomas E., *The history of surgical anaesthesia ... With an introductory essay by Chauncey D. Leake, and a concluding chapter, The future of anaesthesia, by Noel A. Gillespie* (New York, 1945), (revised reprint, 1963).

131. Reprinted in *Br. J. Anaesth.*, 26 (1954) pp.268–81, 337–41, 433–41; 27 (1955) pp.42–6, 105–10, 150–5, 189–95, 264–6, 362–8, 412–17, 464–7, 558–62; 28 (1956) pp.40–5, 90–6, 136–42, 230–6, 385–90, 481–5, 526–31.

132. Hill, A. Bradford, 'Snow – an appreciation', *Proc. Roy. Soc. Med.*, 48 (1955) pp.1008–12; Brown, P. E., 'John Snow, the autumn loiterer', *Bull. Hist. Med.*, 35 (1961) pp.519–28; Bergman, Norman A., 'The legacy of John Snow: an appreciation of his life and scientific contribution on the 100th anniversary of his death', *Anaesthesiology*, 19 (1958) pp.595–606; Pelling, Margaret H., *Some approaches to nineteenth-century epidemiology, with particular reference to John Snow and William Budd* (B. Litt. thesis, Oxford University, 1971–2); Pelling, M., 'Exclusive and inclusive: John Snow and the Committee for Scientific Enquiries', in her *Cholera, fever and English medicine, 1825–1865* (Oxford, 1978) pp.203–49; Thomas, K. B., *DSB*, 25 (1975) pp.502–3.

133. Pelling, Margaret H., op. cit. in note 132 above; Pelling, Margaret H., 'The smallpox analogy: William Budd', in her *Cholera, fever and English medicine, 1825–1865* (Oxford, 1978) pp.203–49; Dolman, C. E. *DSB*, 2 (1970) pp.574–6.

134. Hutchinson, Herbert, *Jonathan Hutchinson: life and letters* (1946); *Medical Classics*, 5 (1940–1) pp.109–245 (contains chronological biography, bibliography etc.). His own interleaved and annotated copy of the *Archives of Surgery* is in the Library of the Royal College of Physicians of London.

135. *Medical Classics*, 3 (1939) pp.889–971 (includes bibliography, pp.890–913); Lassek, A., *The unique legacy of Doctor Hughlings Jackson* (Springfield, Ill., 1970); Engelhardt, H. T., *John Hughlings Jackson and the concept of cerebral localization* (Tulane University of Louisiana thesis, New Orleans, 1972); Smith, C. U. M., 'Evolution and the problem of the mind. Part II: John Hughlings Jackson', *J. Hist. Biol.*, 15 (1982) pp.241–62; Dewhurst, K., *Hughlings Jackson on psychiatry* (Oxford, 1982); Clarke, E. S., *DSB*, 7 (1973) pp.46–50.

136. Sherrington, C. S. [Obituary]. *Proc. Roy. Soc.*, 103B (1928) viii–xvi; Young, R. M., *Cerebral localisation from Gall to Ferrier*, PhD thesis, King's College, Cambridge

(1964–5); Heffner, H. E., 'Ferrier and the study of the auditory cortex', *Arch. Neurol.*, 44 (1987) pp.218–21; Clarke, E. S., *DSB*, 4 (1971) pp.593–5.

137.   Critchley, M., *Sir William Gowers, 1845–1915: a biographical appreciation* (London, 1949).

138.   Ryckewaert, A. and B. Naveau, 'Principaux apports de Charcot et de Pierre Marie à la pathologie ostéo-articulaire', *Rev. Rhum.*, 51 (1974) pp.405–13; Swazey, J. P., *DSB*, 9 (1974) pp.108–9.

139.   Carter, K. C., 'Edwin Klebs' criteria for disease causality', *Med. Hist. J.*, 22 (1987) pp.80–9; Carter, K. C., 'Koch's postulates in relation to the work of Jacob Henle and Edwin Klebs', *Med. Hist.*, 29 (1985) pp.353–74.

140.   Rolleston, Sir Humphry Davy, *The right Honourable Sir Thomas Clifford Allbutt, a memoir* (1929); Fulton, John Farquhar, 'Clifford Allbutt's description of psycho-motor seizures', *J. Hist. Med.*, 12 (1957) pp.75–7; Cohen, H. 1st baron of Birken-head, 'The Rt Hon. Sir Thomas Clifford Allbutt FRS', in *Br. Congr. Hist. Med.*, 7th (1969); *Cambridge and its contribution to medicine* (1971) pp.173–92.

141.   MacDermott, H. E., 'Notes on the early editions of Osler's textbook of medicine', *Ann. Med. Hist.*, N.S.6 (1934) pp.224–40; see also *Medical Classics*, 4 (1939–40) pp.175–283; Nation, E. F., *An annotated checklist of Osleriana* (Kent, Ohio, 1976); Roland, C. G. (ed.), *Sir William Osler, 1849–1919: a selection for medical students* (Toronto, 1982); Golden, R. L. and C. G. Roland, *Sir William Osler: an annotated bibliography with illustrations* (San Francisco, 1988).

142.   Manson-Bahr, Sir Philip, *Patrick Manson, the father of tropical medicine* (London, 1962); Manson-Bahr, Sir Philip, 'Patrick Manson as a parasitologist. "A critical review"', *Internat. Rev. Trop. Med.*, 1 (1961) pp.77–131; Chernin, E., 'Sir Patrick Manson's studies on the transmission and biology of filariasis', *Rev. Infect. Dis.*, 5 (1983) pp.148–66; Chernin, E., 'Sir Patrick Manson: an annotated bibliography and a note on a collected set of his writings', *Rev. Infect. Dis.*, 5 (1983) pp.353–86; Cook, G. C., 'Tropical Sprue: implications of Manson's concept', *J. Roy. Coll. Phycns Lond.*, 12 (1978) pp.329–49; Clarkson, M. J., *DSB*, 9 (1974) pp.81–3.

143.   Sarton, George, 'The discovery of X-rays, with a facsimile reproduction (No. xviii) of Röntgen's first account of them published early in 1896', *Isis*, 29 (1938) pp.349–69 (includes: Weil, E., 'Some bibliographical notes on the first publication on the Roentgen rays', pp.362–65); Glasser, Otto, *Wilhelm Conrad Röntgen and the early history of the Roentgen rays ...* (1933); Glasser, Otto, *Dr. W. C. Röntgen*, 2nd edn (Springfield, Ill., 1958); Etter, Lewis E., 'Some historical data relating to the disco-very of the Roentgen rays', *Amer. J. Roentgen.*, 56 (1946) pp.220–31; Nitzke, W. R., *The life of Wilhelm Conrad Röntgen of the X-ray* (Tucson, 1971); Turner, G. L'E., *DSB* (1975) pp.529–31.

144.   Vaughan, R. B., 'The romantic rationalist: a study of Élie Metchnikoff', *Med. Hist.*, 9 (1965) pp.201–15; Mechnikova, Olga, *Vie d'Élie Metchnikoff 1845–1916* (Paris, 1920), (English translation: *Life of Élie Metchnikoff*, Boston, 1921); Levinson, H. and V. Robinson, 'Metchnikoff', *Med. Life*, 30 (1923) pp.235–64; Frolov, V. A., 'I. I. Metchnikoff's contribution to immunology', *J. Hyg. Epidem. (Praha)*, 29 (1985) pp.185–91.

145.   Cajal, S. Ramón y, *Recuerdos de mi vida*, 3rd edn (Madrid, 1923); Cajal, S. Ramón y, *The structure of the retina*, comp. and trans. by S. Thorpe and M. Glickstein (Springfield, Ill., 1972); Loewy, A. D., 'Ramón y Cajal and methods of neuroanato-mical research, with a translation of part of Histologie du système nerveux, Paris, 1909, vol.1, ch.2', *Perspect. Biol. Med.*, 15 (1971) pp.7–36; Matilla Gomez, V. *et al.*, 'Homenaje a Cajal', *Ann. Roy. Acad. Med.*, 101 (1984) pp.485–512; *Ramón y Cajal, 1852–1934*, 2 vols (Madrid, 1978); 'Symposium "Horizons in Neuroscience" (1982: Valencia), Ramón y Cajal's contribution to the neurosciences ...' (Amsterdam, 1983).

146.   Benedetti, E. L., 'Camillo Golgi', *Sci. Med. Ital.*, 7 (1958) pp.105–32; Golgi Centen-nial Symposium (1973, Pavia–Milan) *Perspectives in neurobiology*, ed. by M. Santini (New York, 1975); Legée, Georgette, 'Évolution de l'histologie du système nerveux au XIXe siècle: l'impulsion donnée par Camillo Golgi (1844–1926)', *Clio Med.*, 17 (1982) pp.15–32; Zanobio, B., *DSB*, 5 (1972) pp.459–61.

147. Absolon, K. B. (ed.), *The intimate Billroth (letters to his confidante: the Billroth–Seeger letters)*, 2nd edn (Rockville, Md, 1986); Rutledge, R. H., 'In commemoration of Theodor Billroth on the 150th anniversary of his birth. I: his surgical and professional accomplishments. II: his personal life, ideas and musical friendships', *Surgery*, 86 (1979) 672–93; Veltheer, W., 'The dawn of gastric resection. [Billroth]', *Neth. J. Surg.*, 33 (1981) pp.107–14; Genschorek, W., *Wegbereiter der Chirurgie: Johann Friedrich Dieffenbach, Theodor Billroth* (Leipzig, 1982); Absolon, K. B., *The surgeon's surgeon: Theodor Billroth, 1829–1894*, 3 vols (Lawrence, Kansas, 1971–87); Absolon, K. B., 'The surgical school of Theodor Billroth', *Surgery*, 50 (1961) pp.697–715.

148. Bett, W. R., 'Sir Frederick Treves, Bart. (1853–1923)', *Ann. Roy. Coll. Surg. Engl.*, 12 (1953) pp.189–93.

149. Marquardt, Martha, *Paul Ehrlich* ... (1949); Dale, Sir Henry, 'Paul Ehrlich, born March 14, 1854', *Br. Med. J.*, (1954) I, pp.659–63; Work, T. S., 'The work of Paul Ehrlich and his position in the history of medical research', *Internat. Arch. Allergy*, 5 (1954) pp.89–114; Bäumler, Ernst, *Paul Ehrlich, scientist for life* (New York, 1984); Parascandola, J., 'The theoretical basis of Paul Ehrlich's chemotherapy', *J. Hist. Med.*, 36 (1981) pp.19–43; Saiter, H., *Paul Ehrlich, Begründer der Chemotherapie: Leben, Werk, Vermächtnis*, 2nd edn (Munich, 1963); Dolman, C. E., *DSB*, 4 (1971) pp.295–305.

150. Singer, Charles, 'A great country doctor. Francis Adams of Banchory (1796–1861)', *Bull. Med. Hist.*, 12 (1942) pp.1–17 (contains a bibliography of his writings, pp.16–17); Craig, John, 'Francis Adams, 1796–1861', *Lancet* (1961) I, pp.441–2; Guthrie, Douglas, 'Dr. Francis Adams of Banchory, died February 26, 1861', *Br. Med. J.* (1961) I, p.585; Malloch, Archibald, 'A letter from Francis Adams of Banchory', *Canadian Med. Assn J.*, 29 (1933) pp.199–201; Richards, R. L., 'Francis Adams of Banchory, 1796–1861: a centennial tribute', *Scottish Med. J.*, 6 (1961) pp.160–3; Tait, H. P., 'A gifted country practitioner. Francis Adams of Banchory', *Practitioner*, 186 (1961) pp.252–5.

151. Keys, Thomas E., 'Some American medical imprints of the nineteenth century', *Bull. Med. Lib. Assn*, 45 (1957) pp.309–18; Annan, Gertrude L., 'Medical Americana', *J. Amer. Med. Assn*, 192 (1965) pp.139–44.

152. See Power, Sir D'Arcy, *British medical societies* (1939).

153. For an interesting history of this Society see Schafer, Sir Edward Sharpey, *History of the Physiological Society during its first fifty years, 1876–1926* (1927).

154. See Hurry, Jamieson B, *A history of the Reading Pathological Society* (1909).

155. See Gough, W. Brian, 'The minute books and the foundation of the Birmingham Medical Institute', *Birmingham med. Rev.*, N.S.20 (1957–8) pp.363–8.

156. See Burke, Michael P., 'The Dublin Surgical Society', *Irish J. Med. Sci.*, no. 344 (1944) pp.333–44.

157. See MacDermot, H. E., *History of the Canadian Medical Association, 1867–1921* (Toronto, 1935); and Graham, Donald C., 'The Canadian Medical Association: its genesis and development', *Med. J. Australia* (1962) I, pp.772–7.

158. See Lewis, D. Sclater, *The Royal College of Physicians and Surgeons of Canada, 1920–1960* (Montreal, 1962).

159. Shaftel, Norman, *et al.*, 'History of the Medical Society of the State of New York, 1807–1957 (The first seventy-five years, by Norman Shaftel; The years between, 1882–1906, by Emerson Crosby Kelly; The last fifty years, by John F. Rogers)', *N.Y. State J. Med.*, 57 (1957) pp.433–532.

160. Jessup, Everett C., *A brief history of the Nassau County Medical Society, Inc.*, (New York, 1961).

161. See Hyslop, Newton E., 'America's oldest student medical society: one hundred and fifty years of Boylston', *New Engl. Med. J.*, 265 (1961) pp.324–7.

162. See Warthen, Harry J., 'The Richmond Academy of Medicine, 1820–1900', *Virginia Med. Monthly*, 89 (1962) pp.559–65; and Williams, Carrington, 'Richmond Academy of Medicine, 1900–1960', *Virginia Med. Monthly*, 89 (1962) pp.566–77.

163. Fishbein, Morris *et al.*, *A history of the American Medical Association* (Philadelphia, 1947).

164. See Hutchinson, Sir Jonathan, *The New Sydenham Society. Retrospective memoranda ... Subject index and index of names, compiled by Charles R. Hewitt* (1911); Meynell, G. C., *The two Sydenham Societies: a history and bibliography of the medical classics published by the Sydenham Society and the New Sydenham Society (1844–1911)* (Acrise, Kent, 1985).

7 The growth of medical periodical literature

Leslie T. Morton

> To insure continuity of interest there must be constant rejuvenation and resti-
> mulation, and in no place of modern activity is it so imperative that the
> scientific spirit should burn and shine like a sacred fire, as in the field of
> medicine. The highest function of the medical journalist today is to introduce
> new currents of scientific ideas and to keep them in circulation.
>
> (Fielding Hudson Garrison)

A periodical may be defined as a publication issued in successive parts at regular or irregular intervals and intended to be continued indefinitely. Such works as annual reviews and the *Advances* series (Academic Press and Year Book Publishers) are regarded as periodicals, as are the proceedings and transactions of societies. Proceedings and transactions of congresses are not periodicals.

Before the advent of scientific journals, communication between scientists was by means of personal correspondence. More extensive work was published in book form, a slow and laborious process, in which the author himself might have to bear the cost of production. William Harvey first announced his discovery of the circulation in lectures in 1616 and published it in a badly-printed book issued in Frankfort 12 years later.

Scientific and medical journals first made their appearance in the latter half of the seventeenth century, and provided a new and revolutionary means of communication. The early journals were of two kinds – the transactions and proceedings of academic bodies, which reproduced the texts of papers delivered at their meetings; and journals published by individuals or societies and containing papers from a variety of sources.

Types of journals

Sir Theodore Fox,[1] a former editor of the *Lancet*, distinguished between two contrasting types of medical journal: the medical recorder and the medical newspaper. The medical recorder, he said, 'is a journal which records new observations and experiments in techniques. As one of the principal means of communication between investigators it is at present necessary for the advancement of medical knowledge'. In contrast, he regarded a medical newspaper as one 'whose function is to inform, interpret, criticize, and stimulate. By telling doctors what other doctors are doing and thinking, it helps to integrate the profession'. Its correspondence columns provide readers with the opportunity to express opinions and air their views; it also publishes book reviews. The *Biochemical Journal and the Journal of Experimental Medicine* are examples of recorders, while the *British Medical Journal, The Lancet, New England Journal of Medicine* and *Klinische Wochenschrift* are both recorders and newspapers. However, Franz J. Ingelfinger,[2] then editor of the *New England Journal of Medicine*, disagreed with this view. He felt that Fox did not take sufficiently into account the fact that technology would affect not only the content of biomedicine but its transmission: 'The results of modern research are jet-diffused'. General medical journals seek news-worthiness but face obstacles because of their usually slow publication schedules and because of contents that readers find either obscure or contradictory to long-held beliefs. In addition, general medical journals now find themselves in competition with the lay press and the controlled-circulation ('giveaway') journals because medical news has become big news. One effect of this escalating public interest in medical news is that general medical journals that are reliable and have maintained their news-worthiness are increasingly cited. These journals thus eventually transmit research findings to the public as well as to the health-care professions.

Some journals such as *Nature, Science*, and *Biochemical and Biophysical Research Communications* are vehicles for preliminary communications, in which their contributors announce what they consider to be some important discovery or stake a claim for priority in this respect.

N. Howard-Jones[3] divided journals into three categories: primary, secondary and tertiary. Primary journals are those reporting first-hand observations made in the clinic, the laboratory or the field. *The Lancet, Wiener medizinische Wochenschrift*, and *La Presse Médicale* are examples. Specialist medical journals may be included in this category. R. J. Dannatt[4] has published a detailed survey of primary sources of information.

Secondary journals are intended to indicate what has been published in the primary journals. They are the abstracting journals and the indexes, for example *Excerpta Medica*, the *Meditsinskij Referativnyi Zhurnal* and *Index Medicus*.

Tertiary journals neither record original observations nor simply list or abstract original papers. They attempt to review present knowledge on a particular subject by reference to the relevant literature. The preparation of such reviews may involve reference first to secondary literature, to find out what has been written on the subject, and then reference to some of this literature in primary journals.

Numerous papers dealing with the history of periodical literature have been published, some of which cannot be relied upon for the presentation of facts. Few can agree upon the date of issue of the earliest periodical, many claims to this title having been made, but two extensive lists can be consulted to advantage. F. H. Garrison's check-list of medical and scientific periodicals of the seventeenth and eighteenth centuries[5] is worthy of careful study and contains references to the earliest writings on the subject. Excluding translations, abridgements and reprints, the list comprises 432 medical titles (10 in the seventeenth and 422 in the eighteenth century) and 349 scientific titles. However a number of the titles cannot really be described as periodicals. D. A. Kronick[6] has published a list of addenda and corrigenda which adds 192 entries and numerous additions and corrections. W. R. LeFanu[7] has produced an extensive chronological survey of medical periodicals published in all British lands from the seventeenth century to 1938, which provides details of editors, title changes, dates of reprinting, amalgamations, indexes, inclusive dates and number of volumes, with location of copies. A continuation of LeFanu's list has been compiled by A. M. Shadrake[8] but covers only titles published in Great Britain and Ireland from 1938 to 1961 and also excludes reports of societies and hospitals. Shadrake's supplement provides an alphabetical list giving title, date and frequency of publication of 262 numbered entries, and has an appendix showing the numbers of journals starting publication in each year from 1938 to 1961.

D. A. Kronick[9] has published an extensive study of the origin and development of scientific and technical periodicals, dealing with the various types (society proceedings, abstracts, reviews, almanacs, annuals etc.) and providing a comprehensive bibliography. This includes much of medical interest and contains several tables indicating comparative numbers of periodicals on various subjects at different dates.

Origins and development

It was the foundation and growth of the scientific societies that promoted the early journals, some of which were issued as their proceedings or transactions. These were in due course followed by independent general and specialist journals. Garrison[10] wrote that the genesis of the medical and scientific periodical is out of the scientific society by the newspaper. E. Chernin[11] put it more bluntly: 'Journals as we know them were spawned in the mid-17th century and arose from the desperation men felt in attending meetings of their "invisible colleges" and in keeping up with their personal correspondence about new discoveries.' Up to the middle of the seventeenth century men of science were dependent on private correspondence between one another to keep abreast of new knowledge.[12] When Henry Oldenburg (?1615–77) became secretary of the Royal Society of London he began extensive correspondence with scientists all over the world. This work soon became so heavy that assistance was required and arrangements were made for a 'Committee of Correspondence'.

Meanwhile a similar state of affairs obtained in France where already in 1663 steps were being taken to publish a literary–scientific periodical that would save time and labour by providing multiple copies of letters. This materialized in the publication in Paris on 5 January 1665 of the *Journal des Sçavans*, a journal concerned preponderantly with book reviews. The *Journal* continued under that title until 1792, was suppressed until 1816, and then reappeared under the auspices of the Institut de France with the more modern title *Journal des Savants*. In England Oldenburg and others concluded that a more truly scientific periodical was needed, and the Council of the Royal Society ordered 'that the *Philosophical Transactions* be composed by Mr Oldenburg, to be printed the first Monday of each month'. The first issue appeared on 6 March 1665. The journal was at first published by Oldenburg as a private venture and at his own expense; the title-page of the first volume gave no reference to the Society: *Philosophical Transactions, giving some accompt of the present undertakings, studies, and labours of the ingenious in many considerable parts of the world,* although it did mention that the printers were 'printers to the Royal Society'. Although the President and Council exercized some supervision, it was not until the 47th volume in 1753 that the Council appointed a Committee of Papers and became officially responsible for publication of the *Transactions*.

Hall[13] has discussed the part played by the Royal Society in the diffusion of information in the seventeenth century, stressing the importance of Oldenburg's correspondence with foreign scientists, the role of the *Philosophical Transactions* and maintaining that the high reputation of English science during that period was due in some measure to the activities of the Society. Porter has described in detail the foundation of both the *Journal des Sçavans* and the *Philosophical Transactions*.

From its commencement the *Philosophical Transactions* contained some items of medical interest and today still includes papers on subjects concerned with the basic medical sciences. This outstanding scientific journal has survived for over 300 years with only a short period of dormancy (1676–83) and its volumes contain some of the most important scientific papers published anywhere in the world.

In Germany the Academia Naturae Curiosorum, still extant under another name, was responsible for the first scientific periodical of that country, *Miscellanea Curiosa Medico-Physica*; 27 volumes were published from 1670–1706. It dealt with anatomy and physiology among other subjects.[14]

The *Acta Medica et Philosophica Hafniensia*, published in Copenhagen from 1673, was founded and edited by Thomas Bartholin (1616–80), the anatomist. Its contents leaned heavily towards medicine, although it cannot be regarded as the first exclusively medical journal. It consisted mainly of short original observations on medical and natural science subjects. Garrison traces its existence until 1829. There is some dispute as to whether or not it was sponsored by the (Royal) Medical Society of Copenhagen, which still exists as Medicinsk Selskab.

The first independent journal devoted exclusively to medicine was *Les*

Nouvelles Descouvertes sur Toutes les Parties de la Médecine, Paris, edited by Nicolas de Blegny. The first issue appeared in January 1679, and the last part of the first volume for December of that year announced a change of title for volume 2. This appeared as *Le Temple d'Esculape, ou les dépositaires des nouvelles descouvertes qui se font journellement dans toutes les parties de la médecine*, for one year only, and in 1681 it appeared until March under the title *Nouveautés Journalières Concernant les Sciences et les Arts qui font Parties de la Médecine*. Publication was transferred to Amsterdam, where it appeared in 1682, for two issues only, as *Le Mercure Sçavant*. It had previously been translated into German and Latin, and was continued in the latter language by Théophile Bonet as *Zodiacus Medico Gallicus*, Geneva, 1680–5.

Le Journal de Médecine, 1681–5, edited by the Abbé Jean Paul de la Roque, was continued by Claude Brunet (1685) who also edited the monthly *Progrès de Médecine*, 1695–1709. Among existing French journals founded in the nineteenth century should be noted *Gazette des Hôpitaux Civils et Militaires* (1828), *Bulletin de l'Académie Nationale de Médecine* (1836), *Le Progrès Médical* (1873) and *La Presse Médicale* (1880).[15]

The first English periodical devoted exclusively to medicine was *Medicina Curiosa: or, a variety of new communications in physick, chirurgery, and anatomy* ..., which was published by Thomas Basset at *The George* in Fleet Street. The first number appeared on 17 June 1684 and the second (and final) issue on 23 October. The first number contained 56 pages and reviewed work published elsewhere, containing nothing original.[16]

Attention was drawn by F. N. L. Poynter[17] to another English journal with a section devoted to medicine. This was the *Weekly Memorials for the Ingenious: or, an account of books lately set forth in several languages, with some curious novelties relating to arts and sciences*, an abstract-review type of journal. It devoted about a third of its space to accounts of medical books and papers but cannot seriously be regarded as a medical journal. It was first published on 16 January 1682, and 50 numbers were issued; and from 20 March of that year a rival journal with the same title was started by the original editor who had quarrelled with the publishers. Four years later appeared *Hippocrates Ridens, or joco-serious reflections on the impudence and mischiefs of quacks and illiterate pretenders to physick*, the four numbers of which were published in 1686. Thus only three English medical periodicals were published during the seventeenth century, all short-lived and none of any importance.

According to Karl Sudhoff the first medical journal published in Germany was the *Acta Medicorum Berolinensum*, Berlin, 31 vols, 1717–31, the text being in Latin.[18] In the same year appeared *Sammlung von Natur und Medicin*, the first medical periodical in the vernacular. Garrison does not record this last but does list *Deliciae Medicae et Chirurgicae*, Leipzig, 1703–5. Other early German journals include *Der patriotische Medicus*,

Hamburg, 1724–6, *Der Arzt*, Hamburg, 1759–64, and *Der Landarzt*, Leipzig, 1765–6.

In 1851 appeared the *Wiener medizinische Wochenschrift*, which is still current, while the *Ärztliches Intelligenz-Blatt*, following in 1854, became the *Münchener medizinische Wochenschrift* in 1885 and represents another contemporary journal. These two periodicals, together with the *Berliner klinische Wochenschrift* (1864, continued in the *Klinische Wochenschrift* in 1922) and the *Deutsche medizinische Wochenschrift* (1875) are among the most widely known of modern German-language medical periodicals. Germany has also produced many specialist periodicals, including Johannes Müller's *Archiv für Anatomie und Physiologie*, commenced in 1834, to become the *Zeitschrift für Anatomie und Entwicklungsgeschichte* in 1921 and anglicized in 1975 as *Anatomy and Embryology; Virchows Archiv für pathologische Anatomie* (1847), now *Virchows Archiv. A. Pathological Anatomy* and *Virchows Archiv. B. Cell Pathology; Langenbecks Archiv für klinische Chirurgie* (1861) and *Pflügers Archiv für die gesamte Physiologie* (1868), now *Pflügers Archiv, European Journal of Physiology*.

W. R. LeFanu[19] notes 37 British medical periodicals founded in the eighteenth century and, although several of these were supported by influential medical men, few survived into the following century. It is difficult to ascertain the reason for this mortality but it is probable that those journals issued by societies were not supported by sufficiently large active memberships, and this type of periodical predominates. The *Medical Transactions of the Royal College of Physicians of London* was published from 1786 to 1820, and represents an important society journal issued during that period.

The first medical journal in Spain was *Efemerides Barométriço-médicas Matritenses*, Madrid, 1737–46. The eighteenth century also saw the birth of medical periodical literature on the American continent. Probably the first was the *Mercurio Volante*, Nos.1–16, published weekly in Mexico City from 17 October 1772 until February 1773. The first medical journal published in the United States was a selection and translation from the *Journal de Médecine Militaire*, Paris, published as *A Journal of the Practice of Medicine, Surgery and Pharmacy in the Military Hospitals of France*. Vol.1, no.1, was published in New York about 1790. The earliest American medical journal was the quarterly *Medical Repository*, New York, July 1797, edited by Edward Miller, Samuel L. Mitchell and Elihu H. Smith; 23 volumes appeared before the journal became extinct in 1824. This was followed by the *Philadelphia Medical Museum*, another quarterly, 1804–11. It was edited by John Redman Coxe (1773–1863), who introduced vaccination into Pennsylvania in 1802. The *Philadelphia Medical and Physical Journal* appeared a few months after the *Museum* but ended in 1809, after the publication of only three volumes. Numerous other periodicals quickly followed, but most were short-lived. These early

American medical journals contained some case reports by physicians and surgeons but consisted mainly of reprints of British articles and reviews of foreign publications.[20]

However the *New England Journal of Medicine and Surgery*, first published in Boston in 1812, has survived to the present day, with certain changes of title. It was founded by John Collins Warren and James Jackson as a quarterly, and the first issue appeared in January 1812. The *Boston Medical Intelligencer* was launched as a weekly on 29 April 1823, and was combined with the *New England Journal of Medicine* in February 1828, to form the weekly *Boston Medical and Surgical Journal*. A hundred years later, in 1928, the title reverted to the original *New England Journal of Medicine*, a journal which now ranks as one of the outstanding medical periodicals of the world. For some years it has been published simultaneously in Boston and London.[21]

Another noteworthy journal, the *American Medical Recorder*, Philadelphia, 1818, shortly afterwards became the *Medical Recorder* and was edited by John Eberle. It contains Beaumont's preliminary papers on Alexis St Martin. In 1829 it was amalgamated with the *Philadelphia Journal of the Medical and Physical Sciences*, which had been founded in 1820. In 1826 Isaac Hays joined the editorial staff and in the following year became sole editor. He changed the title to *American Journal of the Medical Sciences* and continued to edit it for 52 years. This journal still continues its useful career. Numerous other American medical journals published between 1797 and 1850 have been recorded by Myrl Ebert,[22] who mentions that almost 250 were issued during this period and includes alphabetical and chronological indexes of the journals discussed.

The first medical journal to be published in Canada was the bilingual *Journal de Médecine de Québec, Quebec Medical Journal*, which appeared in 1826 and expired in the following year. *La Lancette Canadienne*, Montreal, 1847, lasted for only ten months. The *Canada Medical Journal and Monthly Record of Medical and Surgical Science*, Montreal, ran from 1865 to 1872 (vols 1–8) and was then divided into *Canada Medical and Surgical Journal* and *Canada Medical Record*. The *Record* ceased publication with vol.32, 1904, and the *Journal* was renamed after vol.16 (1888) *Montreal Medical Journal* (vols 17–39, 1888–1910). It was then combined with the *Maritime Medical News*, Halifax, Nova Scotia (vols 1–22, 1888–1910) to become the current *Canadian Medical Association Journal*, 1911–, published in Toronto. The *Union Médicale du Canada*, Montreal, was first published in 1872 and has continued uninterrupted to the present time, incorporating the *Gazette Médicale de Montréal* (vols 1–6, 1887–92) in 1893.[23]

The first medical journal published in Scotland was *Medical Essays and Observations, revised and published by a Society in Edinburgh*, 6 vols 1731. According to Garrison it is an ancestor of the *Edinburgh Medical Journal* via *Essays and Observations, Physical and Literary,* Edinburgh, 1754–65 and *Medical and Philosophical Commentaries, by a Society in Edinburgh,* vols 1–6, 1774–9, continued as *Medical Commentaries,* vols 7–10, 2nd decade, vols 1–10, 1780–1804, continued by *Annals of Medicine,* 8 vols, 1794–1804. This was replaced by the *Edinburgh Medical and Surgical Journal,* 1805–55, which was incorporated with the *Monthly Journal of Medical Science* to form the *Edinburgh Medical Journal,* which sadly ceased publication in 1954. The *Glasgow Medical Journal,* published since 1828, met a similar fate in 1955. Both were replaced by the *Scottish Medical Journal.*

An early Irish medical periodical has been described by J. D. H. Widdess.[24] This is *Collectanea Hibernica Medica,* Dublin, 1783. Only one issue of this has been traced. The *Dublin Medical and Physical Essays* appeared from 1807 to 1808. The first Russian medical journal was the *Sankt-Petersburgskie Vracebnye Vedomosti,* which was published in 52 parts to form one volume, 1792–4.

One of the most significant events in the history of medical journalism occurred on 5 October 1823 (a Sunday) when Thomas Wakley (1795–1862) published the first issue of *The Lancet,* now one of the leading journals in the field. It appeared weekly. The early volumes reported lectures, surgical operations and medical news in general. Wakley was a great reformer who severely criticized prominent members of the profession, urging changes and the removal of abuses in various spheres. He was involved in a number of lawsuits but his fines and expenses were usually defrayed by a sympathetic public and his efforts resulted in considerable improvement. Biographies of Wakley written by Sir Squire Sprigge, a later editor of *The Lancet* and C. W. Brook reveal a forthright character who enjoyed fighting the abuses then encountered in medical and social life.[25] *The Lancet* provides a vivid history of the development of medicine since 1823, and under successive distinguished editors it has upheld the prestige of British medical journalism. For a brief history of *The Lancet* see W. H. McMenemey.[26]

The first entirely medical journal published in the provinces was the *Midland Medical and Surgical Reporter and Topographical and Statistical Journal,* Worcester, August 1828, a quarterly founded by Charles Hastings and others. It appeared until 18 January 1832, when the Provincial Medical and Surgical Association was formed and published its own annual *Transactions* from 1833. The Association also founded the weekly *Provincial Medical and Surgical Journal,* the first number of which was published on 3 October 1840. In January 1853 the title was changed to *Association Medical Journal,* and on 3 January 1857 it assumed its present title, the *British Medical Journal,* as in the previous year the Association had broadened its scope to become the British Medical Association. A prospectus for a monthly *British Medical Journal* was circulated towards the end of 1798 'to be published by R. Phillips, St Paul's Churchyard, on 1 February, 1799', but no issues of this have been traced.[27]

The (Royal) Medico-Chirurgical Society of London was founded in 1805 and began publication of its *Medico-Chirurgical Transactions* in 1809. In 1907 the Society was amalgamated with 14 mainly specialist medical and surgical societies to form the Royal Society of Medicine. Most of the societies published their own journals, and these, too, were amalgamated to form the *Proceedings of the Royal Society of Medicine*, renamed *Journal* in 1978.

The early history of medical journalism in Australia and New Zealand has been surveyed by B. Gandevia and R. Winton.[28] The *Australian Medical Journal* was published in Sydney from August 1846 to September 1847. Another journal bearing the same title was published in Melbourne by the Medical Society of Victoria, first issued in January 1856 and continued under various titles until merged into the *Medical Journal of Australia* in 1914. The *Australasian Medical Gazette* was first published in Sydney in October 1881 as the official organ of the Victorian, South Australian and New South Wales Branches of the British Medical Association. It joined the *Australian Medical Journal* to form the *Medical Journal of Australia*, first published on 4 July 1914. The *New Zealand Medical Journal* was founded by the New Zealand Medical Association in September 1887 and is still current. Numerous specialist medical journals have also been established in Australia during the present century.

A survey of medical journals in India by A. Neelameghan[29] contains sections devoted to problems of early medical journalism in India (suggesting that, between 1820 and 1920, 88 medical journals were founded, but that 60 had merged or disappeared, and by the end of 1920 there remained only 28); a list of societies and periodicals, 1780–1920; an alphabetical list of periodicals and societies; and union catalogues of periodicals in Indian libraries. Early Indian medical journals include the *Transactions* of the Medical and Physical Society of Calcutta, founded in 1823, *India Journal of Medical Science*, Calcutta (1834) and the *Indian Medical Gazette*.

M. A. P. Senadhira[30] has discussed the development of scientific journalism in Sri Lanka and records that the first scientific periodical published in the country was *Medical Miscellany*, issued in 1853. Despite its title it included many articles of a scientific nature.

The earliest known medical journal in South Africa was the *Cape Town Medical Gazette*, first issued in 1847 as a quarterly, but which ceased publication after a brief period. In 1887 the *South African Medical Journal* appeared in East London as a monthly, but after a year it was issued weekly and survived for five years. Another journal with the same title was published monthly in Cape Town from 1893 to 1899. The *South African Medical Record* (Cape Town, 1903) and the *Transvaal Medical Journal*

(Johannesburg, 1905, from 1913 the *Medical Journal of South Africa*) merged in 1927 to form the *Journal of the South African Medical Association*, which in 1932 became the current *South African Medical Journal*.[31]

The history and modern development of Japanese medical periodicals are recorded by S. Onodera.[32] A more recent analysis by M. Taniguchi[33] mentions that in 1963 *Igaku Chuo Zasshi* (founded 1903) abstracted 855 Japanese journals devoted to the medical sciences.

Specialism

Specialist journals were early on the scene. The first noted by Garrison is *Der Arzt der Frauenzimmer*, Leipzig, published weekly from 1771 to 1773. The first specialist journal in Britain was the *Asylum Journal* (1853), renamed *Asylum Journal of Mental Science* with vol.2, *Journal of Mental Science* in 1858, and *British Journal of Psychiatry* in 1963. Today specialism is the rule rather than the exception among new journals, and, as well as broad specialization in such fields as anatomy, biochemistry and surgery, there is now subspecialization, with journals devoted to such subjects as surgery of the hand, cleft-palate repair and biochemical genetics. E. M. Berry[34] is not at all happy about extreme specialization among medical journals.

'One-man' journals may be considered in this group. Several journals were entirely written and conducted by a single person, perhaps because his views were not orthodox at the time, or because his specialty had not been accepted as such, or maybe because he wished to be independent of any editorial control. Among such journals may be mentioned Sir Benjamin Ward's *Asclepiad* (11 vols, 1884–95); Sir Jonathan Hutchinson's *Archives of Surgery* (11 vols, 1889–1900; issue of a final number was delayed until 1911, 'kept back by indecision as to formal announcement of conclusion and preparation of the general index'!); Sir Byrom Bramwell's *Studies in Clinical Medicine* (1889–90), and his *Clinical Studies* (8 vols, 1902–10); and J. W. Ballantyne's *Teratologia* (2 vols, 1894–5).

Abstracting journals

Abstracts may be divided into two types – informative and indicative. An informative abstract gives all the essential details of the publication abstracted and provides all the basic information given by the original writer, making it unnecessary for the reader to consult the original, except for details of methods, techniques, case records and so on. It is particularly useful in the case of a paper published in an obscure journal, an unfamiliar language, or a journal difficult to obtain in the original. An indicative abstract, on the other hand, merely outlines the scope of a paper, helping the reader to determine whether or not it is worth while to read the original.

An abstracting journal may attempt complete coverage of the literature within its scope or it may be selective. A selective service is likely to provide critical and discursive abstracts and will appeal particularly to those who have no time or inclination to examine abstracts of everything published within their subject interest but prefer to be guided by an expert who can select the really important papers.

Almost from the first appearance of periodicals abstracts and digests of their contents were published. Kronick[35] has pointed out the difficulty of classification of certain journals of this period into abstract and reviews journals. Garrison's check-list[36] records a number of items of this type. As the volume of literature grew it became increasingly difficult for readers to cope with the original publications, and digests were a great convenience. Nowadays it would be impossible for a medical scientist to cope with all the literature currently being published on his subject, even if he were able to deal with the many languages represented.

The publication of abstracting journals at first proceeded in a desultory fashion until the nineteenth century and the predominance of German abstracting journals continued into the present century. The various *Berichte* and *Zentralblätter* published by the firm of Julius Springer covered most branches of medicine. Each provided informative abstracts, attempting complete cover of its speciality. Abstracts were in German. During the Second World War these slowly wasted away through lack of material and by 1944 all had suspended publication. Some have reappeared since the war. There was nothing comparable in the English language, although the *British Medical Journal* published a weekly supplement, *Epitome of Current Medical Literature*, from 1892 to 1939 (see also Chapter 8). The *Meditsinskij Referativnyi Zhurnal* was first issued in 1957. Abstracts are in Russian, but authors and titles are given in the language of the original publication. Since 1982 it has appeared in 22 sections, each having monthly parts and an annual index.

Two important abstracting journals of interest in the biomedical field are *Chemical Abstracts* and *Biological Abstracts*. *Chemical Abstracts* first appeared in 1907 and today the literature it covers is so prolific that issues appear weekly. About 8000 journals are screened and 600 000 abstracts are published each year, about a third of them of biochemical interest. The annual indexes are cumulated quinquennially. *Biological Abstracts* commenced publication in 1926. It screens over 8000 journals and its subject coverage includes, among others, genetics, cytochemistry, biophysics, biochemistry, nutrition and physiology. For a fuller account of medical abstracting services, see A. K. Dalby and F. M. Sutherland.[37]

Reviews

Review-type journals are an extension of abstracting journals. In them recently published literature on a particular subject is summarized, usually by an expert in the field. Two annuals of interest in general medicine are the *Medical Annual*, Bristol, and the *Year Book of Medicine*, Chicago. The Year Book Publishers are also responsible for 24 other review annuals covering special branches of medicine and surgery. The *Annual Review* series (Palo Alto, Calif.) includes a dozen annuals of medical interest. A number of other reviews are published annually or irregularly; for further information, see H. Hague.[38] Review articles are often included in journals, general or specialist. They can be of use also by saving time in finding relevant references. Since 1967 the *Index Medicus* has included a section on review material, *Bibliography of Medical Reviews*, arranged under authors and subjects.

Bibliographic control

The most important index to medical periodical literature is the *Index Medicus*, published since 1879 by the National Library of Medicine, Bethesda, Md and its predecessors. In 1989 it indexed the contents of 2750 carefully selected journals and published over 250 000 citations. A full account of the *Index Medicus* since its inception is given by Sutherland.[39] It has also been available on-line since 1964 as MEDLARS (MEDical Literature Analysis and Retrieval System). The on-line files of the database are called MEDLINE (MEDlars on-LINE) and the term MEDLARS is sometimes used to cover the family of databases produced by the National Library of Medicine. For an account of MEDLINE see C. Norris.[40]

Current Contents is published by the Institute for Scientific Information, Philadelphia. It reproduces the contents pages of relevant journals. It is published in several sections; each section appears weekly and includes subject, author and journal title indexes. The sections of medical interest are *Current Contents: Clinical Medicine*, covering about 1200 journals; *Current Contents: Life Sciences*, covering about 1750 journals; and *Current Contents: Social and Behavioral Sciences* (about 1300 journals).

Citation indexing

In recent years a method of information access using citations given in published papers has become available. This is the *Science Citation Index*, an international interdisciplinary index to the literature of science, medicine, agriculture technology and the behavioural sciences. It is produced by the Institute for Scientific Information, Philadelphia. It first appeared for the year 1964 and retrospective volumes later dealt with literature from 1954. It appears six times a year, with annual cumulations. It indexes both journal and non-journal items. In 1989 about 5000 source journals and other publications were covered. Eugene Garfield,[41] founder of the *SCI*, has defined a citation index as an ordered list of references (cited works) in which each reference is followed by a list of the sources (citing works) which cite it. It is based on the principle that there is some meaningful relationship between one paper and some other that it cites or that cites it and thus between the work of the two authors or the two groups of authors who published the papers.

R. K. Poyer[42] made a study of journal article coverage in the pre-clinical sciences by the *Science Citation Index*. Journal article references from 70 dissertations written in anatomy, biochemistry, immunology, microbiology, pathology, pharmacology and physiology were checked against the author section of *SCI* source index. Of the 5795 references cited from 1964 to 1977 *SCI* indexed 5495 (94.8 per cent); of the 300 not indexed, 282 were from journal titles not covered by *SCI* at the time they were published. Thus there were only 18 references that were missed, although the journal titles were covered.

Poyer[43] also attempted to measure the efficiency of various indexing and abstracting services. He examined the extent of journal overlap among four major indexing and abstracting publications: *Index Medicus, Science Citation Index, Biological Abstracts*, and *Chemical Abstracts*. Journal references from 70 dissertations written between 1973 and 1977 were noted and a total of 77 969 articles from 652 journals were examined and verified. He found that 92 per cent were indexed by at least two of these services, 591 covered by only one service and 55 were not indexed. *IM* covered 93.8 per cent, *SCI* 94.8 per cent, *BA* covered 75.8 per cent and *CA* 57.3 per cent. Poyer discusses previous studies in this field. A determination of overlap in coverage of *Excerpta Medica* and *Index Medicus* by J. L. Dolcourt and R. M. Braude[44] showed that 47 per cent of the titles examined were common to both publications, 33 per cent were unique to *EM* and 20 per cent unique to *IM*.

Relevant lists of periodicals include:

British Union Catalogue of Periodicals. A record of the periodicals of the world from the seventeenth century to the present day, in British Libraries, London, Butterworth, 4 vols, 1955–8. Supplement to 1960, 1962. Continued in *New Periodical Titles* until 1980 and then in *Serials in the British Library*, quarterly.

List of Journals Abstracted by Excerpta Medica, Amsterdam (3500 journals listed).

List of Journals Indexed in Index Medicus, Bethesda, Md, National Library of Medicine. Annual; arranged in four sections: alphabetically by abbreviated title followed by full title, by full title followed by abbreviated title, by about 180 subject headings, and by countries (65 countries listed).
World Medical Periodicals, New York, World Medical Association, 3rd edn, 1961, and Supplement 1968. Alphabetical listing with name and address of publisher, frequency of issue, language of publication, and

abbreviated form of title; subject and country indexes. Now rather out of date.

A. N. Brandon has prepared a selected list of books and journals for a small medical library. This first appeared in the *Bulletin of the Medical Library Association* in 1965, and it is revised and published in that journal biennially.

Number and evaluation of periodicals

In 1881 J. S. Billings[45] estimated that there were 864 current medical journals. C. P. Fisher[46] estimated the number in 1912 as 1654. N. Howard-Jones[47] provided evidence that the number of current medical journals has, since 1880, approximately doubled every 30 years. If this is the case, the number today must be around 10 000.

R. J. Dannatt and D. Liepa[48] remind us that there are two components to the rate at which the growth of serials is accelerating: the increase in number and the increase in size. They examined some published estimates and concluded that

> the rate of real growth of the literature is related in the 1970s only to the net increase in the number of new titles published. Reliable information on this is not available but it may be that the net increase figure for serials in all fields of 2.5–3% conceals no increase or a 'steady state' figure for biomedicine, in which case the new biomedical literature is contracting.

D. T. Durack[49] weighed the volumes of the *Index Medicus* from 1879 to 1977 (early volumes listed books as well as journal articles). This remained at approximately 2 kg for over 60 years; during the 10-year period 1946–55 it doubled to about 4 kg and since then has increased more than seven times to about 30 kg (1977) and is still rising. There are several compounding factors. Over the years the paper used in the *Index* has become thinner, but, apart from the increase in the number and size of journals, the number of authors per paper has increased, as has the depth of indexing. A count of the number of authors of original articles published in the *New England Journal of Medicine* and its predecessor, the *Boston Medical and Surgical Journal* between 1886 and 1977 showed that the percentage of articles written by a single author fell from 98.5 per cent to 4 per cent.

R. H. Orr and A. A. Leeds[50] found that the average thickness of a fairly large sample of continuing biomedical serials increased by 28 per cent between 1941 and 1961, the equivalent of a doubling time of 60 years. (However a quarter of this period involved war years which was followed by a post-war literature explosion.)

Many papers have been published concerning the evaluation and 'ranking' of biomedical journals. Because a journal is low on the list of titles borrowed from a national lending library this does not imply that it is unimportant; it may be so important that almost every library stocks it. Estimates of usage have been given by R. J. Dannatt.[51] Five core lists were compared by B. T. Usdin[52] with respect to size, intended users, and content. There is significant agreement among the lists. A table of the 72 journals appearing on four or all core lists is included in Usdin's paper. E. Garfield[53] has reported on which medical journals have the greatest impact.

Editorial control

In recent years the style of publication in many medical journals has been much improved. In 1978 a group of editors of some biomedical journals published in English met in Vancouver to decide on uniform technical requirements for manuscripts submitted to their journals. These laid down rules for the format of papers submitted to their journals, including use of standard units and the form of abbreviation of journal references. These requirements were revised in 1982 and again in 1988.[54] As far as journal abbreviations are concerned it was decided to adopt the style used for *Index Medicus*, which follows the American *National Standard for the Abbreviation of Titles of Publications ANSI 239.5 1985*. More and more biomedical journals are adopting this style of abbreviation, a great convenience to librarians in particular. The Vancouver group evolved into the present International Committee of Medical Journal Editors.

The accuracy of quotations and references in six medical journals published during 1984 was assessed by G. F. de Lacey, C. Record and J. Wade.[55] They found that the original author was misquoted in 15 per cent of all references, and most of the errors would have misled readers. Errors of citation of references occurred in 24 per cent, of which 8 per cent were major errors – that is, they prevented immediate identification of the source of the reference. Some suggestions made by these authors for reducing these high levels of inaccuracy are that papers scheduled for publication with errors of citation should be returned to the author and checked completely and a permanent column specifically for misquotations could be inserted into the journal.

Peer review of manuscripts submitted for publication may be a serious problem for editors and a sore point for would-be authors. P. Morgan[56] has pointed out that peer review improves the quality of published papers and prevents the publication of much poor science: 'The journals with the highest standards extend their influence widely since the papers they reject flow, like water, downhill and along paths of least resistance to lesser journals – but in the process some are purified and others evaporate.' Stephen Lock,[57] editor of the *British Medical Journal*, made a thorough investigation of peer review and how to improve it. While wondering whether the current system is justified, his conclusions make a strong case for something close to it. One weakness in the journal review system is the inability of editors to identify authors who have received useful advice along with the rejection but have not revised before submitting elsewhere.

The future

Lock[58] disagrees with prophecies made by Bernal and Fox that the general journal as we know it would disappear, to be replaced by recorder journals and newspaper journals – the first corresponding to our present-day specialist journal and the second to a kind of amalgam of the non-original parts of the *British Medical Journal, World Medicine,* and *Pulse.* None of this has come about. Lock believes that the superiority of the printed word will go on; predictions about the use of videotape, microfiche and computer print-outs will not be fulfilled. He sees the general journal as continuing to publish original work – but work which will have more immediate relevance to the practising doctor. This will entail more editing in the way of cutting and rewriting, and in selecting shorter articles rather than longer ones. Journals will change with the times but will still be with us at the end of the century.

Notes

1. Fox, T., *Crisis in communication. The functions and future of medical journals* (London, 1965).
2. Ingelfinger, F. J., 'The general medical journal: for readers or repositories?' *New Engl. Med. J.,* 296 (1977) pp.1258–64.
3. Howard-Jones, N., 'Our medical literature – then and now', *Br. J. Med. Educ.,* 7, (1973) pp.70–85.
4. Dannatt, R. J., 'Primary sources of information', in L. T. Morton and S. Godbolt (eds), *Information sources in the medical sciences,* 3rd edn (London, 1984) pp.17–43.
5. Garrison, F. H., 'The medical and scientific periodicals of the 17th and 18th centuries. With a revised catalogue and check-list', *Bull. Inst. Hist. Med.,* 2, (1934) pp.285–343.
6. Kronick, D. A., 'The Fielding H. Garrison list of medical and scientific periodicals of the 17th and 18th centuries; addenda and corrigenda', *Bull. I. ⋅⋅ Med.,* 32 (1958) pp.456–74.
7. LeFanu, W. R., *British medical periodicals: a chronolog⋅ ⋅⋅ lis: ⋅ʃaltimore,* 1938), (reprinted from *Bull. Inst. Hist. Med.,* 5 (1937) pp.735–61, 8∠ι–55; 6 (1938) pp.614–48). Revised edn 1640–1899, together with later additions, ed. by Jean Loudon, Oxford, Wellcome Unit for the History of Medicine, Research Publ. No.6, 1984.
8. Shadrake, A. M., 'British medical periodicals, 1938–1961', *Bull. Med. Lib. Assn,* 51 (1963) pp.181–96.
9. Kronick, D. A., *A history of scientific and technical periodicals. The origins and development of the scientific and technological press, 1665–1790,* 2nd edn (Metuchen, NJ, 1976).
10. *Op. cit.* in note 5 above.
11. Chernin, E., 'A worm's eye view of biomedical journals', *Fed. Proc.,* 34 (1975) pp.124–30.
12. Porter, J. R., 'The scientific journal – 300th anniversary', *Bact. Rev.,* 28 (1964) pp.211–30.
13. Hall, M. B., 'The Royal Society's role in the diffusion of information in the seventeenth century', *Notes Rec. Roy. Soc. Lond.,* 29 (1975) pp.173–92.
14. Cole, F. J., *A history of comparative anatomy. From Aristotle to the eighteenth century* (London, 1944) pp.341–69.
15. Lévy-Valensi, J., 'Les origines de la presse médicale française', *Presse Méd.* (1936) ii, pp.2124–5; Lévy-Valensi, J., 'Histoire de la presse médicale française', *Presse Méd.* (1938) ii, pp.1229–30.

16. Williams, D., '*Medicina Curiosa*: an early medical journal', *Glasgow Med. J.*, 109 (1928) pp.105–9; Johnston-Saint, P., 'The first English medical journal', *Med. Press Circ.*, 201 (1938–9) pp.117–18.

17. Poynter, F. N. L., 'The first English medical journal', *Br. Med. J.*, 2 (1948) pp.307–8.

18. Sudhoff, Karl, 'Das medizinische Zeitschriftwesen in Deutschland bis zur Mitte des 19. Jahrhunderts', *Münch. Med. Wschr.*, 50 (1903) pp.455–63. See also Runge, E., 'Aus dem Anfängen des deutschen medizinischen Zeitschriftenwesens', *Med. Welt* (1937) II, pp.950–2, 984–6, 1019–22.

19. *Op. cit.* in note 7 above.

20. Fye, W. B., 'The literature of American internal medicine: a historical review', *Ann. Intern. Med.*, 106 (1987) pp.451–60.

21. Garland, J., 'A voice in the wilderness. The "New England Journal of Medicine" since 1812', *Br. Med. J.*, 1 (1962) pp.105–8; Morton, L. T., 'The New England Journal of Medicine 1812–1962', *Practitioner*, 188 (1962) pp.128–30.

22. Ebert, M., 'The rise and development of the American medical periodical, 1797–1850', *Bull. Med. Lib. Assn*, 40 (1952) pp.243–76. See also Cassedy, J. H., 'The flourishing and character of early American medical journalism, 1797–1860', *J. Hist. Med. Allied Sci.*, 38 (1983) pp.135–50; Shaftel, N., 'The evolution of American medical literature', *Int. Rec. Med.*, 71 (1958) pp.431–54.

23. Desjardins, E., 'La petite histoire du journalisme médical au Canada', *Union Médicale du Canada*, 101 (1972) pp.121–30, 309–14, 511–18, 1190–6; Roland, C. G., 'Canadian medical journalism in the 19th century', *Canadian Med. Assn J.*, 128 (1983) pp.449–51, 454–5, 458–9.

24. Widdess, J. D. H., 'An unrecognized medical periodical – Collectanea Hibernica Medica', *Irish J. Med. Sci.* (1955) no.356, pp.377–9.

25. Sprigge, S. S., *The life and times of Thomas Wakley, founder and first editor of The Lancet, member of Parliament for Finsbury, and coroner for West Middlesex* (London, 1897). Brook, C. W., *Battling surgeon* (Glasgow, 1945). Reprinted, London, 1962. See also Booth, C. C., 'Medical communication: the old and the new. The development of medical journals in Britain', *Br. Med. J.*, 285 (1982) pp.105–8.

26. McMenemey, W. H., 'The Lancet' 1823–1973, *Br. Med. J.*, 3 (1973) pp.680–4.

27. 'An 18th century *British Medical Journal*', *Br. Med. J.*, (1918) 1, p.183; 'An earlier "British Medical Journal"', *Br. Med. J.* (1936) 2, p.777.

28. Gandevia, B., 'A review of Victoria's early medical journals', *Med. J. Aust.*, 2 (1952) pp.184–8. Winton, R., 'Medical journalism in Australia and New Zealand', *Med. J. Aust*, 1 (1961) pp.723–6.

29. Neelameghan, A., *Development of medical societies and medical periodicals in India, 1780–1920* (Calcutta, 1923).

30. Senadhira, M. A. P., 'The development of scientific journalism in Sri Lanka', in I. Corea (ed.), *Libraries and people: Colombo public libraries 1925–1975* (Colombo, 1975) pp.261–70.

31. 'South African medical journals', *S. Afr. Med. J.*, 30 (1956) pp.311–12, 337–8.

32. Onodera, S., 'Past and present of Japanese medical journals', *Bull. Med. Lib. Assn*, 46 (1958) pp.73–81, 320–34.

33. Taniguchi, M., 'An analysis of Japanese medical periodicals', *Bull. Med. Lib. Assn*, 53 (1965) pp.43–51.

34. Berry, E. M., 'The evolution of scientific and medical journals', *New Engl. J. Med*, 305 (1981) pp.400–2.

35. *Op. Cit.* in note 9 above.

36. *Op. Cit.* in note 5 above.

37. Dalby, A. K., *Medical abstracts and indexes, 1975: a bibliography of abstracting, indexing and current awareness services in medicine and related subjects* (Cambridge, University Library and Librarianship Series, 1975). Sutherland, F. M., 'Indexes, abstracts, bibliographies and reviews', in L. T. Morton and S. Godbolt (eds), *Information sources in the medical sciences*, 3rd edn (London, 1984) pp.44–69.

38. Hague, H., 'Standard reference sources', ibid., pp.72–4.

39. Op. cit. in note 37 above.

40. Norris, C., 'Mechanised sources of information retrieval', ibid., p.102.

41. Garfield, E., '"Science Citation Index" – a new dimension in indexing', *Science*, 144, (1964) pp.649–54; Garfield, E., 'Citation indexing for studying science', *Nature*, 227 (1970) pp.669–71.
42. Poyer, R. K., '*Science Citation Index's* coverage of the preclinical science literature', *J. Amer. Soc. Inform. Sci.*, 33 (1982) pp.37, 317–20.
43. Poyer, R. K., 'Journal article overlap among *Index Medicus, Science Citation Index, Biological Abstracts*, and *Chemical Abstracts*', *Bull. Med. Lib. Assn*, 72 (1984) pp.353–7.
44. Dolcourt, J. L., and R. M. Braude, 'Determination of overlap in coverage of *Excerpta Medica* and *Index Medicus* through SERLINE', *Bull. Med. Lib. Assn*, 64 (1976) pp.324–5.
45. Billings, J. S., 'Our medical literature', in *Trans 7th Int. Med. Congr.* (London 1881) vol.1, pp.54–71.
46. Fisher, C. P., 'Changes in medical periodical literature since January 1909', *Bull. Med. Lib. Assn.*, N.S.2 (1913) pp.21–34.
47. *Op. cit.*, in note 3 above.
48. Dannatt, R. J. and D. Liepa, 'Serials', in M. Carmel (ed.), *Medical librarianship* (London, 1981) p.85.
49. Durack, D.T., 'The weight of medical knowledge', *New Engl. J. Med.*, 298 (1978) pp.773–5.
50. Orr, R.H. and A. A. Leeds, 'Biomedical literature: volume, growth and other characteristics'. *Fed. Proc.* 23 (1964) pp.1310–31.
51. *Op. cit.*, in note 4 above.
52. Usdin, B. T., 'Core lists of medical journals: a comparison', *Bull. Med. Lib. Assn.*, 67 (1979) pp.212–17.
53. Garfield, E., 'Which medical journals have the greatest impact?', *Ann. Intern. Med.*, 105 (1986) pp.313–20.
54. International Committee of Medical Journal Editors, 'Uniform requirements for manuscripts submitted to biomedical journals', *Br. Med. J.*, 296 (1988) pp.401–5; *Ann. Intern. Med.*, 108 (1988) pp.258–65.
55. Lacey, G. F. de, C. Record and J. Wade, 'How accurate are quotations and references in medical journals?', *Br. Med. J.*, 291 (1985) pp.884–6.
56. Morgan, P., 'Peer review in medical journals', *Br. Med. J.*, 292 (1981) p.646.
57. Lock, S., *A difficult balance: editorial peer review in medicine* (London, 1985).
58. Lock, S., 'Medical journals of the future', *J. Roy. Soc. Med.*, 71 (1978) pp.284–5.

8 Medical bibliographies and bibliographers

John Symons

> There is no better float through posterity than to be the author of a good bibliography. Scores know Conrad Gesner by the 'Bibliotheca' who never saw the 'Historia Animalium'. A hundred consult Haller's bibliographies for one that looks at his other works, and years after the iniquity of oblivion has covered Dr Billings' work in the Army ... the great Index will remain an enduring monument to his fame.
>
> (Sir William Osler)

Bibliographies are of vital importance to those searching the vast and constantly growing accumulations of medical literature. They record work done in the past, indicating what has been accomplished, sometimes suggesting paths for future research, and serving as milestones of progress. The contents of thousands of periodicals may be indexed by author and subject in a single volume, presenting the enquirer with a guide to the subject in which he is particularly interested. A good bibliography is of more significance than are most original books, for if comprehensive it can readily be brought up to date, the original definitive contents remaining unchanged. Medicine has received the attention of bibliographers since the sixteenth century, and even today some of the older bibliographies remain of practical value to the historian. Medical bibliographies may be divided into several groups, and their value naturally depends largely upon their accuracy and comprehensiveness. General medical bibliographies attempt to cover the wide range of medical literature in all countries; others are restricted to certain chronological periods, languages, countries, special subjects or types of material. Retrospective bibliographies attempt to cover all the existing literature on a particular subject, whereas current bibliographies, often published in serial form, are concerned only with the most recent literature. To attempt an all-inclusive list of such bibliographies would require an extensive monograph, and this chapter is concerned mainly with general medical bibliographies published in book form, and with the writings of eminent bibliographers whose compilations appear worthy of special note. More complete lists of bibliographies devoted to particular branches of medicine, to special areas and languages will be found in the *Index-Catalogue*, in in Theodore Besterman's *Medicine, a bibliography of bibliographies* (Totowa, NJ, 1971). The latter work consists of the subject-headings of medical interest extracted from Besterman's *A world bibliography of bibliographies*, 4th edn, 4 vols (Lausanne,

1965–6). There is no index of authors, editors, etc., although one is provided in the main work.

A comprehensive survey of medical bibliographies is provided in John B. Blake and Charles Roos, *Medical reference works, 1676–1966: a select bibliography* (Chicago, 1967); *Supplement I, 1967–68* (compiled by M. V. Clark, 1970); *Supplement II, 1969–72* (compiled by J. S. Richmond, 1973); *Supplement III, 1973–74* (compiled by J. S. Richmond, 1975). This work supersedes the section devoted to bibliographies included in the second edition of the Medical Library Association's *Handbook of medical library practice* (Chicago, 1956) but omitted from later editions. John F. Fulton's *The great medical bibliographers* (Philadelphia, 1951) contains a useful historical and biographical account and is well illustrated with reproductions of title-pages. Estelle Brodman's *The development of medical bibliography* (Baltimore, 1954, reprinted Chicago, 1981) contains an invaluable chronological survey of the subject. The current state of the art is well surveyed in L. T. Morton and S. Godbolt (eds), *Information sources in the medical sciences*, 3rd edn (London, 1984).

Several general guides to reference material contain useful surveys of medical topics: Louise Noëlle Malclès, *Les sources du travail bibliographique*, volume 3;[1] Eugene P. Sheehy, *Guide to reference books*;[2] A. J. Walford, *Walford's guide to reference material*, volume 1.[3] Three nineteenth-century French books on medical bibliography also deserve mention. Jean Baptiste Monfalcon's *Précis de bibliographie médicale* (Paris, 1827, see below) contains much general discussion of the subject. The *Essais de bibliographie médicale* (Paris, 1887) of Louis Henri Petit (1847–1900)[4] was intended primarily for the use of medical students and contains interesting bibliographical case-studies. Victor Lucien Hahn (1872–1942)[5] compiled his *Essai de bibliographie médicale* (Paris, 1897) as his doctoral thesis in medicine; it provides details of general and medical bibliographies and of works on medical history and biography, often with useful notes. Petit and Hahn were both on the staff of the library of the Paris Faculté de Médecine and Hahn eventually served as chief librarian from 1920 to 1937. He was appointed in succession to his uncle François Louis Hahn (1844–1921) and was succeeded in his turn by his own son André (1900–75), a rare example of dynastic succession among medical librarians!

In the earliest periods after the invention of printing, publication was essentially limited to monograph form. Periodicals began to appear in the late seventeenth century, gathered strength in the eighteenth, and in the mid-nineteenth century began to overtake the monograph as a publication vehicle for medical and scientific literature. The oldest bibliographies therefore were primarily concerned with monographs, whereas nowadays many current bibliographies list periodical articles only. Bibliographers must also bear in mind the contents of composite works such as symposia, books containing chapters by various authors, historical selected writings, and similar works that are seldom adequately covered by abstracting and indexing organs.

It is not always easy to give a precise definition of a bibliography. Biographical dictionaries, for example, are often as valuable for their bibliographical as for their biographical content. Catalogues of libraries and personal collections cannot be overlooked as important items in medical bibliography. Some describe general collections of national or international importance and the catalogue of even a small collection devoted to a specific subject is often an important contribution to the bibliography of that subject.

Bibliographies of individuals have been noted in the appropriate chapters. Modern bibliographies are seldom bare lists of the works of an author but, following the 'humanistic' bibliographies of Sir Geoffrey Keynes, provide biographical details of the subject, evaluate his work, and provide information on his contemporaries and the printers of his books. General medical bibliographies are no longer attempted, except in periodical form, but the following account outlines the development of bibliographies of medicine, from the period when a slim volume listed the entire output of medical literature to the present day of innumerable current periodical medical bibliographies. Covering all branches of the subject, they are published monthly, quarterly and yearly, none entirely comprehensive, many overlapping despite a certain amount of cooperation, and none up-to-date enough for the research worker who appears to want to know what was published yesterday, and what will appear next month! In recent years conventional publication has begun to give way to the computerized database and to on-line information retrieval.

One of the earliest printed general bibliographies was *Liber de scriptoribus ecclesiasticis* (Basle, 1494) compiled by Johannes Trithemius (1462–1516), Abbot of Sponheim, who achieved that position in 1483 when twenty-one years of age. He reorganized and catalogued the library, which grew from 48 to 2000 books and manuscripts. Because of unpopularity he left Sponheim in 1506 and spent the rest of his life as abbot at Würzburg. His bibliography of ecclesiastical writers includes certain men who influenced medicine, listing almost a thousand writers and seven thousand books chronologically. It was also printed in Paris, 1512 and Cologne, 1531 and 1546. Among other bibliographies, Trithemius also wrote a *Catalogus illustrium virorum Germaniae* (Mainz, 1495). His scholarly annotations add to the value of his useful compilations.[6]

Several sixteenth-century authors produced biographical histories of medicine which can, in a sense, be regarded as attempts at medical bibliographies. Such is the *De medicine claris scriptoribus* of the Lyons physician Symphorien Champier (1472–1539), included in his *Libelli duo* ..., [Lyons, 1506?]. Later examples are the *Catalogus illustrium medicorum* (Strasbourg, 1530) of Otto Brunfels (1488–1534), the *Illustrium medicorum, qui superiori saeculo floruerunt, ac scripserunt vitae* (Paris, 1541) of Remaclus Fuchs (1510–87) and the *Chronologia sive temporum supputatio, omnium illustrium medicorum* (Frankfort-on-Oder, 1556) of Wolfgang Jobst (Guolphgangus Justus) (died 1575).

The name of Conrad Gesner is usually associated with the title 'Father of Bibliography', and his monumental *Bibliotheca universalis* justly earns him that distinction. Although by no means the first bibliographer, his pioneer efforts overshadowed all previous attempts, and his work formed the basis of bibliographical work for many years after his death. Conrad Gesner (more correctly Gessner) was born on 26 March 1516, at Zurich. After an education in the humanities at Strasbourg, Paris and Bourges he turned to medicine, studying first at Montpellier and then at Basle, where he graduated in 1541. Having married early he was forced to devote much of his time to literary and teaching work, in addition to his medical practice. He was professor of Greek at Lausanne from 1537 to 1540, and from 1541 until his death on 13 December 1565 taught at the Collegium Carolinum in Zurich. In 1554 he became town physician at Zurich and in 1558 was granted the title and income of a canon, which gave him a measure of financial security. Throughout his life he was an enthusiastic naturalist and formed a fine collection of fossils and other specimens.[7]

Gesner's numerous published works ranged over medicine, natural history, classical studies and bibliography. His first publication was a Greek dictionary, *Lexicon Graecolatinum* (Basle, 1537). His most popular work was a book on medicines and distillation, *Thesaurus Euonymi Philiatri*, first published at Zurich in 1552 and frequently reprinted and translated into English, German, French and Italian. Four volumes of his *Historia animalium* were published at Zurich between 1551 and 1558, and a fifth volume was added posthumously in 1587. The manuscript of his unpublished *Historia plantarum* is now in the University of Erlangen; two volumes entitled *Opera botanica*, edited by Casimir Christoph Schmiedel, were published at Nuremberg in 1751–71 and a facsimile edition of the illustrations from the manuscript, edited by Heinrich Zoller, Martin Steinmann and Karl Schmid, has recently been published (*Conradi Gesneri Historia plantarum*, 8 vols, Zurich, 1972–80).

His *Bibliotheca universalis* (Zurich, 1545) is a general rather than a strictly medical bibliography. It consists of an alphabetical listing, by forename, of writers in Latin, Greek and Hebrew on all subjects, with an index of surnames. Both published and unpublished works are included, with biographical and bibliographical data. Although Gesner was only 28 when he compiled the work, he was already able to devote nearly seven folio pages to his own life and writings.

A subject approach was provided by the publication of his *Pandectarum sive partitionum universalium ... libri XXI* (Zurich, 1548), which forms the second volume of his *Bibliotheca universalis*. In it the contents of the first volume are rearranged into subject divisions. Although the title refers to 21 classes, only 19 are included. Medicine, which was to have formed class 20, was never published and theology, class 21, appeared as a separate volume in 1549, entitled *Partitiones theologicae, pandectarum universalium ... liber ultimus*. It includes an index covering also the preceding volume.

Conrad Lycosthenes (Wolffhart) (1518–61) published an abridgement of Gesner's *Bibliotheca* as *Elenchus scriptorum omnium ... in compendium redactus* (Basle, 1551), including some additional material, and a similar work by Josias Simler (1530–76) was published as *Epitome bibliothecae Conradi Gesneri* (Zurich, 1555). The additions by Lycosthenes and Simler were also published separately as *Appendix bibliothecae Conradi Gesneri* (Zurich, 1555), constituting a fourth volume of the *Bibliotheca*.

Gesner's *Bibliotheca universalis* and *Appendix* (without the two subject volumes) have been reprinted by Otto Zeller (Osnabrück, 1966) with postscript by H. Widmann. Gesner's major work did not proceed to any further editions (although Gesner continued to collect additional material until his death) but two enlarged editions of Simler's abridgement appeared as *Bibliotheca instituta ... primum a Conrado Gesnero ... in epitomen redacta* (Zurich, 1574 and 1583), the latter edited by Johannes Jacobus Frisius (1547–1611). This last edition has been reprinted by Georg Olms, Hildesheim.

Gesner never produced the exclusively medical bibliography which he was so well qualified to have compiled, but a list of surgical writers and their works is appended to his *Chirurgia, De chirurgia scriptores optimi* (Zurich, 1555), a collection of surgical texts, which he edited. Nevertheless, his *Bibliotheca* deserves inclusion here as a landmark in bibliographical technique and an indispensable foundation for later compilers. His attitude to bibliography is exemplified in the words, attributed to Virgil, printed on the verso of the title-page of his *Bibliotheca*: 'Non mihi sed studiis communibus ista paravi; sic vos non vobis mellificatis apes.' ('Not for myself but for general scholarship have I prepared this, as you bees, do not make honey for yourselves alone.')

Pascal Le Coq (Paschalis Gallus) (1566–1632) drew heavily on Gesner for his *Bibliotheca medica, sive catalogus illorum qui ... artem medicam scriptis illustrarunt* (Basle, 1590), which has some claim to be regarded as the first true strictly medical bibliography. The bulk of the work consists of an alphabetical list of medical authors writing in Latin. This is followed by separate lists of French and German writers and of writers on various special subjects, such as surgery, anatomy and plague. A reprint (from a defective copy), with introduction by G. M. Obinu, was published by Don Bosco (Genoa, 1970) (Scientia Veterum, no. 151–2). Le Coq, a native of Villefagnan in Poitou, studied at Basle and Montpellier; in 1597 he became professor of medicine at Poiters and served as dean of the Faculty there from 1616 until his death.

A first attempt at a medical subject bibliography was provided by Israel Spach (1560–1610), a native of Strasbourg who became professor of medicine there after graduating at Tübingen. His *Nomenclator scriptorum medicorum. Hoc est: elenchus eorum qui artem medicam suis scriptis illustrarunt, secundum locos communes ipsius medicinae* (Frankfort, 1591) is arranged under very broad subject headings with indexes of authors and subjects. He edited an important collection of classic gynaecological texts, *Gynaeciorum, sive, de mulierum ... affectibus et morbis libri* (Strasbourg, 1597) and compiled a parallel volume to his medical bibliography, *Nomenclator scriptorum philosophicorum atque philologicorum* (Strasbourg, 1598), which covers a wide range of non-medical subjects.

Johann Georg Schenck von Grafenberg (died *c.*1620), physician at Haguenau in Alsace, published, in addition to numerous medical writings, *Biblia iatrica* (Frankfort, 1607). It is an author bibliography, arranged alphabetically by forenames and with occasional annotations (such as references to portraits or notes of manuscripts in Schenck's library). Schenck planned further volumes to deal with authors writing in languages other than Latin and with subjects ancillary to medicine, such as chemistry, but no more was published.

Johannes Antonides van der Linden (1609–64) is the best known of seventeenth-century bibliographers, and his compilation is still of value, although not of the standard set by his successors of the eighteenth century. Van der Linden was born on 13 January 1609 at Enkhuizen, and studied philosophy and then medicine at Leyden. He completed his medical studies at Franeker, where he graduated in 1630, and then practised in Amsterdam. In 1639 he returned to Franeker as professor of medicine, moving in 1651 to a professorship at Leyden which he held until his death on 5 March 1664. His *De scriptis medicis libri duo* (Amsterdam, 1637) consists of an alphabetical arrangement by first names of authors, with a rudimentary subject list in systematic order and an index of surnames. Anonymous works and collections of texts appear under the letter A as 'Autores ... incerti' and 'Autores ... varii'. Second and third editions appeared in 1651 and 1662, the latter including a few biographical notes.

The book was later brought up to date and much improved by Georg Abraham Mercklin (1644–1702) as *Lindenius renovatus* (Nuremberg, 1686). This edition is the most useful. It retains van der Linden's arrangement by forenames but the sections of anonymous works and collections are transferred to a separate appendix. Periodical articles are included as well as monographs. The biographical notes are much increased and the subject list is replaced by a usable subject index. New and revised entries are marked by special symbols.

Van der Linden was the author of several medical works, including editions of the writings of Hippocrates (*Opera omnia*, Leyden, 1665), Celsus (*De medicina*, Leyden, 1657) and the seventeenth-century anatomist Adrianus Spigelius (*Opera quae extant omnia*, Amsterdam, 1645, which contains the fifth printing of Harvey's *De motu cordis*).[8]

The *Bibliotheca medici eruditi* (Padua, 1654) of Pedro de Castro (1603–c.1657) is an attempt at a critical medical bibliography, listing a small selection of books with extensive discussion. Later editions were published at the Hague in 1712 (as an appendix to Johann Gerhard Meuschen's *Bibliotheca medici sacri*) and at Bergamo in 1742 (edited by Andrea Pasta). The author was a member of a Jewish family converted to Christianity and practised medicine in France and Italy. In 1640 he embraced Judaism and took the name Ezekiel, but returned to Christianity and to his original name some ten years later. His publications under the two names have been a source of confusion ever since![9]

Martin Lipen (Martinus Lipenius) (1630–92) studied theology at Wittenberg and worked as a schoolmaster successively at Halle, Stettin and Lübeck. He published a series of subject bibliographies under the title *Bibliotheca realis universalis*, 6 vols (Frankfort, 1679–85), covering theology, law, medicine and philosophy, the medical volume appearing in 1679 as *Bibliotheca realis medica*. The subjects are arranged alphabetically with an author index. The work is generously printed with ample space for notes and was intended for the use of booksellers as well as students.

Cornelius à Beughem (1638–1722), a bookseller and councillor of Emmerich, compiled a series of bibliographies of the current literature of his time in various subjects, concentrating on books published after 1650. The medical volume in this series was published as *Bibliographia medica et physica novissima* (Amsterdam, 1681), giving an interesting survey of the productions of a limited period. Another compilation of medical interest was his *Syllabus recens exploratorum in re medica, physica et chymica* (Amsterdam, 1696), which lists the contents of the transactions of societies and of other periodicals. Medical works are also to be found in his *Apparatus ad historiam literariam novissimam*, 5 vols (Amsterdam, 1689–1710), an attempt at a general current bibliography.[10]

Jean Jacques Manget (1652–1742), a native of Geneva, compiled a general medical bibliography, *Bibliotheca scriptorum medicorum, veterum et recentiorum*, 2 vols in 4 (Geneva, 1731). Based on Mercklin's edition of van der Linden, this is arranged alphabetically by authors, though by surname rather than forename, and is not simply a listing of titles but also includes the full text of some periodical articles, reviews and biographical memoirs. There is no subject approach. In an attempt to improve the work's coverage, Manget had inserted an appeal for information in various journals; this attracted a good response from Italy but little or none from elsewhere.

Manget was also responsible for a series of collections of classic texts on various subjects, to which, confusingly, he also gave the title *Bibliotheca*. These are *Bibliotheca anatomica* (compiled jointly with the medical historian Daniel Le Clerc), 2 vols (Geneva, 1685); *Bibliotheca medico-practica*, 4 vols (Geneva, 1695–7); *Bibliotheca chemica curiosa*, 2 vols (Geneva, 1702); *Bibliotheca pharmaceutico-medica*, 2 vols (Geneva, 1703); *Bibliotheca chirurgica*, 4 vols (Geneva, 1721). Some of these went into later editions or were translated into other languages.[11]

The two-volume *Bibliotheca medica* (Jena, 1746) of Christoph Wilhelm Kestner (1694–1747), a native of Kindelbrück, is a subject bibliography with an author index and extensive critical notes. His medical biographical dictionary *Medicinisches Gelehrten-Lexicon* (Jena, 1740, reprinted by G. Olms, Hildesheim, 1971) can be used as a companion volume for a direct author approach. Kestner also wrote a short history of medicine, *Kurzer Begriff der Historie der medicinischen Gelahrtheit überhaupt* (Halle, 1743).

An eighteenth-century example of critical medical bibliography is the *Bibliographie médicinale raisonnée* (Paris, 1756, reissued in 1783), of Pierre Antoine Joseph Du Monchaux (1733–66). Another bibliographical item of the same period is *Enumeratio librorum praecipuorum medici argumenti* (Leipzig, 1773) by Johan Anders Murray (1740–91), a Swede who became professor of medicine at Göttingen. Most of his other writings are on botany and materia medica.

We now meet a figure whose bibliographies completely overshadow those of his immediate predecessors, and who has been acclaimed as the founder of medical and scientific bibliography. His scholarly compilations have proved amazingly complete and reliable, and Sir William Osler was responsible for the phrase 'Haller is the greatest bibliographer in our ranks'. Albrecht von Haller (1708–77) attained prominence as a writer on anatomy, botany, physiology and surgery; he also wrote historical fiction and poetry. A native of Berne, he studied medicine at Leyden under Boerhaave and Albinus and graduated in 1727. He visited London and Paris and practised for some years at Berne before going to the University of Göttingen in 1736 as professor of anatomy, surgery and botany. In 1753 he retired from teaching and took an administrative post at his native Berne, devoting much of his time to his scientific and literary activities. Haller's many papers and printed books range over the wide fields of science and medicine.[12]

Haller's first bibliographical work appeared while he was still at Göttingen. In 1742 he was invited by the Amsterdam publisher Wetstein to prepare a revised edition of Boerhaave's *Methodus discendi medicinam*, first published in 1726. This was a short, basic introduction to the study of medicine with notes of recommended authors; although published under Boerhaave's name, it was in fact an unauthorized compilation based on his lectures. Haller's 'revision' occupied him for nine years! He retained the original text but expanded and updated the bibliographical content beyond recognition, completely changing the character of the work. It was published as *Hermanni Boerhaave ... Methodus studii medici, emaculata et accessionibus locupletata ab Alberto ab Haller*, 2 vols (Amsterdam, 1751). The original pocket-sized volume of 458 pages was swollen to two quarto volumes of 1118 pages in all, constituting a scholarly, annotated medical bibliography arranged in systematic order. There was, however, only a very sketchy author index and no subject index; to make matters worse, there were over 100 pages of additions and corrections at the end. A revised edition published at Venice in 1753 improved matters by incorporating the additions and corrections into the main text. Full author and subject indexes were later compiled by Cornelis Pereboom (*Index auctorum et rerum maxime memorabilium Methodi studii medici*, Leyden, 1759) with page references relating to the Amsterdam edition.

Haller's main reputation as a bibliographer rests on the four substantial subject bibliographies published towards the end of his life. These are: *Bibliotheca botanica*, 2 vols (Zurich, 1771–2, also with London imprint); *Bibliotheca anatomica*, 2 vols (Zurich 1774–7, also with London and Leyden imprints); *Bibliotheca chirurgica*, 2 vols (Berne and Basle, 1774–5); *Bibliotheca medicinae practicae*, 4 vols (Berne and Basle, 1776–88); his *Bibliotheca physica* was never published, but remains in manuscript in the Burgerbibliothek at Berne.[13] All the published volumes are large quartos of anything from 539 to 870 pages each, and their exhaustive nature has done much to facilitate the researches of later bibliographers. They are particularly valuable because they are not mere lists, but are critical. Each one is divided into sections representing historical periods, and subdivided by authors. Details of their lives, writings and editions, with notes on the contents of the books, are provided. Their disadvantage is the lack of a subject approach; all have author indexes but the subject indexes cover the anonymous works only.[14] An improved index to *Bibliotheca botanica*, compiled by J. C. Bay, was published on the bicentenary of Haller's birth (*Bibliotheca botanica ... index emendatus*, Berne, 1908). Christoph Gottlieb von Murr (1733–1811) published additions and corrections to the four bibliographies as *Adnotationes ad Bibliothecas Hallerianas* (Erlangen, 1805).

Haller collected together a library of about 15 000 volumes, which was acquired by the Emperor Joseph II, and is now for the most part in Milan.[15] His original papers are preserved in the Burgerbibliothek at Berne, and include 67 bound volumes of correspondence; a large collection of unpublished manuscripts and interleaved copies of his published works, with corrections and additions; and abstracts of books he had read, covering 1731 to 1776, bound in 20 volumes.[16]

An eighteenth-century medical biographical dictionary of value for its bibliographical content is the *Dictionnaire historique de la médecine* of Nicolas François Joseph Éloy (1714–88), a physician of Mons. The first edition was published at Liège in two volumes in 1755 and was reprinted

at Frankfort in the following year. These were superseded by a much
enlarged edition entitled *Dictionnaire historique de la médecine ancienne et
moderne*, 4 vols (Mons, 1778). Two useful nineteenth-century works lean-
ing heavily on Éloy are the *Biographie médicale*, edited by Antoine Jacques Louis Jourdan (1788–1848), 7 vols (Paris, 1820–5, supplement to
Dictionaire [*sic*] *des sciences médicales*, 1820–2) and the *Dictionnaire historique de la médecine ancienne et moderne* of Jean Eugène Dezeimeris
(1799–1851) and others, 4 vols in 7 (Paris 1828–39). Both are heavily
overweighted to the early part of the alphabet!

A few other eighteenth-century medical bibliographies are worthy of
brief mention, for example that by Joseph Barthélemy François Carrère
(1740–1802) entitled *Bibliothèque littéraire, historique et critique de la
médecine ancienne et moderne* (Paris, 1776) of which only the first two
volumes covering the letters 'A–Coi' were published. Carrère's bibliographical expertise is demonstrated by his exhaustive bibliography of mineral
waters, *Catalogue raisonné des ouvrages qui ont été publiés sur les eaux
minérales en général et sur celles de la France en particulier* (Paris, 1785).
Johann Friedrich Blumenbach (1752–1840), among his numerous medical
and scientific writings, was the author of *Introductio in historiam medicinae
litterariam* (Göttingen, 1786), which is in effect a chronologically arranged
medical bibliography. Johann Daniel Metzger (1739–1805) was the author
of *Skizze einer pragmatischen Literärgeschichte der Medizin* (Königsberg,
1792), to which a supplement was published in 1796. Although this is
primarily set out as a narrative, it contains a substantial bibliographical
element.

The Swiss physician, politician and journalist Paulus Usteri (1768–
1831) compiled an annual bibliography of recent publications entitled
Repertorium der medicinischen Litteratur des Jahres 1789 [*–1793*], 5 vols
(Zurich, 1790–5); this was continued as *Medicinische Litteratur des Jahres
1794* (Leipzig, 1796–7). It is arranged by subjects, with annotations, and
there is an author index. Usteri graduated in medicine at Göttingen in
1788 but the French Revolution diverted him from a medical to a political
career.

Ernst Gottfried Baldinger (1738–1804) was the author of numerous
medical works, including a bibliography of therapeutics entitled *Littera-
tura universa materiae medicae, alimentariae, toxicologiae, pharmaciae, et
therapiae generalis, medicae atque chirurgicae, potissimum academica*
(Marburg, 1793). Karl Gottlob Kühn (1754–1840), best known for his
editions of Galen and other classical medical authors, commenced a
*Bibliotheca medica, continens scripta medicorum omnis aevi, ordine metho-
dico disposita*; only the first volume was published, at Leipzig in 1794. A
subject bibliography with historical notes was published by Immanuel
Vertraugott Rothe as *Handbuch für die medizinische Litteratur nach allen
ihren Theilen* (Leipzig, 1799). Immanuel Gottlieb Knebel's *Versuch einer*

chronologischen Uebersicht der Literärgeschichte der Arzneiwissenschaft
(Breslau etc., 1799) contains some bibliographical notes but is essentially a
chronological history of medicine.

By the end of the eighteenth century, the subject approach was generally
supplanting arrangement by authors or by periods. The first important
subject catalogue of medicine was the work of Wilhelm Gottfried Ploucquet (1744–1814), a native of Württemberg, who was professor of medicine at Tübingen. His *Initia bibliothecae medico-practicae et chirurgicae*,
Tübingen, was published in eight volumes between 1793 and 1797. This
was followed by a continuation and supplement, issued in four volumes as
Bibliotheca medico-practica et chirurgica realis recentior (Tübingen, 1799–
1803). These two series were then superseded by a revised and enlarged
version entitled *Literatura medica digesta*, 4 vols (Tübingen, 1808–9). A
supplement was published in 1814. Ploucquet's bibliographies list articles
in periodicals, books and dissertations, and are arranged by subject.

Jeremias David Reuss (1750–1837), professor and university librarian
at Göttingen, compiled a subject index to the publications of learned
societies in all disciplines up to the end of the eighteenth century, *Repertorium commentationum a societatibus literariis editarum, secundum discip-
linarum ordinem*, 16 vols (Göttingen, 1801–21, reprinted by Burt Franklin,
New York, 1961). Volumes 10 to 16 are devoted to medicine and surgery.

A specifically medical subject bibliography is *Die Literatur der Heilwis-
senschaft*, 2 vols (Gotha, 1810–11) compiled by Karl Friedrich Burdach
(1776–1847). A supplementary volume covering the years 1811 to 1820
appeared in 1821.

Johann Samuel Ersch (1766–1828), professor and librarian at Halle,
compiled a number of general bibliographies. The medical section of his
*Handbuch der deutschen Literatur seit der Mitte des achtzehnten Jahrhun-
derts bis auf die neueste Zeit*, 2 vols (Amsterdam and Leipzig, 1812–14)
was issued separately as *Literatur der Medizin* ... (1812). A revised edition,
edited by Friedrich August Benjamin Puchelt (1784–1856), was published
at Leipzig in 1822. It is systematically arranged, with a comprehensive
index of subjects; it gives a very thorough coverage of publications of the
German-speaking countries from the mid-eighteenth century to the early
nineteenth.

The writings of Thomas Young (1773–1829) cover several branches of
knowledge, and he has been called 'the most highly educated physician of
his time'. He made important contributions in physics, physiological
optics and Egyptology.[17] His work on medical bibliography was entitled
*An introduction to medical literature, including a system of practical nos-
ology* (London, 1813) and consists of a selection of books necessary to a
complete medical library, those of primary importance to students and
those of established value being specially indicated. A systematic arrangement is adopted, which is also intended as an attempt at an improved

classification of diseases. There is a subject index, and contents of certain (mainly British) periodicals are included, but generally only those published since 1750. Entries are very brief, but the book was extremely popular, a second edition, considerably enlarged, appearing in 1823. The work also includes several of Young's medical papers.

The Berlin publisher Theodor Christian Friedrich Enslin (1787–1851) was responsible for a number of subject bibliographies, listing works published from 1750 onwards in the German-speaking countries. Some of these passed through several editions and were later carried on by his pupil Wilhelm Engelmann (1808–78) in Leipzig. The *Bibliotheca medico-chirurgica et pharmaceutico-chemica* (Berlin, 1817) went through three further editions under Enslin's supervision in 1821, 1823 and 1825. Engelmann produced the fifth edition (Leipzig, 1838) with a supplement in 1841. The sixth edition, 1848, was entitled *Bibliotheca medico-chirurgica et anatomico-physiologica*, with a supplement in 1868 (reprinted Hildesheim, Olms, 1964). Meanwhile a separate *Bibliotheca pharmaceutico-chemica* had appeared in 1846. A *Bibliotheca veterinaria* was published by Enslin (Berlin, 1825) and a second edition was published by Engelmann (Leipzig, 1843).

The career of Robert Watt (1775–1819) is of great interest and, although his *Bibliotheca Britannica* is by no means confined to medicine, the circumstances attending its origin are worthy of note. Watt was a native of Ayrshire, his early years being spent as a ploughboy, labourer and carpenter. He read avidly in his spare time and in 1793 began to attend classes at the University of Glasgow, and later also at Edinburgh. He eventually decided to take up medicine, became a licentiate of the Glasgow Faculty in 1799, and went into general practice at Paisley. He became a member of the Faculty in 1807 and in 1810 gained an MD from King's College, Aberdeen. He then practised in Glasgow, and established a subscription library for the use of students attending his lectures. His *Catalogue of medical books, for the use of students attending lectures on the principles and practice of medicine* (Glasgow, 1812) is now very rare, but has been reprinted in facsimile in a bibliographical study of Watt by Francesco Cordasco.[18] The Catalogue includes over a thousand entries, and the library also included a similar number of theses. This was the beginning of Watt's monumental *Bibliotheca*.

Watt served as president of the Glasgow Faculty in 1812–16, became physician to the Royal Infirmary and was the author of several medical books and articles, but in 1817 for reasons of health he retired from practice to Campvale, where he settled down to concentrate on his bibliography, assisted by his sons and others. He died on 12 March 1819, just as the first sheets were printed, the work being issued in parts. Parts 1–4 were printed at Glasgow, 1819–20, and parts 5–9 at Edinburgh, 1821–4. The completed work is in four volumes, and was published as *Bibliotheca*

Britannica: or a general index to British and foreign literature (Edinburgh, 1824). The first two volumes are arranged alphabetically by authors and the last two by subjects, constituting an index to the author sequence. The work includes periodical articles and is particularly useful for medical items. It remains a worthy monument to a painstaking bibliographer.

Constables, the publishers, went bankrupt in 1826 in a famous crash, which also ruined Sir Walter Scott, and Watt's widow never received the promised payment. On the death of Watt's youngest daughter Mary, in 1864, in Govan parish lunatic asylum, most of the manuscript slips for the *Bibliotheca* were discovered in two sacks and are now preserved in Paisley Public Library, mounted in 69 volumes.[19]

Johann Ludwig Choulant (1791–1861) was the author of several medical bibliographies, mainly of an historical nature, but he was also an expert in several branches of medicine. A native of Dresden, he graduated at Leipzig in 1818, and eventually became Director of the Chirurgisch-Medicinische Akademie at Dresden, from which he retired in 1860. He translated many works from English into German, and edited the writings of several other authors. Choulant's bibliographical writings include a bibliographical study of Celsus, *Prodromus novae editionis Auli Cornelii Celsi librorum VIII de medicina* (Leipzig, 1824); *Handbuch der Bücherkunde für die ältere Medicin* (Leipzig, 1828), which is recognized as his greatest bibliographical work, and of which a second edition was published in 1841 (reprinted Graz, 1956); *Bibliotheca medico-historica sive catalogus librorum historicorum de re medica et scientia naturali systematicus* (Leipzig, 1842, reprinted Hildesheim, Olms, 1960), to which a supplement in two parts was added by Julius Rosenbaum (Halle, 1842–7); and *Die anatomischen Abbildungen des XV. und XVI. Jahrhunderts* (Leipzig, 1843), which was an introduction to his *Geschichte und Bibliographie der anatomischen Abbildung, nach ihrer Beziehung auf anatomische Wissenschaft und bildende Kunst* (Leipzig, 1852). Additions and corrections are included in his *Graphische Incunabeln für Naturgeschichte und Medicin* (Leipzig, 1858, reprinted Munich, 1924 and Hildesheim, Olms, 1963).

Choulant's work on anatomical illustration was later published in much improved form as *History and bibliography of anatomic illustration in its relation to anatomic science and the graphic arts ... Translated and edited ... by Mortimer Frank* (Chicago, 1920). It includes a life of Choulant and additional essays by Fielding H. Garrison and Edward C. Streeter. Mortimer Frank (1874–1919) died before publication. A revised edition, with a new historical essay by Charles Singer and a bibliography of Mortimer Frank by J. Christian Bay, was published at New York in 1945 (reprinted New York, Hafner, 1962). Choulant has been described as 'author of sterling bibliographies', and his compilations are all valuable productions worthy of study by historians and bibliographers.[20]

The *Précis de bibliographie médicale* (Paris, 1827) of Jean Baptiste

Monfalcon (1792–1874) has already been mentioned. It is an attempt at a select medical bibliography, arranged by authors, with subject and chronological tables and a useful introductory essay covering such topics as bibliographical method, the history of printing, and library design. An earlier edition (Paris, 1826) was entitled *Précis de l'histoire de la médecine et de bibliographie médicale*. Monfalcon was a native of Lyons and spent his working life there as physician and librarian.

Kurt Polykarp Joachim Sprengel (1766–1833) is best known for his monumental *Versuch einer pragmatischen Geschichte der Arzneikunde*, 5 vols (Halle, 1792–1803, also later editions and translations). His *Literatura medica externa recentior* (Leipzig, 1829) covers works published outside Germany from 1750 onwards. It is arranged by subjects, with an author index.

A worthy successor to Haller was found in Adolph Carl Peter Callisen (1786–1866), an army surgeon who became professor and librarian at the Koneglige Kirurgisk Akademi at Copenhagen in 1830. Callisen was a native of Glückstadt and graduated at Kiel in 1809. His author catalogue covers the years from 1780 onwards, and contains over 99 000 items. The work is entitled *Medicinisches Schriftsteller-Lexicon der jetzt lebenden Aerzte, Wundärzte, Geburtshelfer, Apotheker und Naturforscher aller gebildeten Völker*, 33 vols, privately printed (Copenhagen and Altona, 1830–45, reprinted Nieuwkoop, De Graaf, 1962–5). Each author and each book is numbered, and material incorporated includes articles in journals, as well as monographs, with prices and notes of reviews. Biographical information is given, including portraits. The first 21 volumes cover an alphabetical sequence of authors and are followed by four volumes devoted to anonymous works and to an exhaustive treatment of periodicals and miscellaneous writings. This sequence is repeated in eight supplementary volumes. The work as it stands is limited to authors known, or believed, to be living. Callisen had originally intended a further series covering deceased authors and a subject index. His work is most useful on account of its wide scope and reliability. Its author arrangement supplemented the subject catalogue of Ploucquet until both were superseded by the *Index-Catalogue*.

A bibliography of little scientific value, but full of wit and obscure information, was compiled by James Atkinson (1759–1839) when he was almost 75 years of age. Atkinson practised as a surgeon at York, following a long family tradition. His *Medical bibliography, A and B*, was printed at York, 1833, with another issue from London in 1834. It consists of an alphabetical arrangement by authors, with discursive and amusing annotations, and there is nothing to indicate that Atkinson intended to continue the work beyond the letter B. In fact he light-heartedly tackled the task with the words: 'What blockhead but myself would have chosen such a subject for relaxation?' Atkinson possessed a large collection of medical portraits and an extensive library, which was sold by Sotheby's in 1851. The catalogue bears the title *Catalogue of the valuable and curious medical and miscellaneous library of the late James Atkinson, Esq., author of 'Medical Bibliography'.*[21]

Sir John Forbes (1787–1861) published *A manual of select medical bibliography* (London, 1835) as an appendix to *The cyclopaedia of practical medicine* (4 vols, 1833–5), of which he was one of the editors. The bibliography consists of an alphabetical arrangement of subjects, under which books and articles are arranged in chronological order. Entries are abbreviated, and references to articles in periodicals are not complete, but this constituted the most comprehensive English attempt to date at a subject classification of medical literature. Forbes entered the Navy as assistant surgeon in 1807, after securing a diploma as surgeon at Edinburgh; he took his MD there ten years later. He afterwards practised at Penzance and Chichester, and in 1821 published a translation of Laënnec's work on auscultation, followed in 1824 by a translation of Auenbrugger's writings on the same subject. In 1840 Forbes removed to London to edit the *British and Foreign Medical Review*, and became a Fellow of the Royal College of Physicians in 1845. He was knighted in 1853.[22]

The *Bibliographie des sciences médicales* (Paris, 1874, reprinted London, Verschuyle, 1954) of Alphonse Pauly (1830–1909) is an accurate tool, giving sources of information where the compiler was unable to consult the originals. It includes articles in periodicals, and is divided into bibliography, biography, history, epidemics, medical geography, and so on, a detailed table of contents and author index adding to its value. Pauly was on the staff of the Bibliothèque Nationale.

Richard Neale (1827–1900) began work on his *Medical digest* as a student and devoted some 50 years of his life to it. The first edition, published by the New Sydenham Society, was entitled *The medical digest, being a means of ready reference to the principal contributions to medical science during the last thirty years* (London, 1877). Second and third editions were issued under the title *The medical digest, or busy practitioner's vade-mecum* in 1882 and 1891; appendices appeared in 1886, 1895 and 1899. The *Medical digest* is selective and deals with a limited number of journals; entries are drastically abbreviated and are arranged in classified order with an extensive index. The work was popular in its day and partially fills the gap between Watt and the *Index Medicus*.[23]

Some of our most valuable bibliographical tools have originated in the United States of America, and medicine in general is particularly indebted to the bibliographers of that country responsible for the *Index-Catalogue*, the *Index Medicus* and their successors, which originated in the last century, and mainly owed their success to the efforts of John Shaw Billings. Born on 12 April 1838 in Cotton Township, Indiana, Billings was

educated at Miami University and at the Medical College of Ohio, where
he graduated in 1860 and became a demonstrator in anatomy. During the
Civil War he joined the Union Army as a surgeon and did not return to
civilian life. In December 1864, Billings was assigned to the Surgeon-
General's Office in Washington and took charge of the 1365 books then
comprising the Library. This he developed into the most useful medical
library in the world,[24] purchasing books from Europe and cataloguing his
acquisitions, with a view to publication. In 1876 he issued his *Specimen
fasciculus of a catalogue of the National Medical Library*, and this was
soon followed by the publication of the *Index-Catalogue of the Library of
the Surgeon-General's Office*. The first series was published in 16 vols
(Washington, 1880–95); the second series, 21 vols (1896–1916); the third
series, 10 vols (1918–32); and the fourth series, 11 vols (1936–55). This last
ceased when it reached the letters 'Mn'. These four series are in dictionary
form, and include entries for monographs under both authors and subjects but articles in journals under subjects only. Each item receives only a
single subject-entry. Full names of authors, dates of birth and death, and
references to biographical material and portraits are included. A supplementary fifth series in three volumes was published in 1959–61 to include
the more important literature from the accumulation of arrears up to
1950. One volume contains authors and titles and two are devoted to
subjects.

With Robert Fletcher, Billings inaugurated the *Index Medicus* in 1879,
and when he retired from the Surgeon-General's Office in 1895 to occupy
the Chair of Hygiene and Bacteriology at the University of Pennsylvania,
he left behind three progressive monuments, the *Index-Catalogue*, the
Index Medicus and the activated Surgeon-General's Library, any one of
which might serve as a memorial to one man. After a year at Pennsylvania
Billings became Director of the New York Public Library, and built it up
into a comprehensive system serving an extensive community. Billings
received numerous honours during his lifetime and has been revered by
successive generations of medical bibliographers.[25]

A native of Bristol, Robert Fletcher (1823–1912) was closely associated
with Billings in his bibliographical work and in the launch of the *Index
Medicus* in 1879. Fletcher qualified in medicine in 1844 and in 1847 went
to America, settling in Cincinnati. He saw active service during the Civil
War and, after working in the War Department, was transferred to the
Surgeon-General's Library in 1876, where he served as Principal Assistant
Librarian for almost 35 years, dying in harness at the age of 89. In spite of
his heavy bibliographical commitments he found time to teach classes in
medical jurisprudence and maintained a serious interest in anthropology.[26]

Fielding Hudson Garrison (1870–1935), who with Billings and Fletcher
makes up a remarkable bibliographical trio, was educated at the Johns

Hopkins University, Baltimore, and joined the Surgeon-General's Library as a clerk in 1891. He took instruction in medicine in the evenings at Georgetown University, Washington, and obtained an MD degree in 1893. In 1899 he became Assistant Librarian under Fletcher and succeeded him as Principal Assistant Librarian in 1912. He found time for substantial historical and bibliographical work. He was the author of *An introduction to the history of medicine*, first published in Philadelphia in 1913 and reprinted in 1914, with three further editions in 1917, 1921 and 1929. The last of these was reprinted in 1961. He gave a course on the history of military medicine, which was published in book form in 1922, and contributed an excellent history of paediatrics to Isaac A. Abt's *Pediatrics by various authors*, vol. 1 (Philadelphia, 1923). This was reprinted as *Abt–Garrison history of pediatrics ... with new chapters on the history of pediatrics in recent times, by Arthur F. Abt* (Philadelphia and London, 1965). Garrison's other publications include *John Shaw Billings: a memoir* (New York and London, 1915), and the original check-list for Garrison–Morton (see below). In 1930 Garrison retired from the Surgeon-General's Library, and became librarian of the Welch Medical Library at Johns Hopkins.[27]

Index Medicus. A monthly classified record of the current medical literature of the world was initially conceived by Billings as a by-product of his work on the *Index-Catalogue*.[28] It was a commercial rather than an official publication. The first series, edited at first by Billings and Fletcher and then by Fletcher alone, was published initially by Leypoldt of New York and later by Davis of Boston and Chicago. It ran for 21 volumes, 1879–99 and then collapsed from lack of funds. It was revived in 1903 with the support of the Carnegie Institution of Washington: second series, edited by Fletcher and Garrison, 18 vols (1903–20); third series, edited by Garrison, 6 vols (1921–7). Meanwhile an alternative publication, the *Quarterly Cumulative Index to Current Medical Literature* had been established by the American Medical Association. This ran for 12 volumes, 1916–26 and then amalgamated with the *Index Medicus* to form the *Quarterly Cumulative Index Medicus*, published under the auspices of the American Medical Association.

The gap between the first and second series of *Index Medicus* (1900–2) was partially filled by *Bibliographia Medica*, 3 vols (Paris, 1900–2) and by *Index Medicus Novus (Die medicinische Weltliteratur)* (Vienna, 1899–1900). A British publication to fill the gap was proposed by J. Y. W. MacAlister of the Royal Medical and Chirurgical Society; much indexing work was done, but publication was delayed by difficulty in raising funds and the revival of *Index Medicus* in 1903 led to the abandonment of the project.[29]

The *Quarterly Cumulative Index Medicus*, 60 vols (1927–56) was published quarterly until the outbreak of war, when it appeared belatedly as half-yearly bound volumes. The backlog increased until publication ceased in 1959 with the issue of volume 60 covering July–December 1956. This bibliography lists under authors and subjects the contents of journals issued during six-monthly periods, books being listed separately. It was relied upon as the most authoritative and comprehensive index to this material, but prompt publication is essential to the needs of modern research, and other tools were encroaching upon the field previously held by the *Quarterly Cumulative*, and were filling its functions more speedily, if not more effectively.

Meanwhile the cessation of publication of the *Index-Catalogue* had not terminated the publication of lists of books added to the Army Medical Library (formerly the Surgeon-General's Library, afterwards the Armed Forces Medical Library, and finally the National Library of Medicine, formerly of Washington, but since 1962 situated in Bethesda, Maryland). Books added to the library were listed as author entries as a supplement to the Library of Congress *Cumulative Catalog* for 1948 and entries for 1949 and 1950 appeared as supplementary volumes to the Library of Congress *Author Catalog*, that for 1950 having a subject index. Author and subject entries for additions in 1951 were included in the *Army Medical Library Catalog* published in 1952, to be followed by similar schemes for 1952 and 1953. These were superseded by *Armed Forces Medical Library Catalog: a cumulative list of works represented by Armed Forces Medical Library cards, 1950–1954*, 6 vols (Ann Arbor, Michigan, 1955). Authors and subjects each have three volumes. Annual volumes were issued for 1955 to 1958, which in turn were superseded by *National Library of Medicine Catalog: a list of works represented by National Library of Medicine cards, 1955–1959*, 6 vols (Washington, 1960). The final series covering 1960–5, again in 6 vols, was published in 1966, in January of which year appeared the first issue of the computer-generated *National Library of Medicine Current Catalog*. This was at first produced twice monthly, with quarterly and annual cumulations. Publication became monthly in 1970 and quarterly in 1974. A sexennial cumulation, covering 1965 to 1970, was published in 8 vols and a quinquennial cumulation for 1971–5 in 5 vols; subsequent cumulations have appeared on microfiche.

We have to take certain circumstances into consideration when consulting the *Index-Catalogue* and its successors. It only covers literature housed in the one library, which although very comprehensive, obviously does not contain everything. The volumes of each series appeared over a number of years, certain letters of the alphabet recurring at intervals of up to 20 years. In 1926 subject entries were dropped for material published after 1925, but were resumed in 1932. This covers letters 'Ge-Z' of the third series, and the gap must be filled by consulting the *Quarterly Cumulative Index*, the *Index Medicus*, and the *Quarterly Cumulative Index Medicus*.

Furthermore all series should be consulted, as historical material added in recent years will obviously appear in recent volumes of the catalogue.[30]

Author, but not subject, approaches to the National Library of Medicine's historical collections are provided by a series of specialized catalogues: *A catalogue of incunabula and manuscripts in the Army Medical Library*, by Dorothy M. Schullian and Francis E. Sommer (New York, 1950); *A catalogue of sixteenth-century printed books in the National ' ˙ ıry of Medicine*, by Richard J. Durling (Bethesda, Md, 1967); *A catalogue of incunabula and sixteenth-century printed books ... first supplement*, by Peter Krivatsy (Bethesda, Md, 1971); *Short-title catalogue of eighteenth century printed books in the National Library of Medicine*, by John B. Blake (Bethesda, 1979). It should also be noted that the fourth series of the *Index-Catalogue* contains two specialized bibliographies, which are easily overlooked: vol. 3 (1938) contains a bibliography of medical congresses, to which a supplement was added in vol. 4 (1939); vol. 6 (1941) contains the first fascicule (A-Alberti) of *Bio-bibliography of XVI century medical authors*, by Claudius F. Mayer, but this ambitious project was halted by the Second World War.

The Index-Catalogue has been described as 'America's greatest contribution to medicine'. Its value is inestimable, and no medico-historical bibliographical research can be completed without reference to these records of the contents of the most influential medical library in the world.

News that the *Quarterly Cumulative Index Medicus* was to cease publication in 1959 was received with dismay by every medical librarian. Fortunately a new index to the contents of medical journals had commenced publication during the war, partially to fill the gap caused by delays in the publication of the *Quarterly Cumulative*. This was the *Current List of Medical Literature*, begun in 1941 as a weekly publication, and taken over in 1945 by the Armed Forces Medical Library, to be greatly improved; from 1950 it was published monthly, with author and subject indexes, which greatly facilitated its use. Entries were arranged under titles of journals, so that these indexes were essential, but the *Current List* never gave as good a service as the *Quarterly Cumulative*. However it constitutes the sole coverage between 1957 and 1959. Although librarians tend to overlook the *Current List* for the years covered by the *Quarterly Cumulative*, each indexed journals not covered by the other, so that they are complementary.

In January 1960 the National Library of Medicine published an enlarged monthly *Index Medicus* to replace the *Current List*, and research workers were not left without an index to the medical literature of the world. Until 1965 the annual *Cumulated Index Medicus* was published by the American Medical Association but since 1966 the National Library of Medicine has issued both the *Cumulated Index Medicus* and the *Index Medicus*. The process is automated, and based on a computerized system of information retrieval known as MEDLARS (Medical Literature Analysis and Retrieval System). Subject headings have been drastically altered and standardized, being based on a simple classification system. Allied to MEDLARS we have GRACE (Graphic Arts Composing Equipment), a computer-driven photo-typesetter, which prints the *Index*, and which has resulted in great improvements in layout, with variations in type size which make for easier consultation. These developments have led to the creation of one of the world's largest databases in the medical field. The on-line files are known as MEDLINE (MEDlars onLINE).

Abstracts and digests are frequently of more value than index entries, particularly where the original articles are in foreign languages or in obscure journals, and several organs containing abstracts as prominent features have been published during the nineteenth and twentieth centuries. The *Jahrbücher der in- und ausländischen gesammten Medicin*, generally known as *Schmidts Jahrbücher*, after Karl Christian Schmidt (1792–1855), the founder, was published in 336 volumes between 1834 and 1922. C. F. Canstatt's *Jahresbericht über die Fortschritte der gesammten Medicin in allen Ländern* appeared between 1841 and 1916, and the *Centralblatt für die medicinischen Wissenschaften* was published from 1865 to 1915.

Turning to British examples, the *Retrospect of practical medicine and surgery* was founded by William Braithwaite (1807–85) and 123 volumes appeared between 1840 and 1901 (the title being changed to *Retrospect of medicine* from vol. 13). An American edition was also published in New York. Braithwaite was succeeded as editor by his son James. The *Half-yearly abstract of the medical sciences*, 58 vols (1845–73) was founded by William Harcourt Ranking (1814–67); this also was reprinted in America (New York, 1845–51 and Philadelphia, 1866–74). The Medical Research Council (formerly Committee) published *Medical Science Abstracts and Reviews* between 1919 and 1925, and the *Bulletin of War Medicine* from 1940 to 1946. The British Medical Association published *Abstracts of World Medicine* from 1947 to 1977; *Abstracts of World Surgery, Obstetrics and Gynaecology* was issued as a separate publication from 1947 to 1952 but the two were then combined. It was selective but authoritative.

The National Library of Medicine began to publish the *Bibliography of Medical Reviews* as an annual in 1956. The first five issues were cumulated in vol. 6, 1961. In March 1965 it began to be included as a section in the monthly issues of *Index Medicus* and, since 1967, an annual cumulation has been part of the *Cumulated Index Medicus*. Five-year cumulations have also continued to appear. It is of particular value in literature searches, as review articles generally contain useful lists of references.

The *Medical Annual*, published by Wright of Bristol, has appeared every year since 1883, and provides useful summaries of the literature published in the previous year. These were arranged alphabetically by subjects until 1958, when broad subjects were divided into sub-sections, and original articles were included. Classified lists of new books and details of new preparations and appliances are included, and the *Medical Annual* enables medical men without ready access to libraries to maintain themselves up-to-date. It is not consulted often enough, tending to be overlooked in preference for consultation of the more comprehensive bibliographies but is a valuable source for ready reference.

A major abstracting organization is the non-profit-making Excerpta Medica Foundation, established at Amsterdam in 1946. Its publication, *Excerpta Medica*, first appeared in 1947 and is now the most comprehensive abstracting tool devoted to medicine, covering over 3500 journals. Its computerized database, EMBASE, is comparable to MEDLARS. It is divided into 45 sections, devoted to different branches of the biomedical field, and each section is issued monthly. Abstracts are arranged in classified order, with subject and author indexes, and there is an annual cumulation. The series is of particular value to the large medical library, which can afford to subscribe to the complete set, and to the small specialized library which can cover its entire field with one, or possibly two sections. The small library in a medical school or general hospital may find that it can take none of the sections, as otherwise departments not being served would consider themselves neglected.

Annual review publications are of value as bibliographical sources; *Annual Reviews, Year Books* and *Advances* are published for many subjects.

Two selective bibliographies containing abstracts and arranged under specific subject headings, with chronological treatment under these headings, have been compiled by Arthur L. Bloomfield. *A bibliography of internal medicine. Communicable diseases* (Chicago, 1958) and *A bibliography of internal medicine. Selected diseases* (Chicago, 1960) both have author but not subject indexes, and contain details of bibliographies, histories, classic descriptions and review articles under the specific headings.

The *British Medical Book List*, mainly intended for the overseas reader, was established by the British Council in 1950 as a guide to recently published books. It was replaced in 1972 by an expanded version entitled *British Medicine*, which, since 1980, has been published by Pergamon Press. The London medical booksellers and publishers, H. K. Lewis, long maintained a valuable subscription library. Quarterly and annual lists of recent publications were issued and general catalogues of the Library's holdings were published from time to time. The last complete edition, containing publications up to the end of 1972, was published in 1975 and triennial supplements were issued until the shop and library closed in 1989.

Fielding Hudson Garrison has previously been mentioned in this chapter in connection with his work at the National Library of Medicine, but his name is more closely associated by modern bibliographers and librarians with *Garrison and Morton's Medical bibliography: an annotated check-list of texts illustrating the history of medicine*, first printed in this form in London in 1943. This was originally printed in the *Index-Catalogue* (Series 2, vol. 17, 1912, pp.89–178), and was later published as 'Revised student's check-list of texts illustrating the history of medicine, with references for collateral reading' (*Bull. Inst. Hist. Med.*, 1, 1933, pp.333–434). Leslie T. Morton completely revised this latter, classifying and annotating the entries, and improving the work beyond recognition. The chronological arrangement of entries under subjects provides an historical outline of the main events in the development of each topic. Complete forenames of authors, dates of birth and death, and useful annotations enhance the value of this essential tool in every medical library. The second edition, published in 1954, contains 6808 entries and provides sections devoted to medical bibliography, historical periodicals and collective biography. It was reprinted with minor additions in 1961 and 1965. The third edition, published in 1970 under the title *A medical bibliography (Garrison and Morton)*, contains 7354 entries and in the fourth edition, 1983, the total has risen to 7830.

Garrison–Morton is used extensively by medical booksellers and the citations from periodicals have been rearranged under titles of journals by Lee Ash in *Serial publications containing medical classics. An index to citations in Garrison–Morton* (New Haven, Conn., 1961). A second edition, based on the third edition of Garrison–Morton, compiled by Lee Ash and Michael A. Murray, was published at Bethany, Conn., 1979. The first edition contains Leslie Morton's own account of the genesis of the project. Entries are arranged alphabetically by titles of journals, then chronologically with the names of authors and their Garrison–Morton numbers. This enables booksellers and librarians to identify those issues containing classic articles.

Another useful tool for tracing original descriptions of diseases, eponymous literature, and other historical information is Emerson Crosby Kelly's *Encyclopedia of medical sources* (Baltimore, 1948). The compiler also edited *Medical Classics*, 5 vols (Baltimore, 1936–41) which reprinted many of the most significant classics in the history of medicine, with English translations and much biographical and bibliographical material.

A currently produced index of special value to those interested in the history of medicine and science is published quarterly by the Wellcome Institute for the History of Medicine. *Current Work in the History of Medicine* has appeared since 1954, and items are indexed under subjects, with author indexes, and with addresses of authors. Lists of books recently published and forthcoming are included, and this publication has proved of inestimable value to medical historians and librarians; it has been indispensable both to the original author of this book and to his successors. It was distributed gratis for some 20 years, but sadly, this is no longer the case!

A cumulation of *Current Work* on cards has been maintained at the Wellcome Institute Library and this was reproduced by Kraus International Publications as *Subject-catalogue of the history of medicine and related sciences*, 18 vols (Munich, 1980). It incorporates *Current Work* up to 1976. There are nine subject volumes, four topographical and five biographical. There is no author approach, but the coverage is more comprehensive than that of *Current Work*. Monographs, which in *Current Work* are listed only by author, are entered under subjects, and much material from before *Current Work's* starting date of 1954 is included, both monographs and journal articles. Entries for monographs are for the most part based on the Wellcome Library's holdings, but journal articles are based on citation in *Current Work* and it therefore cannot be assumed that they will be held by the Library.

Bibliography of the History of Medicine has been published annually by the National Library of Medicine since 1965 (covering publications of 1964) and is cumulated every five years. It began as a by-product of *Index Medicus* and is now prepared from HISTLINE, the Library's database in the history of medicine. It is divided into biographical and subject sections with an author index.

The journal *Isis*, founded in 1913, has always included bibliographies of recent publications in the history of science and these have now been published in cumulated form as *Isis cumulative bibliography. A bibliography of the history of science formed from Isis critical bibliographies* (London, 1971–). Six volumes, edited by Magda Whitrow, covering material listed from 1913 to 1965, appeared between 1971 and 1984; vols 1–2 cover personalities and institutions, vol. 3 subjects (in classified order), vols 4–5 civilizations and periods and vol. 6 is an author index. A further series covering 1965 to 1974, edited by John Neu, was published in 2 vols, 1980– 5 and follows the same arrangement. The work contains much material relevant to the history of medicine and its comprehensive retrospective coverage is especially valuable. A useful feature is the citation of reviews.

Two useful single-volume bibliographies of use for the history of medicine are Pieter Smit's *History of the life sciences, an annotated bibliography* (Amsterdam, 1974) and S. A. Jayawardene's *Reference books for the historian of science, a handlist* (London, 1982). Jonathon Erlen's *The history of the health care sciences and health care 1700–1980, a selective annotated bibliography* (New York, 1984) is limited to works in the English language.

Paul T. Durbin (ed.), *A guide to the culture of science, technology and medicine* (New York and London, 1980) contains essays on the history and philosophy of various subject areas with surveys of current trends and basic bibliographies. A similar work with a stronger bibliographical emphasis is Pietro Corsi and Paul Weindling (eds), *Information sources in the history of science and medicine* (London, 1983).

Biographical information, and also bibliographies of the writings of individuals, are frequently useful to librarians in answering readers' queries. Many of the bibliographies are mentioned throughout this book and others are included in biographical studies. Biographies published in English in the nineteenth and twentieth centuries are recorded in *A bibliography of medical and biomedical biography* (1989), compiled by Leslie T. Morton and Robert J. Moore (supersedes John L. Thornton's *A select bibliography of medical biography*, 2nd edn, 1970). A comprehensive list of biographical material is also contained in *Catalog of biographies in the Library of the New York Academy of Medicine* (Boston, 1960).

There are innumerable bibliographies of special branches of medicine, and it is not intended to attempt to mention them all in this chapter, but a few examples must be recorded. Anatomy was an early subject to attract the attention of bibliographers. The *Bibliographiae anatomicae specimen* of James Douglas (1675–1742) was first published in London in 1715, with a second edition at Leyden in 1734. Haller's monumental bibliography of the subject has been mentioned above. The *Histoire de l'anatomie et de la chirurgie*, 6 vols in 7 (Paris, 1770–3) of Antoine Portal (1742–1832) could equally well be described as a chronological bibliography of those subjects. It contains indexes to the literature of specific topics. George Edward Day (1815–72), professor of medicine at St Andrews, published an *Anatomical and physiological bibliography from 1849 to 1852 inclusive* [privately printed, 1853?], of which few copies seem to have survived.[31] K. F. Russell's *British anatomy, 1525–1800: a bibliography* (Melbourne, 1963) is comprehensive and an invaluable study within the limits of the title. Containing numerous illustrations it is a model of its kind, and is a good example of an extensive study of an important subject, which might be followed up by similar bibliographical studies of other topics. An enlarged second edition was published at Winchester in 1987, shortly after Professor Russell's death at the age of 76.

Surgery, as mentioned above, was covered by Portal and by Haller's *Bibliotheca chirurgica*, 1774–5, the former with a subject approach, the latter without. Comprehensive subject coverage was provided a few years later by Stephan Hieronymus de Vigiliis von Creutzenfeld (1749?–88). His *Bibliotheca chirurgica in qua res omnes ad chirurgiam pertinentes, ordine alphabetico ... exhibentur*, 2 vols (Vienna, 1781) covers the literature to 1779; it is arranged alphabetically by subjects and has an author index. Entries are annotated.

E. Alan Baker and D. J. Foskett's *Bibliography of food. A select international bibliography of nutrition, food and beverage technology and distribution, 1936–56* (London and New York, 1958) is arranged under subject headings, with an author index, but does not include articles in journals.

Otto Neubauer's *Bibliography of cancer produced by pure chemical compounds. A survey of the literature up to and including 1947* (London, 1959) is arranged alphabetically by authors, followed by a subject arrangement in 32 sections, subdivided according to the chemical nature of the carcinogen, under which entries are arranged chronologically.

W. J. Bishop compiled a *Bibliography of international congresses of medical sciences* (Oxford, 1958) which is invaluable in tracing the proceedings of these organizations. Within its limits it supersedes the more general bibliography included in the *Index-Catalogue* in 1938–9 (see above).

The catalogue of *The Evan Bedford Library of Cardiology*, published by the Royal College of Physicians of London in 1977, is systematically arranged, with indexes of names and subjects. It thus constitutes a bibliography of the subject.

Joan Stuart Emmerson has compiled a useful list of 'translations of medical works of classical interest and importance published before 1900' which was published by the University Library, Newcastle upon Tyne as *Translations of medical classics: a list* (1965). This covers a wide field and the entries are arranged alphabetically by authors, with full names and dates, titles of the original works, and short titles of the translations into English.

Bibliographies of special branches of medicine are published by certain libraries, by drug firms and other organizations. The National Library of Medicine at Bethesda has issued many such lists of references, some being distributed gratis, and others being remarkably cheap.

In conclusion, something may be said of national medical bibliography. America and Australia, where a culture has developed comparatively recently, following European colonization, are particularly suitable areas for such study. Francisco Guerra has described some of the early bibliographies containing medical Americana.[32] His survey covers the entire American continent and discusses general bibliographies containing medical material, as well as those specifically concerned with medicine, with biographical information on the compilers.

The medical bibliography of the United States has been covered in detail by Francisco Guerra, Robert B. Austin and Francesco Cordasco. Francisco Guerra's monumental *American medical bibliography, colonial period and revolutionary war 1639–1783* (New York, 1961) attempts to record not only directly medical books and periodicals but also material of medical interest in almanacs, magazines and newspapers. It is a mine of information although, inevitably with such an ambitious and wide-ranging project, there are errors of detail to be found.[33] The basic arrangement is chronological, with indexes of authors and subjects.

Robert B. Austin's *Early American medical imprints. A guide to works printed in the United States, 1668–1820* (Washington, 1961) was commenced in 1946 when the National Library of Medicine was segregating its Americana. The 2106 numbered entries are arranged alphabetically by authors, and a chronological index gives the item numbers published in each year. Locations of copies and some annotations are provided. Austin's work has recently been continued by Francesco Cordasco's *American medical imprints 1820–1910* (Totowa, N.J., 1985). This is arranged by decades, with an author index, and includes locations. Neither Austin nor Cordasco has a subject approach.

Detailed coverage of Australia's much smaller output is provided in Edward Ford's *Bibliography of Australian medicine 1790–1900* (Sydney, 1976). A total of 2567 items are described with full collations, biographical data and locations. The arrangement is alphabetical, with a chronological list of publications to 1850 and a subject index. There is also a small section of addenda not covered by the index.

Medical bibliography is certainly far from dead and the development of new technologies for the storage and retrieval of information offers exciting possibilities for the future.

Notes

1. Malclès, Louise Noëlle, *Les sources du travail bibliographique*, 3 vols in 4 (Geneva, Paris, 1950–8, vol. 3, Sciences exactes et techniques).
2. Sheehy, Eugene P., *Guide to reference books*, 9th edn (Chicago, 1976), *Supplement*, 1980.
3. Walford, A. J., *Walford's guide to reference material*, 4th edn, 3 vols (London, 1980–7, vol. 1, Science and technology).
4. See obituary by V. L. Hahn, *Janus*, 5 (1900) p.324.
5. See obituary in *Mém. Soc. franç. Hist. Méd.*, 1 (1945) pp.80–3.
6. See Guenther, Ilse, 'Johannes Trithemius', in P. G. Bietenholtz (ed.), *Contemporaries of Erasmus* (Toronto, 1985–7) vol. 3, pp.344–5; Arnold, Klaus, *Johannes Trithemius (1462–1516)* (Würzburg, 1971); Steffen, Christel, 'Untersuchung zum "Liber de scriptoribus ecclesiasticis" des Johannes Trithemius', *Arch. Gesch. Buchwesens*, 10 (1969) cols 1247–1354.
7. See Wellisch, Hans, 'Conrad Gessner: a bio-bibliography', *J. Soc. Bibliog. Nat. Hist.*, 7 (1975) pp.151–247 (includes full bibliography of literature about Gesner, with a section on his work as a bibliographer); Fischer, Hans, 'Conrad Gessner (1516–1565) as bibliographer and encyclopedist', *Library*, 5th ser., 21 (1966) pp.269–81; Schazmann, Paul Émile, 'Conrad Gesner et les débuts de la bibliographie universelle', *Libri*, 2 (1952) pp.37–49; see also Thornton–Tully.
8. See Sarton, George, 'Johannes Antonides van der Linden (1609–1664), medical writer and bibliographer', in E. A. Underwood (ed.), *Science, medicine and history. Essays ... in honour of Charles Singer* (London, 1953) vol. 2, pp.3–20.
9. See Friedenwald, Harry, *The Jews and medicine* (Baltimore, 1944) vol. 2, pp.452–3; also Modena, A. and E. Morpurgo, *Medici e chirurghi ebrei dottorati e licenziati nell' Università di Padova dal 1617 al 1816* (Bologna, 1967) pp.19–22.
10. Lynn Thorndike has published an analysis to determine what subjects were being discussed during the period, basing his enquiry on Beughem's bibliography; see 'Another glimpse of medicine in the seventeenth century: Beughem's bibliography', *Ann. Med. Hist.*, N.S.6 (1934) pp.219–23.
11. See Portmann, Marie Louise, 'Jean Jacques Manget (1652–1742), médecin, écrivain et collectionneur genevois', *Gesnerus*, 32 (1975) pp.147–52.
12. See Thornton–Tully; also Hintzsche, Erich, '(Victor) Albrecht von Haller', *DSB*, 6 (1972) pp.61–7. Haller's publications are listed in Lundsgaard-Hansen-von Fischer, Susanna, *Verzeichnis der gedruckten Schriften Albrecht von Hallers* (Berne, 1959).

13. *Bibliotheca botanica, Bibliotheca anatomica* and *Bibliotheca chirurgica* have all been reprinted by Olms, Hildesheim; *Bibliotheca botanica* has also been reprinted by Forni, Bologna, and Johnson, New York.

14. *Bibliotheca medicinae practicae*, which was left unfinished at Haller's death, has only an author index; vols 3 and 4 were published posthumously, edited respectively by F. L. Tribolet and J. D. Brandis.

15. The bulk of the collection is at the Biblioteca Nazionale Braidense, but a number of volumes were distributed to other libraries in Lombardy, including the University of Pavia. Many of the manuscripts were returned to Switzerland in 1928. See Pecorella Vergnano, Letizia, *Il fondo halleriano della Biblioteca Nazionale Braidense di Milano. Vicende storiche e catalogo dei manoscritti* (Milan, 1965). A catalogue of the collection, so far as it could be identified in the Braidense and other libraries in Milan, has been published as Monti, Maria Teresa, *Catalogo del fondo Haller della Biblioteca Nazionale Braidense di Milano*, 9 vols (Milan, 1983–7, Part 1, 3 vols in 4, printed books and manuscripts; Part 2, 5 vols, dissertations).

16. See Thormann, Franz, *Register zur Briefsammlung von Albrecht v. Haller in der Berner Stadtbibliothek. (Beilage zum Bericht der Stadtbibliothek über die Jahre 1933–1935.)* A number of selections from the correspondence have been published. The Albrecht von Haller-Stiftung was established at Berne in 1977 to promote the study of Haller and his work.

17. See Wood, Alexander, *'Thomas Young', natural philosopher 1733–1829. Completed by Frank Oldham. With a memoir of Alexander Wood by Charles E. Raven* (Cambridge, 1954); Morse, Edgar W. 'Thomas Young', *DSB* 14 (1976) pp.562–72; also Thornton–Tully.

18. Cordasco, Francesco, *A bibliography of Robert Watt, M.D., author of the Bibliotheca Britannica. With a facsimile edition of his Catalogue of medical books, and a preliminary essay on his works. A contribution to eighteenth century medical history* (New York, 1950, reprinted Detroit, 1968).

19. See Goodall, Archibald L. and Thomas Gibson, 'Robert Watt: physician and bibliographer', *J. Hist. Med.*, 18 (1963) pp.37–50; Goodall, Archibald L., 'Robert Watt, physician and bibliographer', *Proc. Roy. Soc. Med.*, 54 (1961) pp.809–12; and Finlayson, James, *An account of the life and works of Dr Robert Watt* (London, 1897).

20. See Laage, Rodolphine J. Ch. V. ter, 'Reflections on Johann Ludwig Choulant and his medico-historical bibliographies', in P. Smit and R. J. C. V. ter Laage (eds), *Essays in biohistory ... presented to Frans Verdoorn* (Utrecht, 1970) pp.115–33.

21. See Rolleston, Sir Humphry, 'The two James Atkinsons: James Atkinson of York (1759–1839); James Atkinson the Persian scholar (1780–1852)', *Ann. Med. Hist.*, 3rd ser., 3 (1941) pp.175–82; and Ruhräh, J., 'James Atkinson and his medical bibliography', *Ann. Med. Hist.*, 6 (1924) pp.200–21.

22. See Bishop, P. James, 'The life and writings of Sir John Forbes (1787–1861)', *Tubercle*, 42 (1961) pp.255–61; also in *Brompton Hosp. Rep.*, 30 (1961) pp.255–64; Sakula, Alex, 'Sir John Forbes (1787–1861), a bicentenary review', *J. Roy. Coll. Phycns Lond.*, 21 (1987) pp.77–81.

23. The obituaries of Richard Neale in *Lancet* (1900) II, p.1617, and *Br. Med. J.*, (1900) II, pp.1617–18, testify to the esteem in which his *Digest* was held by his contemporaries.

24. Miles, Wyndham D., *A history of the National Library of Medicine* (Bethesda, Md, 1982) contains a detailed history of the Library, with accounts of the work of Billings, Fletcher and Garrison and also of the *Index-Catalogue* and *Index Medicus*.

25. See *Selected papers of John Shaw Billings. Compiled, with a life of Billings, by Frank Bradway Rogers* ([Chicago], 1965); Garrison, Fielding Hudson, *John Shaw Billings: a memoir* (New York and London, 1915); Lydenberg, Henry Miller, *John Shaw Billings* (Chicago, 1924).

26. See Brodman, Estelle, 'Memoir of Robert Fletcher', *Bull Med. Lib. Assn*, 46 (1961) pp.251–90.

27. See Cope, Sir Zachary, 'Fielding Hudson Garrison', *Ciba Symposium*, 10 (1962) pp.98–103; Kagan, Solomon R., *Life and letters of Fielding H. Garrison* (Boston, 1938).

28. See Blake, John B. (ed.), *Centenary of Index Medicus 1879–1979* (Bethesda, Md, 1980); includes Blake, John B., 'Billings and before: nineteenth-century medical bibliography'

(pp.31–52) and Rogers, Frank B., '"Index Medicus" in the twentieth century' (pp.53–61).

29. See Godbolt, Shane and W. A. Munford, *The incomparable Mac. A biographical study of Sir John Young Walker MacAlister* (London, 1983).
30. See Mayer, Claudius Francis, 'The Index-Catalogue as a tool of research in medicine and history', in E. A. Underwood (ed.), *Science, medicine and history. Essays ... in honour of Charles Singer* (London, 1953) vol. 2, pp.482–93.
31. See Marmoy, C. F. A. and J. L. Thornton, 'The anatomical and physiological bibliography of George E. Day (1815–1872)', *Ann. Sci.*, 28 (1972) pp.285–91.
32. Guerra, Francisco, 'Some bibliographers of early medical Americana', *J. Hist. Med.*, 17 (1962) pp.94–115.
33. See reviews in *Bull. Hist. Med.*, 37 (1963) pp.481–7 (John B. Blake) and *Library*, 5 ser., 18 (1963) pp.310–12 (Richard J. Durling).

9 Private medical libraries

Alain Besson

A scholar's library is to him what a temple is to the worshipper who frequents it. There is the altar sacred to his holiest experiences. There is the font where his new born thought was baptized and had a name in his consciousness. There is the monumental tablet of a dead belief, sacred still in the memory of what it was while yet alive.

(Oliver Wendell Holmes)

It would be difficult to determine when medical men started to make private collections of books, manuscripts and specimens, but it was not until the seventeenth century that extensive museums and libraries became recognized possessions of wealthy intellectuals. Even at that period such collections were esteemed as novelties, rather than as having an educational value, and were frequently formed in a haphazard manner, much as a jackdaw collects attractive objects. In fact John Hunter is recognized as having initiated the scientific collection of specimens for research purposes, and it is only in comparatively recent years that this material has been used extensively for teaching purposes. L. W. G. Malcolm wrote a lengthy article on medical collectors of the seventeenth and eighteenth centuries, confining his study almost entirely to museum specimens, and it is interesting to note that many of the persons considered also possessed extensive collections of books.[1]

The acquisition of a few textbooks does not imply the possession of a library, and we are mainly concerned with medical men who systematically purchased books, not merely as 'furniture' but for educational purposes. In addition to catalogues compiled during the lifetime of collectors, records of book collections abound in various forms. Probate inventories and, later, auction catalogues form monuments to one-time collections of books, and many auction catalogues can be traced by means of the *Index-Catalogue* and the British Library Catalogue. Priced catalogues are of particular interest, and the early lists contain many rare items that are now unobtainable. An even more precious form of catalogue is that of a complete library which has been presented to, or otherwise acquired by, an institution. In many cases, however, one finds it impossible to trace evidence of certain medical men having collected books, because the collections have been dispersed without bearing any signs of ownership. Equally frustrating are the early library catalogues of unknown physicians. The *c.*1627 inventory in British Library Sloane MS 580 (fols 3v–36r) is but one example, and it is interesting that the majority of its 368 entries are classed under 28 medical subject headings – an unusually detailed classification for a private library catalogue of the period.

When no inventory is to be found, and the collection has been dispersed, it is sometimes possible to reconstruct a personal library from signs of ownership such as bookplates and inscriptions in books. The importance of provenance studies is now firmly established and is well illustrated in a paper by Nellie B. Eales[2] on indications of former ownership of early medical and biological books in the library of Francis Joseph Cole (1872–1959), Professor of Zoology in the University of Reading. The first bookplates came from Germany, the earliest known being the Hans Igler Plate, which has been dated as early as 1450. During the sixteenth and seventeenth centuries bookplates became more numerous, and the earliest medical bookplate known is a label recording the gift of books to St John's College, Cambridge, in 1634, by John Collins, Regius Professor of Physic at Cambridge. George C. Peachey mentions bookplates having been used by Thomas Fuller, Alexander Cuninghame, William Oliver, Charles Lucas, Erasmus Darwin and John Coakley Lettsom, among others (see Plates 1–2 for more recent examples).[3]

A brief review of the literature on the libraries of physicians has been written by Philip J. Weimerskirch,[4] who is also engaged in the compilation of a bibliography of catalogues of scientists' libraries. Ellen B. Wells has published a long list of printed sources relating to the personal libraries of scientists, with clear indications of physicians' collections.[5] Medical bibliophiles have been the subject of studies by W. J. Bishop, Robert Herrlinger and Herman H. Henkle, and Thomas E. Keys has written about the development of private medical libraries.[6] More specialized sources of information on physicians' libraries include a study of the book collections of Tudor doctors, by Eric Sangwine;[7] a paper by John L. Thornton on eminent bibliophiles connected with St Bartholomew's Hospital, London, including William Harvey, Francis and Charles Bernard, Edward Browne, John Radcliffe, Richard Mead, Anthony Askew and Sir D'Arcy Power;[8] articles by Thomas E. Keys on American bibliophile physicians and major bookmen – collectors, booksellers and publishers – of recent times;[9] and a series of surveys of German collectors by Bernd Lorenz.[10]

Before printing became firmly established, books were of necessity in manuscript form, and taking into account the rarity of this material, it will be appreciated that the possessor of even a score of manuscripts was considered to own an extensive library. Giovanni de' Dondi (1330–89), one of the most eminent physicians of the fourteenth century and a significant figure among the early Paduan humanists, pos   ed one of the strongest humanist collections of the time, yet a 1389 .   tory of his library lists only 111 titles.[11] Dondi spent much of his career teaching medicine at Padua, where he also lectured on astronomy, philosophy and logic. Later he became physician to the Visconti family of Milan. His book collection reveals his dual interest in astronomy and the humanities.

In the following century, the French physician Jacques de Pars, Physician to Charles VII, built up a valuable collection of scientific and medieval manuscripts, which he bequeathed to the College of Medicine at Paris. Giammetto Ferrari da Grado, professor of medicine at Pavia from 1432 to his death in 1472, possessed 89 manuscripts of which 25 were non-medical, and this is one of the largest fifteenth-century collections of medical books known. The *c*.1454 inventory of the books of Giovanni di Maestro Nicola of Norcia (died 1455) lists 64 items, and there are only 45 entries in the list of the books of the Florentine physician Simone di Cinozzo di Giovanni Cini (died 1481),[12] yet both documents provide useful indications of the interests of ordinary physicians of the time. A collector on a larger scale was Amplonius Ratingk (*c*.1363–1435), founder of the Collegium Amplonianum at Erfurt. Ratingk travelled extensively collecting books, and employed a number of copyists. He was physician to the city of Cologne, and the catalogue of his library compiled by himself lists 640 manuscripts comprising about 2000 separate works. Both the catalogue and the books are still preserved at Erfurt.

One of the finest collections of the fifteenth century was that of the Schedels.[13] Hermann Schedel (1410–85) was city physician of Nuremberg, and most of his eminent library survives intact. It went to his cousin the physician Hartmann Schedel (1440–1514) after Hermann's death, becoming part of an even more significant collection, which is still preserved in Munich. Hartmann Schedel used his library while compiling the Nuremberg Chronicle, published in 1493, and it contains a large proportion of medical books and manuscripts. His friend Hieronymus Muenzer (1438–1508) also built up a remarkable library,[14] but he had wide interests and medical literature is not strongly featured among the volumes in libraries throughout Europe and America identified as formerly belonging to him. Muenzer had studied medicine in Pavia, and practised medicine in Nuremberg, having been born in Feldkirchen. Ulrich Ellenbog (c. 1430–99) also studied medicine at Pavia, and his library was bequeathed to the Benedictine Abbey at Ottobeuern, where one of his sons had become Prior. The collection was dispersed this century, and some of the books can be identified in Cambridge University Library and at Yale.

Nicolaus Pol (*c*.1470–1532) was a physician and theologian who collected a remarkable library, which at his death numbered about 1500 items. These have been scattered among monastic libraries in the Tyrol, but some 40 items have found their way to the Cleveland Medical Library. Max H. Fisch has made an intensive effort to locate Pol's books and manuscripts, and his scholarly study lists 467 items, there being 30 manuscripts, 251 incunabula, and 186 early sixteenth-century publications.[15] Most of these are in the Collegiate Church at San Candido (Innichen) in the Tyrol, but 40 are at Cleveland and 15 at Yale. Pol was physician to the Emperor Maximilian I, and his books in their original bindings are boldly lettered inside the covers 'Nicolaus Pol Doctor 1494'. He was the author of *Libellus de cura morbi Gallici per lignum Guaycanum*, which was written in 1517 but not printed until 1535.

The libraries of sixteenth-century Cambridge medical men have been discussed by W. M. Palmer,[16] and full transcripts of the post-mortem inventories of their collections have been published in an important work by Elisabeth Leedham-Green.[17] John Perman (died 1545), a Cambridge surgeon, owned over 200 books, about half of which were medical. Another Cambridge medical man, Robert Pickering (died 1551), owned nearly 150 volumes, 43 of which were medical. They included books by Hippocrates, Celsus, Rhazes, Mondino, Mesue, Fernel and several of Galen's works. John Hatcher (1512?–87) was Regius Professor of Physic at Cambridge and owned an extensive library of over 500 books, a substantial number of which were medical. Some of Hatcher's books were bequeathed to his son-in-law, Thomas Lorkin (*c.*1529–91). Lorkin, also Regius Professor of Physic at Cambridge, built up a collection as large as Hatcher's, but his was very much a gentleman's, as well as a physician's, library.[18] Smaller libraries owned by Cambridge physicians and surgeons of the time include those of John Thomas (1490?–1545), John Seward (died 1552), Henry Walker (died 1564) and John Caius.[19] Inventories of the libraries of some Oxford medical men of the time, such as Robert Barnes (died 1604), have been published by A. B. Emden.[20] Nicholas Gibbard or Gibbert (died 1593) is also on record as having left a 'row of books' to Magdalen College, Oxford, where he was a Fellow. R. T. Gunther published a list consisting of 33 items, few of which remained in their original bindings.[21]

Dr John Clement (died 1572), elected President of the Royal College of Physicians in 1544, left an inventory of his sizeable collection. Compiled in 1546, this inventory lists 180 titles. It has been published by A. W. Reed.[22]

Alchemy and astrology were wholeheartedly embraced by many six-teenth-century physicians, such as Myles Blomefylde or Blomefield (1525–1603), a physician and alchemist of Bury St Edmunds and Chelmsford.[23] Only 24 books are thought to have been owned by him, yet his collection gives useful evidence for the stock of learning of a physician and alchemist of the period, and for the last days of popular religious drama in East Anglia. A much more prominent figure of the time was Dr John Dee (1527–1608), who acquired a very miscellaneous collection of books and manuscripts. A mathematician and astrologer, Dee was born on 13 July 1527, and the library housed in his residence at Mortlake was assembled over a period of many years. In 1583 he travelled in Bohemia and Poland, being awarded the degree of doctor of medicine by the University of Prague, and he returned to Mortlake in 1589. During his absence abroad, a mob broke into his house, destroying or stealing much of his property, although he was able to recover about three-quarters of the total number of his books. Montague Rhodes James[24] has provided interesting material on Dee's library, printing the three known catalogues of his manuscripts, two of which contain the works he owned about 1556, while the third was compiled on 6 September 1583. List A contains 45 items, list B 32 and list C (1583) about 201, together with several others probably belonging to Dee, but not mentioned in the catalogue. In his *Compendious rehearsal*, Dee informs us that he had nearly 4000 items, a quarter of which were written books, but M. R. James doubts this, as the catalogue lists nothing near this number. The manuscripts are mainly concerned with medieval science, alchemy, astrology, astronomy, physics, geometry, optics and mathematics, and Dee was often forced to sell his books to purchase food. The remains of his library were sold some years after his death, some of the volumes finding their way to Corpus Christi College, Oxford. Certain of Dee's manuscripts were purchased by Sir Simonds D'Ewes, and the identification of some of these, and of others not recorded by James, has been established by Andrew G. Watson.[25] An eagerly awaited new edition of the catalogues of Dee's manuscripts and printed books, with facsimile reproductions, by R. J. Roberts and A. G. Watson, is in press. Dr John Dee had earned fame as an alchemist, and on 10 March 1575, Queen Elizabeth paid him a visit, but as his wife had been buried on that day, the Queen did not enter his house. It is ironical that he died in poverty in December 1608, at Mortlake, where he had retired four years previously.

The author of *The anatomy of melancholy*, Robert Burton (1577–1640) was not medically qualified, yet his book is of great interest in the history of psychiatry. Burton bequeathed his books to the Bodleian Library at Oxford, with the stipulation that duplicates should go to Christ Church. There were only 86 medical volumes in his donation; an edition of his library was recently published by Nicolas K. Kiessling.[26]

William Harvey (1578–1657) built a library and museum for the College of Physicians, and he bequeathed his books and papers to the College. Many of these were unfortunately destroyed during the Civil War, and most of the remainder perished during the Great Fire of 1666. Apart from the only copy in the College of Physicians which can be certainly identified as Harvey's, books known to have belonged to him are in the British Library, Uppsala University, the Pybus Library in Newcastle, and the University of Indiana. Harvey's friend, George Ent, presented his library to the Royal Society, a catalogue of the collection being printed in 1680. Ent was born on 6 November 1604, and was educated at Rotterdam and at Sidney Sussex College, Cambridge. He then studied medicine at Padua for five years, graduating MD there in 1636 and receiving the same degree at Oxford two years later. He held many appointments at the College of Physicians, becoming a Fellow in 1639. Ent was knighted by Charles II in the Harveian Museum, following a lecture attended by the King. The writings of Ent include *Apologia pro circulatione sanguinis, contra Æmilium Parisanum* (London, 1641) in which he defended Harvey's doctrines, while his *Opera omnia medico-physica* was printed in Leyden in 1687. Ent was an original Fellow of the Royal Society and died on 13 October 1689. He is probably best known for obtaining Harvey's manuscript of *De generatione* from the author, and supervising its publication. One might consider the possibility of his having had other Harvey manuscripts at the same time, and the chance that they may have survived unrecognized in some repository, perhaps even as part of Ent's library.

Jean Riolan the Younger (1580–1657) owned a good collection of sixteenth- and seventeenth-century books, which was sold in 1655 by John Martin and James Allestrye in St Paul's Churchyard. There is a copy of the sale catalogue in the Bodleian Library at Oxford and another, incomplete, in the British Library. Interestingly there also exists a partial catalogue of Riolan's library, but published in Paris in 1654. John L. Thornton has suggested that the printing of the 1654 Paris catalogue was interrupted when it was decided to sell the collection in London instead of in Paris, and that copies of the incomplete Paris catalogue may have been acquired for insertion in the London version.[27]

The seventeenth century saw an increase in the number of private collectors, but as a rule little is known of their libraries. Most medical men possessed books, but at their deaths these were usually dispersed with their belongings. Gui Patin (1601 72) was a great book-lover and collected a library of 10 000 volumes. He had studied medicine at Paris, became professor at the Collège Royal de France, and was founder of the École de Médecine. Patin contributed little or nothing to the literature of his profession, but he was a brilliant Latin orator, and his letters were published in numerous editions.

Gabriel Naudé (1600–53) began to study medicine at Paris, and at the age of 20 became librarian to President Henri de Mesmes. In 1626 he went to Padua to continue his medical studies, but returned to librarianship in charge of the libraries of Cardinals Bagni, Barberini and Richelieu successively. His greatest work, however, was in connection with the library of Mazarin, for whom he travelled in Flanders, Italy, Germany and England, collecting 45 000 books and manuscripts in eight years. In 1651 Mazarin's property was confiscated, the library being put up for sale. Naudé pleaded in vain against this, and paid 3000 livres for the medical books. He then went to take charge of Queen Christiana's collection at Stockholm but, upon Mazarin's return to power, the latter purchased Naudé's private collection of 8000 volumes. Naudé died on 29 July 1653, on his way to assist Mazarin to begin afresh in amassing his collection, which in 1660 contained 45 000 volumes. It was bequeathed to the Collège Mazarin, and later taken over by the State. Naudé wrote at least 86 books and pamphlets, his book on librarianship being translated into English by John Evelyn as *Instructions concerning erecting a library* (1661). His other books were mainly concerned with history, religion and politics.

Vopiscus Fortunatus Plempius (1601–71) was professor of medicine at Louvain University and collected together a large working collection of books which was sold in Louvain in 1672. The sale catalogue lists 1074 titles, of which there are 768 medical works.

In 1710 a catalogue of the libraries of Sir Thomas Browne (1605–82) and his son was printed, and a facsimile reproduction with an introduction and notes was recently published.[28] The greater part of the books probably belonged to Sir Thomas. There were 2377 lots, these being classified by subject, and subdivided by size. Very few of these books can be identified today. The catalogue itself is very rare,[29] there being only three copies known, one in the British Library, another being among the books bequeathed to McGill University by Sir William Osler,[30] and the third, formerly in the possession of John F. Fulton, is at Yale. Edward Browne (1642–1708) was the eldest son of Sir Thomas and was born at Norwich. After studying medicine at Cambridge, he went to London in 1664, and thence travelled on the continent, visiting Paris and keeping a journal recording the occasion, of which the original manuscript is in the British Library.[31] Elected FRS in 1667, Edward Browne resumed his travels in 1668, visiting Holland, Belgium, Germany, Austria, Hungary, etc., and keeping an account of everything he saw. He wrote *A brief account of some travels in Hungaria, Servia, Austria, Styria, Corinthia, Carniola and Frivli* (London, 1673) and *An account of several travels through a great part of Germany in four journeys* (London, 1677) and the items of particular bibliographical and medical interest in these have been abstracted.[32] Edward became a Fellow (1675) and then President (1704–8) of the College of Physicians, and was Physician to St Bartholomew's Hospital, London from 1682 to 1708.

Thomas Bartholin (1616–80) is considered in this chapter because his library was destroyed by fire, and he vividly described the occurrence, but he also came from a distinguished family. His father, Caspar Bartholin (1585–1629) was born at Malmo, and became professor of medicine at Copenhagen. He was the author of *Anatomicae institutiones* (Wittenberg, 1611), which went into several editions and translations. The younger Caspar Bartholin (1655–1738) is the one associated with Bartholin's duct and Bartholin's glands.[33] Thomas Bartholin was born in Copenhagen, graduated in medicine at Basle, and travelled extensively before returning to Copenhagen to occupy the chair of mathematics, and then of anatomy. He founded the *Acta Medica et Philosophica Hafniensia* (1672–80) and lived at Hagestedgaard, where he collected together a library. While he was attending the funeral of his former teacher, Poul Moth, his house was destroyed, together with his books and manuscripts. Thomas Bartholin described the grievous tragedy, mentioning other collections destroyed by fire, and providing details of 27 manuscripts, several of which he was preparing for publication, and listing 129 printed items. This was first published in Copenhagen in 1670, and has been translated into English by Charles D. O'Malley, together with Bartholin's travelogue.[34]

Nathan Paget (1615–79) was a native of Cheshire, graduated MA at Edinburgh in 1638, and in the following year obtained a medical degree from Leyden with his thesis *Disputatio de peste*. He became a Fellow of the College of Physicians where he acted as Censor and delivered the Harveian Oration (1664), and was physician to the Tower of London. Paget amassed a very considerable library, less than half of which was medical, but it contained the writings of Hippocrates, Galen, Averroes, Harvey, and a collection of plague tracts. The collection was auctioned by William Cooper, and the catalogue was printed as *Bibliotheca medica viri clarissimi Nathanis Paget, M.D. Cui adjiciuntur quamplurimi alii libri theologici philosophici, &c. Quorum omnium auctio habebitur Londini, ad insigne Pelicani in vico vulgo dicto Little-Britain 24 die Octobris. Per Gulielmum Cooper bibliopalam* (1681). This contains 2178 lots, among which there are numerous valuable items of both medical and literary interest. Paget was associated with Francis Glisson in his report on rickets, and was also a friend of Milton.[35]

Sir Charles Scarburgh (1616–94) is chiefly remembered for his influence on mathematics and on the Royal Society, but he was also a physician to Charles II, to James II and to William III. He collected a magnificent library of 2500 books on a wide range of subjects, including more than 400 medical works, but the collection was dispersed after Scarburgh's death.[36]

Francis Bernard (1627–98) lived in Little Britain and was physician to St Bartholomew's Hospital, London. He collected together an extensive library and is reputed to have read every volume. He was famed as a scholar, and as the introductory to the auction catalogue has it,

> We must confess that being a Person who Collected his Books for Use, and not for Ostentation or Ornament, he seem'd no more solicitous about their Dress than his own; and therefore you'll find that a gilt Back or a large Margin was very seldom any inducement to him to buy.

His library was the most extensive to be sold by auction during the seventeenth century, and the catalogue lists many interesting items.[37] It contains 14 747 works and 39 bundles, there being 869 books on Theology, 277 on Law, 938 on Mathematics, 4484 on Medicine, 4950 on Philology, etc., 1163 on Italian, Spanish and French, and 2066 devoted to Divinity, History, etc. Bernard was acquainted with French, Italian and Spanish, in addition to Greek and Latin, and was deeply interested in astrology, poetry and theology. The Catalogue contains several Caxtons, which fetched small sums at the auction, but as there are many printer's errors and obscure items, it is difficult to assess the true value of certain entries. Elton states that there were 13 Caxtons which were sold for less than two guineas; De Ricci gives 16 Caxtons which sold at from four to five shillings each; Lawler lists 22 Caxtons with their prices; Fletcher says 'about a dozen Caxtons' and Sir Norman Moore gives the number as sixteen. Lawler gives the total for the sale as about £5000, while Fletcher states £1920. There is a priced catalogue in the British Library, should one be disposed to total up almost 15 000 lots! Francis Bernard, who was physician to James I, was very popular as a physician, and remained in London during the Plague. As the contents of his library indicate, he was a true scholar, and it is a pity that the auction catalogue is the sole monument to a library that might have graced one of the contemporary institutions.

Charles Bernard (1650–1711), traditionally said to be a much younger brother of Francis, was also a great book-collector. He was Serjeant-Surgeon to Queen Anne, and Surgeon to St Bartholomew's Hospital. Unlike Francis, Charles Bernard collected as a bibliophile, but his library also ended at an auction sale, with a catalogue as a monument. The books are grouped under theology, medicine, history, classical, miscellaneous, mathematics, French, Italian, English, prints and manuscripts, each subject being subdivided by size. There are 1234 numbered octavo items, 953 quartos and 686 folios.[38]

John Locke (1632–1704) the physician and eminent philosopher, possessed a library of some 3675 volumes, about 10 per cent of which were devoted to medicine. Locke catalogued his books in duplicate, arranged and press-marked them to his own method, and although they were dispersed, many of them, together with a large collection of his papers and manuscript material are now in the Bodleian Library at Oxford.[39]

William Croone (Croune) (1633–84) bequeathed his medical books to the College of Physicians, London and had intended to found two lectureships, one at the College, and the other at the Royal Society, but he failed to make provision for these in his will. This was remedied by his widow, afterwards Lady Sadleir, in her will dated 25 September 1701. Croone was professor of rhetoric at Gresham College, and in 1662 was created doctor of physic by royal mandate at Cambridge. In 1670 he was appointed by the Barber Surgeons' Company as anatomical lecturer on muscles, which post he held until his death. Croone had a large practice in the City of London and was elected a Fellow of the College of Physicians in 1675, to become a Censor four years later. He made many reports to the Royal Society, of which he was at one time secretary, and was keenly interested in physics, meteorology, embryology and blood transfusion. Croone was the author of *De ratione motus musculorum* (London, 1664), first published anonymously, which was afterwards issued in association with Willis's *Cerebri anatome* from Amsterdam in 1664, 1667 and 1676.[40]

Robert Hooke (1635–1702) was a passionate book-collector, and his numerous purchases at auction or from booksellers were meticulously recorded in his diary. His library of over 3000 volumes, the large majority of which were scientific and medical, was sold by auction on 29 April 1703, and a facsimile reproduction of the sales catalogue was recently published.[41]

Although considered to be a quack, similar in character to Nicholas Culpeper, William Salmon (1644–1713) was no ordinary charlatan, but a cultivated man with an enquiring mind. He collected books for use in his writings, not for their rarity, so that he acquired a working library. This was sold on 16 November 1713, and a catalogue was printed as *Bibliotheca Salmoneana, pars prima. Or, a catalogue of part of the library of the learned William Salmon, M.D., deceas'd ... Which will begin to be sold by auction at St. Paul's Coffee-House ... by Thomas Ballard.* This lists 3571 books, 656 of which are medical. Salmon was the author of several books, tracts and translations, some of which went into numerous editions. They include *Synopsis medicinae* (1671); *Select physical and chirurgical observations* (1687); *Practical physick* (1692); *The family dictionary* (1693), a work on domestic medicine; *Ars chirurgica* (1699); and *Ars anatomica* (1714). Salmon also possessed two microscopes, a collection of mathematical instruments, and also paintings and curiosities.[42]

Founder of the Royal College of Physicians of Edinburgh, Sir Robert Sibbald (1641–1722) collected books all his life, and gave some of them to the College about 1682. His library was auctioned on 5 February 1723, when the major portion was purchased by the Faculty of Advocates, but he had previously sold some 900 volumes in 1707.

Edward Tyson (1650–1708) had intended to bequeath his books to the College of Physicians, but he eventually left them to his nephew, Richard Tyson. Some manuscripts and printed books have found a place in the College, but he also presented a collection to the Bodleian Library at Oxford.

The numerous book-collectors of the eighteenth century have retreated into insignificance before the figures of men such as Sloane, Mead, Askew and William Hunter. These men dominated the scene throughout the greater part of the century, amassing wonderful libraries, those of William Hunter and Sir Hans Sloane avoiding the auctioneer's hammer.

Sir Hans Sloane was born at Killyleagh, County Down, on 16 April 1660, and in his nineteenth year came to London to study medicine. He became friendly with Robert Boyle, and was a frequent visitor to the Physic Garden at Chelsea, which belonged to the Society of Apothecaries. Sloane was deeply interested in botany, which brought him into contact with John Ray. In 1683 Sloane went to Paris to continue his medical studies, before proceeding to the University of Orange to take an MD. On his return to London he went to live with Thomas Sydenham, assisting him in his practice, and Sloane soon became a Fellow of the College of Physicians and of the Royal Society. In 1687 he went to Jamaica as a physician to the Duke of Albemarle, where Sloane spent 15 months studying the natural history of the island, but, on the death of the Duke, Sloane returned to England and published *A voyage to the islands of Madeira, Barbados, Nieves, St Christopher and Jamaica, with the natural history of the last of those islands*, two volumes (1707–25). This had been preceded by his *Catalogus plantarum quae in insula Jamaica sponte proveniunt* (London, 1696), in the preparation of which he had been assisted by Ray. He became physician to Christ's Hospital, and took a house in Great Russell Street. He also married Elizabeth Langley, an heiress with a large fortune, and was created baronet upon the accession of George I. Sir Hans Sloane held many prominent positions, including those of President of the College of Physicians (1719–35), and of the Royal Society, in which he succeeded Newton. Sloane collected antiquities, coins, medals, crystals, seals and gems, as well as botanical and zoological specimens. He had over 40 000 printed books, in addition to prints, pictures and drawings, while his manuscripts numbered 3700, and included autograph writings by Francis Glisson, Sir Thomas and Edward Browne, and William Harvey. He bought entire collections, including that of Francis Bernard, as indicated by marked sales catalogues in the British Library. Sloane had spent fantastic sums on the acquisition of this material, but on his death, in 1753, instructed his executors to offer the entire collection to the nation for the sum of £20 000. A lottery was held in order to raise this sum, and in 1754 Montague House was purchased to house it, with several other collections, which formed the nucleus of the library of the British Museum and hence of the British Library.[43] Soon after its entry into the British Museum, the collection ceased to exist as a separate entity, but Sloane's own catalogues of his books and manuscripts make it possible to identify many of them. In 1978 it was discovered that Sloane had catalogued his own medical books in his interleaved copy of G. A. Mercklin's eight-volume edition of J. A. van der Linden's *Lindenius renovatus ... de scriptis medicis libri duo* (Nuremberg, 1686).[44]

John Woodward (1665–1728) is best known for his important contributions to geological, mineralogical and botanical science. Besides being a naturalist, however, he was also a medical practitioner and a professor of medicine, and he was appointed Professor of Physick at Gresham College, in the City of London, in 1692. His only medical work, *The state of physick: and of diseases ... more particularly of the small-pox* (1718) resulted in controversy with the eminent physicians John Friend and Richard Mead, which culminated in a duel between Woodward and Mead in 1719. Woodward amassed a vast collection of fossils, minerals and objects of antiquarian interest, as well as a large working library of books rich in early scientific and natural history, as well as works of classical authors. This library was put up for sale on 11 November 1728, and the auction catalogue included 4755 lots of books.[45]

Further afield, one of the cornerstones of the Russian Academy of Sciences Library was formed in the early eighteenth century by the acquisition of the personal libraries of two Scottish physicians. The dramatis personae of this unusual tale were Drs Robert Erskine (1677–1718) and Archibald Pitcairne (1652–1713). Pitcairne had learnt medicine mainly at Paris in the 1670s, became a medical professor at Leyden University for a brief period of time (1691–2), and lived in Edinburgh thereafter, practising medicine. He was a founder member of the Royal College of Physicians of Edinburgh. His friend and colleague Robert Erskine graduated MD at Utrecht in 1790, was elected a Fellow of the Royal Society of London three years later, and in 1704 left for Russia. There Erskine pursued a brilliant career, becoming chief physician to the Tsar and occupying the highest position in the Russian medical hierarchy. He was also appointed, by Peter the Great, Chief librarian of the collections which were to become the Museum and Library of the Russian Academy of Sciences, and he negotiated the purchase of Pitcairne's personal library. This was a large working library for an up-and-coming physician, and most of the volumes are medical, although there is also a large number of books on mathematics, as well as books on other subjects. Erskine's own collection was much larger, comprising over 1000 medical items and as many books on other subjects. It too eventually passed to the future library of the Russian Academy of Sciences. Transcripts of the catalogues of both collections were recently presented to the National Library of Scotland.[46]

In France, Camille Falconet (1671–1762) collected books for 70 years, a catalogue being printed in 1763.[47] This represents a very important eighteenth-century scientific library, and Falconet was also interested in philosophy, mathematics, history and literature. He possessed 50 000 volumes at one time, bequeathing to the Bibliothèque Royale the books it did not already house.

Richard Mead was born in Stepney on 11 August 1673, and at the age of 16 went to the Universities of Utrecht and Leyden. In 1693 he made a tour of Italy and took a degree at Padua. On his return to England, Mead set up in practice in Stepney. He was elected a Fellow of the Royal Society in 1703, and became Physician to St Thomas's Hospital the same year. He received an MD from Oxford in 1707, and in 1716 was elected a Fellow of the College of Physicians. Richard Mead built up a most lucrative practice, and spent his money freely. He acquired many of his books, all of which were beautifully bound, in Rome. He also collected statues, coins, gems, prints, drawings and manuscripts, and possessed at one time over 10 000 printed books. The entire collection was sold after Mead's death, the books realizing over £5500 in a sale which began on 18 November 1754 and lasted 28 days. The catalogue lists 6827 items, and bears the title

Bibliotheca Meadiana; sive catalogus librorum Richardi Mead, M.D. qui prostabunt venales sub hasta, apud Samuelem Baker: in vico dicto York Street, Covent Garden, Londini, die lunae 18vo Novembris, MDCCLIV. Iterumque die lunae 7mo Aprilis, MDCCLV, [London, 1754]. The anatomical section has been the subject of an interesting study by K. F. Russell, who provided information on Mead's books and papers, and lists the books in his collection devoted to human anatomy.[48] Mead's pictures, coins, medals and so on were sold separately for £10 550 18s 0d, the Greek manuscripts being sold to Anthony Askew.

Mead financed the publication of several prominent works, including De Thou's *Historia sui temporis*, seven volumes (London, 1733) and was always ready to support scholarship. He was himself the author of *A mechanical account of poisons in several essays* (London, 1702); *De imperio solis ac lunae in corpora humana et morbis inde oriundis* (London, 1704); *A short discourse concerning pestilential contagion and the methods to be used to prevent it* (London, 1720), of which seven editions appeared in one year, followed by an eighth in 1722, and a ninth in 1744; *De variolis et morbillis liber. Huic accessit Rhazis de iidem morbis commentarius* (London, 1747), of which an English translation appeared the same year; and *Monita et praecepta medica* (London, 1751). Mead also edited William Cowper's *Myotomia reformata* in 1724, while the best collected editions of Mead's medical works are those published in London, 1762, and in three volumes at Edinburgh in 1765. Dr Johnson once said: 'Dr. Mead lived more in the broad sunshine of life than almost any man,' and when he died on 16 February 1754, he had certainly lived a very comfortable existence throughout his career.

Little is known about Dr Edward Worth (1678–1733), but his personal library of over 4500 books, which he left to Dr Steevens' Hospital in Dublin at his death, is of interest because it represents an almost unique eighteenth-century Irish doctor's library exactly as he collected it.[49] The collection is notable for its beautiful bindings, and it includes 21 incunabula. The only catalogues of the collection in existence today are in manuscript form. Another example of a general practitioner's library of the eighteenth century is preserved at Preston, and is known as Dr Shepherd's Library. Richard Shepherd was born at Sizergh, Kendal, in 1694, and after qualifying practised in Preston, where he twice became Mayor. He died on 4 December 1761 and bequeathed his library to the Corporation of Preston in trust for the benefit of the inhabitants. His will, dated 18 June 1759, left the interest on £200 for the librarian, £40 for shelving and fittings, and after the death of his brothers the interest on the estate (about £1000) was to be spent on books, none of which was to be borrowed. The collection was rehoused on several occasions and is now in Harris Public Library. It contains nearly 10 000 volumes, more than double the original bequest, including many early books from notable printers, and houses writings by Paré, Felix Platter and Harvey, together with numerous non-medical items. A printed catalogue was issued in 1870.[50]

William Smellie (1697–1763) made a will dated 5 December 1759 and added four codicils, leaving his books to the grammar school at Lanark, in his time one of the most famous in Scotland. In 1769, following the death of his widow, the trustees commenced carrying out the provisions of the will. The books were transferred to the new school opened in 1820, and remained locked up until 1884. They became dilapidated and their removal to Glasgow was suggested, but not carried out. In 1934 the books were temporarily removed to the Lindsay Institute, Lanark and remained there until 1941. Miles H. Phillips was responsible for the renovation of the library between 1936 and 1939, and it now consists of 407 volumes, excluding Glaister's *William Smellie* (1893) and Miles Phillips' gift of Peter Camper's *Itinera in Angliam* (1748–85). The collection has been described by Haldane P. Tait and Archibald T. Wallace.[51]

The mantle of Mead fell upon Anthony Askew (1722–74), who succeeded him in the book world. Askew had already purchased Mead's Greek manuscripts, and at the sale of the latter's library acquired many other items. Askew had spent two years visiting Italy, Hungary, Athens and Constantinople, during which time he laid the foundations of his library. Rare manuscripts and choice editions in exquisite bindings abounded in his library and Askew has been credited with having made bibliomania fashionable. He possessed a 1632 folio of Shakespeare containing writing of Charles I, a volume that had belonged to General Monk, Cicero's *Of old age and friendship*, printed by Caxton in 1481, and a special collection of the editions of Æschylus. Askew owned the first printed editions of many of the classics, but his library contained very few medical items, not more than 150 volumes. After the death of Askew, the library was sold at an auction which lasted from 13 February to 7 March 1775. The catalogue of the collection was sold at one shilling and sixpence, with a few copies on royal paper at four shillings, and is arranged in four alphabetical sequences, English, French, Italian and Spanish, and Greek and Latin. Entitled *Bibliotheca Askeviana, sive catalogus librorum rarissimorum Antonii Askew M.D. Quorum auctio sint apud S. Baker & G. Leigh, in vico dicto York Street, Covent Garden, Londini, die lunae 13 Februarii MDCCLXXV, in undeviginti sequentes dies*, it 'contains the best, rarest and most valuable collection of Greek and Latin books that were ever sold in England', there being 3750 numbered lots. Books were purchased by the French bookseller De Bure (£500), George III (£300), the British Museum (£300), Dr Hunter, physician to His Majesty (£500), the Bodleian Library, and Cambridge University, in addition to many private buyers. A manuscript note in the sale catalogue states that the 'whole library amounted to £4,090 10s.'[52] A copy of the sale catalogue in the University of London Library has the prices of all the items inserted in ink, showing that Huxham's *Essay on fevers* (1750) fetched 1s 6d; Mead, *On the plague* (1744) large paper, 1s; and Mead, *On poisons* (1745) large paper, 3s 6d. The same copy has 'Dr. Hunter' written against several items. Anthony Askew was better known as a scholar than as a physician, and contributed nothing to the literature of medicine. He consorted with the eminent scholars of his day, and his house was frequented by most foreigners visiting this country. Askew succeeded to the gold-headed cane, which had previously been carried by Radcliffe and Mead, and was to be passed on to William Pitcairn and Matthew Baillie, before it was presented to the College of Physicians by the widow of the last named.

The library of John Douglas (died 1758) was catalogued with the title *Bibliotheca anatomica-medico-chirurgica, a catalogue of the genuine library of Mr. John Douglas ... Which will be sold by auction ... on Thursday and Friday the 3rd and 4th of this instant August 1758*, and the 373 items in the catalogue were grouped by size. The priced catalogue in the Royal College of Surgeons Library indicates that the books fetched very little, some commanding as little as sixpence. The larger collection belonging to Robert Nesbit (died 1761) was sold, there being 1632 numbered entries in the catalogue entitled *A catalogue of the large and valuable library of Robert Nesbit, M.D. ... Which ... will be sold by auction, by Samuel Paterson, ... on Wednesday the 29th of July, 1761, and the eight following evenings*. This catalogue included the copyright, with plates and original drawings, for Nesbit's *Human osteogony*, first printed in 1736. According to the catalogue at the Royal College of Surgeons, this item went for £2 6s to 'Dr. Brisbane'.

William Hunter (1718–83) has been overshadowed as a scientist by his brother John, but as a scholar the latter was unable to approach him. John Hunter's museum was acquired by the Royal College of Surgeons, while William Hunter's collection went to Glasgow, and it has been suggested that, had these locations been reversed, William Hunter would occupy the position to which John has been raised largely as the result of his collection being in London, and in the hands of the influential Royal College of Surgeons. Whatever the verdict, William Hunter as a scholar and collector of coins, manuscripts and rare books was supreme, and the fact that he bequeathed this material to the University of Glasgow, to found the Hunterian Museum, ensures his continued remembrance even should his anatomical and gynaecological work be forgotten. In 1807 Hunter's collections were transferred from Great Windmill Street, London, to Glasgow, for at his death, on 30 March 1783, he had left his Museum to trustees for 30 years, after which it was to go to Glasgow, together with £8000 towards its upkeep. A special building was erected in the University grounds, and the collection was eventually removed to the new Museum. The collection includes over 600 volumes of manuscripts, some of which were formerly in monastic libraries. A catalogue of this material was printed in 1908,[53] and contains invaluable information on the material listed, including bibliographical notes on authors, details of owners, illuminations and inscriptions. The printed books had to wait even longer before they were listed in printed form, but the resultant catalogue[54] indicates a remarkably rich collection. There are over 10 000 volumes, of which 534 are incunabula, 2300 were printed in the sixteenth century, and about half the collection is medical.[55]

The library of John Coakley Lettsom (1744–1815) has been described by the biographer James Johnston Abraham[56] as a room 39 feet long, 20 feet broad, and divided into 16 compartments, over each of which was the bust of a distinguished personage connected with the subject shelved therein. Lettsom divided his books as follows:

1.	Tracts and pamphlets	Bust of John Wesley
2.	Miscellanies	„ „ Dryden
3.	Reviews	„ „ Addison
4.	Surgery and Chemistry	„ „ Pott
5.	Antiquities and Medals	„ „ Stukeley
6.	Prints and Maps	„ „ Hogarth
7.	Arts and Science	„ „ Newton
8.	Divinity and Law	„ „ Locke
9.	Dictionaries and Classics	„ „ Bacon
10.	History and Biography	„ „ Voltaire
11.	Poetry	„ „ Milton
12.	Voyages and Geography	„ „ Raleigh
13.	Natural History	„ „ Boyle and Franklin
14.	Medicine	„ „ Sydenham
15.	Medicine and Botany	„ „ Fothergill
16.	Hortus Siccus and Manuscripts	„ „ Mead

The library contained about 6000 volumes, and was open to the medical profession on Saturdays. Lettsom also possessed an extensive museum and elaborate gardens. After his death his collections were sold by auction, a large number of the books going to the British Museum.

The collection of John Crawford (1746–1813) forms part of the Medical Library of the University of Maryland, his books having been sold in 1813. The number of these in the sale is unknown, as is also the amount raised. Crawford was born in Northern Ireland, and educated at Trinity College, Dublin, obtaining an MD from St Andrews in 1791. He had previously served as physician to a hospital in Barbados, returning to England in 1782, but in 1790 we find him as a Surgeon-Major to the Colony in Demerar. In 1794 he was again in England, and went to Leyden, where he graduated MD. Crawford went to Baltimore in 1796, and became friendly with Benjamin Rush. He introduced vaccination into Baltimore in 1800, and held several public appointments. Crawford's library was very extensive for the period and he freely loaned his books, presenting a number of them to the Library Company of Baltimore. He died on 9 May 1813, and selected titles from the Crawford Collection now at Maryland indicate the extent of his collection.[57]

The three Alexander Monros held the chair of anatomy at Edinburgh from 1720–1846, and during that period the medical school achieved recognition as the foremost teaching establishment for medical students in the British Isles. The Royal College of Physicians, Edinburgh, houses 12 volumes of lectures given by Monro primus (1697–1767), and the introductory surgical lecture devoted to history has been published by R. E. Wright-St Clair, who has also written an interesting biographical study of the Monros.[58] The University of Otago Medical School Library, Dunedin, New Zealand contains a 46-page manuscript life of Alexander primus copied down by himself, and also houses about 300 volumes of manuscripts and printed material appertaining to the Monros. These were taken to New Zealand by David Monro, son of Alexander Monro tertius (1773–1859), who became Speaker in the House of Representatives there. His son-in-law, Sir James Hector acquired this material, and after his death Lady Hector deposited them in the Parliamentary Library at Wellington. Later Sir James's son, Charles Monro Hector arranged for their transfer to the University of Otago Medical School.[59] The term 'foramen of Monro' has been named after Alexander Monro secundus (1733–1817), but it has been suggested that there is no justification for the retention of this eponym.[60]

The library of Johann Friedrich Blumenbach (1752–1840) of Göttingen is mainly intact, and in 1955 was in the possession of Robert M. Herbst at Michigan State College.[61] He received this through his grandfather, Ernst Friedrich Gustav Herbst (1803–93), who had been a pupil of Blumenbach, and was his colleague at Göttingen. Herbst received the library in 1840, some of the items having been collected as early as 1767. It consists of several hundred volumes, uncatalogued, and many of the books contain annotations by Blumenbach, particularly the copies of his own publications.

Caleb Hillier Parry (1755–1822) bequeathed his collection of 555 medical books to Bath Hospital, and they were later presented to the city, where they are housed in the Victoria Art Gallery and Municipal Library. They include writings by Guy de Chauliac, Andrew Boorde, Hippocrates, Thomas Vicary, Peter Lowe, William Clowes and many other outstanding authors. The collection has been described by Reginald W. M. Wright.[62]

By his will, Matthew Baillie (1761–1823) left 'all his Medical, Chemical and Anatomical books' to the library of the Royal College of

Physicians. Baillie's collection was essentially a modern medical library –
48 per cent of the 900 printed books it consisted of were published in the
first 23 years of the nineteenth century – and as such it was truly
remarkable. A manuscript catalogue of the collection was made in 1823,
and is preserved in the library of the Royal College of Physicians.[63]
Another important gift to the Royal College of Physicians was that of
about 1000 books belonging to one of its Fellows, Arthur Farre (1811–
87). More than half of these books were not previously in the College
Library, and there is a manuscript catalogue of the collection in Farre's
own hand, entitled 'Catalogue of about 1,000 books presented to the
College Library by Arthur Farre, M.D., F.R.C.P., 1877'. Farre was for
most of his life professor of obstetric medicine at King's College, London, and lectured for two years on comparative anatomy at St Bartholomew's Hospital.

Georg Franz Burkhard Kloss (1787–1854) owned a remarkable
library of manuscripts and early printed books, his collection having
been made for a revision of Panzer's *Annalen*. Osler stated that the
'Kloss library was the most important collection of early printed books
ever made by a medical man'. Kloss was born at Frankfort-on-Main on
31 July 1787, and graduated at Göttingen in 1809. He became head of
the Rochus-Hospital for smallpox, scabies and syphilis, and began collecting books in 1816, concentrating on incunabula and early printed
books. His library was sold at Sotheby's, the catalogue being entitled
*Catalogue of the library of Dr. Kloss ... including many original and
unpublished manuscripts, and printed books with MS annotations, by
Philip Melanchthon ... Which will be sold by auction by Sotheby & Son, ...
May 7th, and nineteen following days ...* (1835). Despite this title only
three items were associated with Melanchthon, and Kloss protested to
Sotheby. This catalogue lists 4623 items, mostly printed before 1537,
with a few manuscripts. The books contain his book label, and many of
them are now in the Bodleian, the British Library, the Waller Library,
and the Osler and Cushing Collections.[64]

The name of Peter Mark Roget (1779–1869) is of course associated
with his *Thesaurus of English words and phrases*, but he was also a
physician, having gained his MD at Edinburgh in 1798. Roget enjoyed a
lifelong interest in both science and language. He was physician to the
Royal Infirmary at Manchester from 1805 to 1808; physician and lecturer in London, 1808–48; an officer, and in 1829–30, President of the
Medical and Chirurgical Society; and held many other offices in the
medical and scientific world. Among the 4089 volumes listed in sale
catalogues of his library, dispersed after his death, there were no less
than 1732 works on medicine and science.[65]

Thomas Radford (1793–1881), a native of Manchester, became an
obstetrician, after studying at Guy's and St Thomas's Hospitals. In 1818

he returned to his native city as surgeon to the Manchester and Salford Lying-in Hospital, and Radford also became prominently connected with St Mary's Hospital. In the year 1853 he presented his valuable library to the institution, later giving money towards its upkeep, and in 1877 a catalogue of the Radford Library was compiled by C. J. Cullingworth. Thomas Radford was a founder of the school of medicine at Manchester, and among other qualifications was a Member (1817) and Fellow (1852) of the Royal College of Physicians, and was awarded an MD from Heidelberg in 1839.

Harvard Medical School Library houses the Warren Library which was accumulated by five generations of physicians, the 2000 books and pamphlets having been bequeathed to the School by John Warren (1874–1928). The first John Warren (1753–1815) had been professor of anatomy and surgery to the Medical School, and his son John Collins Warren (1778–1856) added to the collection of books. Jonathan Mason Warren (1811–67), J. Collins Warren (1842–1927) and John Warren also augmented the library to form a remarkable collection of valuable material. This is described in an article by Thomas E. Keys on twentieth-century American medical bibliophiles.[66]

Samuel D. Gross (1805–84) bequeathed his library to the Philadelphia Academy of Surgery which he had founded, and it was deposited in the College of Physicians of Philadelphia in 1885, most of it being now housed in the Gross Room. There are about 2400 volumes representing the best medical literature of the period, mainly European, with a valuable historical collection chiefly devoted to surgery.

Oliver Wendell Holmes (1809–94) gave his working collection of medical books to the Boston Medical Library in 1889, and the 908 volumes include many association copies from his friends.[67]

Another personal collection added to Boston Medical Library was that of William Read (1820–89). Read founded the Obstetrical Society of Boston in 1861, and three years later was elected physician to the City. He was the author of *Placenta praevia: its history and treatment* (Philadelphia, 1861), in which he abstracted reports of over 1000 cases. His library reflected his particular interest in obstetrics, and Henry R. Viets has provided information on Read's book-collecting activities.[68]

Samuel Lewis (1813–90) was born in Barbados, qualified at Edinburgh, and practised in Philadelphia, where he became an ardent supporter of the College of Physicians. In 1864 he gave that library over 2400 volumes, and continued with his friends to add to the collection until it grew to 13 899 volumes. Some of the rarer items are housed in the Samuel Lewis Room, but the collection of early printed items, fine bindings and classic writings in all branches of medicine, together with complete sets of numerous medical journals, must represent the greatest contribution to the growth of any medical library of the nineteenth century.

A native of Manchester, William Worrall Mayo (1819–1911) emigrated to the United States in 1845, and finally settled in Rochester, Minnesota. With his two sons, W. J. Mayo and C. H. Mayo, he founded the Mayo Clinic, and his books are preserved in the library there. Thomas E. Keys has provided a short-title check-list of the medical items, and has also contributed a paper on Charles N. Hewitt (1836–1910), whose medical books, with those of Mayo, form the nucleus of the Mayo Clinic Library.[69]

Jean Martin Charcot (1825–93) owned an extensive collection of books which, after his death, was presented by his son J. B. Charcot to the Salpêtrière, Paris. It is arranged with the library furniture as left by Charcot, and contains his notes for his lectures, classic medical texts, books on the history of medicine, numerous reprints and periodicals, together with some general literature.[70]

David Lloyd Roberts (1835–1920) was a student at Manchester Medical School, at the Royal Infirmary, and also studied in London for a short period. In 1858 he became surgeon to St Mary's Hospital for Women and Children, and was elected FRCP in 1878. Lloyd Roberts published an edition of Sir Thomas Browne's *Religio Medici* in 1898, and later presented his fine Browne collection to the John Rylands Library, Manchester, while his medical books are now at Manchester University and the Royal College of Physicians, London. Lloyd Roberts also collected glass, water-colours, mezzotints and other material, and gave generously of his collections to the Welsh University and its colleges, particularly that at Bangor. His *Student's guide to midwifery* (1876) went into three editions, and he endowed five lectureships, three in London and two in Manchester.

Joseph Frank Payne (1840–1910), the physician and historian, amassed a considerable collection of books which was sold in the year following his death. Osler intended to secure the entire library on behalf of the Johns Hopkins Medical School, but it was sold before he realized the fact. It went to the Wellcome Historical Medical Library, London, and the remaining books, chiefly herbals and Miltoniana, were sold separately. Osler managed to secure certain of these items. The catalogues were issued by Sotheby & Co. as *Catalogue of the ... collection of early medical works ... also ... books & tracts on pestilence, the property of John [sic] Frank Payne ... which will be sold by auction ... July, 1911,* and *Catalogue of the remaining portion of the library of ... Joseph Frank Payne ... which will be sold by auction ... Jan., 1912.*

Joseph Lister (1827–1912), the celebrated scientist and surgeon, assembled a great library which fell into oblivion in the course of time, and was painstakingly traced a few years ago by Owen and Sarah

Wangensteen, who have published a detailed analysis of its contents.[71] It appears that Lister had assembled 3000 books, largely scientific and medical.

Sir John Williams (1840–1926) was the principal founder and first president of the National Library of Wales, Aberystwyth. He had been educated at University College Hospital, London, and served for a time as house surgeon at the Children's Hospital, Great Ormond Street, before he became a general practitioner at Swansea. He returned to University College in 1872, finally to become Professor of Obstetrical Medicine in 1887. Williams was a sound teacher and a successful consultant, but retired in 1893, and returned to Wales ten years later. He collected Welsh books and manuscripts and presented about 1200 manuscripts to the National Library of Wales. Williams also donated over 25 000 printed books, in addition to prints, drawings and portraits. Throughout his life he donated books to the Library, and at his death bequeathed £43 000 to the institution.[72]

Probably the best-known medico-historical collection of this century is that made by Sir William Osler (1849–1919). This is owing not only to the fact that his library is maintained intact at McGill University, but also that the magnificent catalogue of the library has attracted the attention of every medical bibliographer, librarian and historian. Furthermore Osler inspired others to collect, by his writings and his example, and stimulated an interest in medical history by presenting valuable books to numerous medical libraries. Surely no other medical man has had so many clubs, societies and medals named in his honour, or has had such influence upon historians and bibliographers, many of whom only know him through his writings and by means of biographical studies of various aspects of his career. William Osler was born on 12 July 1849, at Bond Head, Ontario, and in 1868 went to Toronto Medical School before proceeding to McGill, where he graduated in 1872. Following postgraduate work in Great Britain and on the continent he returned to McGill as lecturer on the institutes of medicine (1874–6). He became pathologist to Montreal General Hospital in 1876, and physician two years later. In 1878 Osler returned to London, qualified MRCP, and became a frequent visitor to Britain. He was appointed professor of clinical medicine at Pennsylvania and, in 1889, physician-in-chief to Johns Hopkins Hospital. Finally he was appointed Regius Professor of Medicine at Oxford in August 1904.

Osler wrote numerous articles and books,[73] among the more important being *The principles and practice of medicine* (1892) which went into 16 editions, and numerous reprintings and translations; *The evolution of medicine* (1921), being the Silliman Lectures delivered at Yale in 1913; *The cerebral palsies of children* (1889); and *On chorea and choreiform affections* (1894). William Osler began collecting books at an early age, his first acquisition being the Globe Shakespeare, and his second an 1862 Boston edition of Sir Thomas Browne's *Religio medici*. When at Montreal he collected Canadian medical and scientific journals, which he presented to the Medical Library on leaving in 1884. He purchased books on all his travels, presenting numerous items to other libraries.[74] The Academy of Medicine at Toronto, the College of Physicians of Philadelphia, and the Medical and Chirurgical Faculty of the State of Maryland were among the many institutions benefiting by his interest.[75] Osler gave his collection on the heart and lungs to the Johns Hopkins Hospital, and the Johns Hopkins University received the books dealing with English literature, in memory of Osler's son, Revere. At his death on 29 December 1919, Sir William Osler bequeathed his books to McGill University, but, as the catalogue of these was incomplete, he provided for it to be finished before the books were sent to Canada. The Osler Library at McGill was officially opened on 29 May 1929.

Probably the most readable catalogue ever compiled is that of the Osler library, which was edited after Osler's death by W. W. Francis, R. H. Hill and Archibald Malloch, and published as *Bibliotheca Osleriana; a catalogue of books illustrating the history of medicine and science collected, arranged and annotated by Sir William Osler, and bequeathed to McGill University* (Oxford, 1929). This lists about 7600 bound volumes and the collection is particularly rich in first editions and the early classics of medicine, but the arrangement of the catalogue needs a more adequate index than is provided. Bibliotheca Prima represents Osler's idea of fundamental contributions to medicine and science, their chronological position being determined by the original date of an author's chief contribution to the subject, followed by later works, commentaries, biographies and bibliographies. Bibliotheca Litteraria consists of literary works by physicians, medical works by laymen, medical poems, and any literature featuring medicine. Bibliotheca Historica includes historical works, and literature on medical institutions. Further sections are devoted to Bibliotheca Biographica and Bibliotheca Bibliographica, the latter being particularly rich and important. The Incunabula section contains 106 items, with cross-references to 30 others included in Bibliotheca Prima. This is followed by Manuscripts and Addenda. Osler's book-collecting career is outlined in an incomplete preliminary essay on 'The collecting of a library', while Appendix I describes 'A record day at Sotheby's' and Appendix II records books bequeathed to libraries other than McGill.

Sir William Osler held several prominent positions, was president of the Classical Association and of the Bibliographical Society, curator of the Bodleian Library, and a delegate of the Clarendon Press. He was prominent in establishing the Medical Library Association in the United States, and in forming the Medical Library Association of Great Britain, although the latter did not function for long. His love of books was infectious, and he stimulated his colleagues by his example. It is impossible to record his numerous activities, but Harvey Cushing's brilliant biography provides full information, while publications on various aspects of Osler's career abound.[76] In accordance with his wishes the ashes of Sir William Osler repose at McGill University among the books he had collected with such loving care.[77]

William Willoughby Francis (1878–1959) was librarian of the Osler Library from 1929 until his death, and had previously been engaged in editing the catalogue. His mother was first cousin to Osler, and W. W. Francis was the fount of information relating to Osler and his library. Francis was born in Montreal, qualified at Johns Hopkins University, and studied on the continent before setting up in practice in Montreal. He was demonstrator in pathology at McGill, but gave up practice owing to ill-health. He will be remembered as custodian of the Osler Library, and as the friend of everybody interested in that collection.[78]

A specialized collection on hypnotism, consisting of approximately 900 books, was assembled by the prominent Berlin neurologist Albert Moll (1862–1939). Moll studied at Breslau, Freiburg, Jena and Berlin, where he received his MD in 1885. He started to practise neurology in Berlin in 1887 and became one of the pioneers in hypnotic psychotherapy in Germany, while developing a strong interest in the field of sexology. His book collection, which ranges from a copy of Johannes Argenterius's *De sommo et vigilia libri duo* (Florence, 1556) to Moll's own works, was sold before his death and is now based at Vanderbilt Medical Center Library.[79]

When Sir D'Arcy Power died on 18 May 1941, at the age of 85, he had already made arrangements for the sale of his library, as his house in London was rendered unsafe for its storage. He had entered St Bartholomew's Hospital as a student in 1878, and was intimately connected with the institution at his death. He wrote *A short history of St Bartholomew's Hospital, 1123–1923* (1923) and contributed many other books and articles on the history of medicine. He was a successful surgeon, but it is as a historian of medicine that he will be remembered. Sir D'Arcy edited *Memorials of the craft of surgery* (1886), wrote an outstanding biography of William Harvey (1897) in the Masters of Medicine Series, edited John Arderne's *Treatise of fistula in ano* (1910) and *De arte phisicali et de chirurgia* (1922), while his lectures delivered at the Institute of the History of Medicine of the Johns Hopkins University were published as *The foundations of medical history* (1931). In that year the Osler Club issued a volume of his *Selected writings*, consisting mainly of historical material published between 1877 and 1930, together with a bibliography of his writings numbering 609 items. His final volume appeared in 1939 as *A mirror for surgeons: selected readings in surgery*. Sir D'Arcy was one of the editors responsible for revising Plarr's *Lives of the Fellows of the Royal College of Surgeons of England*, published in 1930 in two volumes, and he also wrote 200 lives for the *Dictionary of National Biography*. The sale catalogue of his books was issued by Sotheby & Co. as *Catalogue of valuable books, manuscripts, autograph letters, etc., comprising the property of Sir D'Arcy Power* (1941) and lists many early texts on medicine, surgery and medical bibliography, but a large number of the books were eventually exposed for sale on a stall in Farringdon Road Market, London. The Royal College of Surgeons of England houses Sir D'Arcy's typescripts and manuscript material.[80]

Henry Barton Jacobs (1859–1939) presented over 5000 books, 2500 prints, 1000 medals and 400 letters to the Johns Hopkins University, where they are shelved in the Henry Barton Jacobs Room of the Welch Medical Library. The collection is particularly rich in items relating to tuberculosis and bacteriology.

LeRoy Crummer (1872–1934) was educated at Omaha High School, the University of Michigan, and obtained his MD from the North-western University Medical School, Chicago, in 1896. He visited European clinics on several occasions, and later made frequent trips to Europe on book-hunting expeditions. In 1919 Crummer was appointed professor of medicine at Nebraska University, which position he held for six years. He was eminently successful as a physician, and equally so as a bibliophile. Accompanied by his wife, he made periodic tours of the main book centres of Europe, amassing a remarkable library of which two catalogues were prepared. The first, *A list of old medical books, books on the history of medicine, and medical bibliography, and a list of medical portraits in the possession of LeRoy Crummer, Omaha, Nebraska. Together with some bibliographical notes, catalogued and compiled by Myrtle A. Crummer, Mimeographed edition* (1925) contains a foreword by LeRoy Crummer describing some of his experiences in book-collecting, and lists 936 books and 257 portraits. The second, *A catalogue: manuscripts and medical books printed before 1640, in the library of LeRoy Crummer, Omaha, Nebraska. Privately printed at Omaha, April 15, 1927*, lists 422 items arranged alphabetically under manuscripts, incunabula and books printed during the sixteenth century. Crummer made some very interesting discoveries during his book-collecting tours, including an unpublished manuscript of William Heberden. His books were donated to the University of Michigan, the University of Nebraska and to numerous other libraries in the United States and in England.[81]

One of the finest medical collections of this century was that made by Axel Erik Waller (1875–1955) who was born at Önum, Västergötland on 29 November 1875, and died at Linköping, Sweden on 28 January 1955. Waller collected widely and wisely, and acquired 150 incunabula, over 20 000 books, almost the same number of letters, together with manuscripts and autographs. In 1950 Waller presented his magnificent collection to the Royal University of Uppsala where it is preserved at the Bibliotheca Walleriana. Hans Sallander prepared the catalogue, which was published as *Bibliotheca Walleriana. The books illustrating the history of medicine and science collected by Dr. Erik Waller and bequeathed to the Library of the Royal University of Uppsala*, two volumes (Stockholm, 1955). This reveals something of the richness of the collection, many of the items being very rare, with some unique copies of printed books not recorded elsewhere. The writings of Vesalius, Paré and Harvey are particularly well represented, and there are numerous association items.[82]

The American College of Surgeons houses 2600 volumes donated by Hiram Winnett Orr (1877–1956)[83] over many years, and he also made gifts to several other libraries. Born at West Newton, Pennsylvania, Winnett Orr graduated at the University of Michigan School of Medicine in 1899, and was associated with the Nebraska Orthopedic Hospital for 50 years. He was an advocate of the closed plaster method of treating open fractures, and wrote *Osteomyelitis, compound fractures and other infected wounds* (St Louis, 1929); *Wounds and fractures* (Springfield, Ill., 1941); and *On the contributions of Hugh Owen Thomas, Sir Robert Jones and John Ridlon, M.D. to modern orthopedic surgery* (Springfield, Ill., 1949). Winnett Orr formed an Anne of Brittany Collection of almost one thousand items, which is now in the Love Memorial Library of the University of Nebraska. His medical books are listed in *A catalogue of the H. Winnett Orr Historical Collection and other rare books in the Library of the American College of Surgeons* (Chicago, 1960), edited by L. Marguerite Prime and Kathleen Worst. It is arranged alphabetically by authors within two main sections, and includes illuminating annotations and a number of interesting illustrations.

Logan Clendening (1884–1945) of Kansas City collected together a remarkable medico-historical library which he used in connection with his lectures as professor of medical history at the University of Kansas. In 1936 his wife gave him a fine collection on anaesthesia containing many rare items, which now number over a thousand. At his death about 3500 volumes, with a handsome endowment, went to the University, and the History of Medicine Collection contained 8000 items in 1960.[84] Some of the rarest items, association and presentation copies have been described by Richard J. Durling and Phoebe Peck.[85] Logan Clendening was the author of *The human body* (1927) and *Source book of medical history* (1942). The Clendening Medical Library, University of Kansas Medical Center was named after him in September 1957.

It would be difficult to assess the influence of Sir William Osler on medical book-collecting and bibliography. It was Osler who inspired Harvey (Williams) Cushing (1869–1939) to form his own notable collection, which eventually went to Yale with the libraries of Arnold C. Klebs and John F. Fulton.[86] Osler collected widely over the fields of medicine and science, but Harvey Cushing carefully selected his literature so that it did not overlap with the collections being formed by Klebs and Fulton, having persuaded them eventually to donate their books to Yale. Cushing wrote *The life of Sir William Osler*, two volumes (1925) an ideal biography unequalled in its class. He was eminently successful as a brain surgeon, and his writings indicate the wide range of his knowledge.[87] A catalogue of his collection was published as *The Harvey Cushing collection of books and manuscripts* (New York, 1943). This consists of a short-title catalogue of all the printed books and manuscripts bequeathed to Yale University by Cushing, but not his personal correspondence. When Harvey Cushing retired from the Peter Bent Brigham Hospital in 1932, he disposed of his files of surgical periodicals, and also modern text-books on medicine, surgery and neurology, so that this material is lacking.

The Catalogue is divided into I. Manuscripts, II. Orientalia, III. Incunabula, IV. General works, and V. Cushing memorabilia. The third section contains 168 numbered entries. In these divisions entries are arranged alphabetically by authors, dates of birth and death being provided, except for classical writers. Each entry bears a letter governing its arrangement in the alphabetical sequence, followed by a figure, thus facilitating cross-reference. Titles are arranged alphabetically under authors' names, but many reprints of articles in journals are indistinguishable from books. The Catalogue indicates a remarkably rich collection and is well worthy of a place beside the *Bibliotheca Osleriana*, although it lacks the informative annotations provided in the latter. John Fulton wrote the standard biography of Cushing, another was contributed by Elizabeth H. Thomson, and there have been numerous shorter studies of various aspects of his career.[88] A diary of his experiences during the war was published as *From a surgeon's journal, 1915–18* (London, 1936).

Following a visit to the Osler Library Cushing decided to leave his books to Yale, and he approached Klebs and Fulton to do likewise. Fulton became the leader in the project and the correspondence between these three concerning the plan was printed for John Fulton's sixtieth birthday.[89]

Arnold Carl Klebs (1870–1943) was born at Berne on 17 March 1870, the son of Edwin Klebs, and graduated from Zurich and Basle. In 1896 he went to the United States of America, practising in Chicago until 1909, when he returned to Europe and devoted the remainder of his life to medical history. He paid several lengthy visits to the States, and was the friend of Osler, Cushing, Welch, Sudhoff and later of John Fulton. Klebs was particularly interested in incunabula, and although only 20 years were represented in his collection, the incipit and colophon of every fifteenth-century book on medicine and science in the libraries of Europe and the United States which he visited are represented in facsimile, with notes on the contents of each by Klebs. His short-title list was first published in 1938,[90] but he did not complete his detailed bibliography, the notes for which are at Yale. The collection of about 22 000 items is particularly rich in herbals, plague tracts, smallpox tracts, and the history of tuberculosis.

John Farquhar Fulton (1899–1960) was born at St Paul, Minnesota, and became an eminent physiologist, bibliophile and medical historian. Graduating at Harvard Medical School, he became a Rhodes Scholar at Oxford, and in 1929 was appointed professor of physiology at Yale. He held that chair until his appointment in 1951 to the newly created position of Sterling Professor of the History of Medicine. Fulton presented his library to Yale in 1940. It is particularly rich in the literature of physiology and neurology, seventeenth- and eighteenth-century writers being particularly well represented. His historical writings include *Selected readings in the history of physiology* (Springfield, Ill., 1930); *Physiology* in the Clio Medica series (New York, 1931); *Harvey Cushing: a biography* (Springfield, Ill., 1946); and *The great medical bibliographers: a study in humanism* (Philadelphia, 1951). A bibliography of his writings by Madeline E. Stanton and Elizabeth Thomson lists 520 numbered items, and his historical and bibliographical work has been admirably surveyed by William LeFanu.[91] It is not only by his writings that John Fulton is remembered, but through his friendship with everyone interested in medical history and bibliography. An article on the subject by a student, a librarian or a fellow historian attracted a lengthy letter of encouragement from John Fulton, and he was always ready with advice and assistance. His death was deeply regretted throughout the world by his numerous friends, but he left his writings, his library at Yale, and his example as a worthy successor of Osler.[92]

The Duke School of Medicine Library, Durham, North Carolina houses the Josiah C. Trent Collection, built up by Josiah C. Trent (1914–48) during a very brief lifetime. He wrote 43 papers on the history of medicine, and assisted by Henry Schuman built up a collection of 4000 books and 2000 autographs and manuscripts within ten years. These include editions of Vesalius, Paré, Beaumont, Culpeper, Harvey, Holmes and a manuscript diary of Edward Jenner covering the years 1810 to 1812. The collection has been described by Henry Schuman and Martha Alexander.[93]

Despite the fact that so many historical medical books are being added to the larger medical libraries, either by individual purchase or by donations as collections, there are still a large number of private collectors. Probably few are in the Osler, Cushing or Fulton category, but book-collecting remains a fascinating hobby for medical men. It is more necessary to specialize if one would acquire a large collection, and the library built up by Davis Evan Bedford (1898–1978) is an outstanding example. Comprising over 1000 rare books on the heart and circulation, it is a unique collection in the field of cardiology. Dr. Bedford a founder member of the British Cardiac Society and an international authority on cardiology in his lifetime, ensured that his collection would not be dispersed by presenting it to the Royal College of Physicians of London. The published catalogue of the collection is enriched by annotated entries by Bedford and remains an invaluable bibliographical tool.[94] Bedford also contributed an interesting description of the landmarks in the history of cardiology, as represented in his collection.[95] Another specialized collection, that of early obstetrical books acquired by Alfred M. Hellman (1880–1955) was described by the owner in a well-illustrated catalogue published in 1952, and his daughter described later additions in 1958.[96] This contained numerous editions of Rösslin's *Rosengarten*, together with many other outstanding books in the history of obstetrics.

In 1965, the University of Newcastle acquired as a donation the remarkable collection of medical books, portraits and engravings collected during more than 40 years by Frederick Charles Pybus (1883–1975), formerly professor of surgery in the University of Durham. Mainly devoted to the history of surgery, anatomy and medical illustration, the library consists of about 2500 volumes, 2000 engravings, and 50 portraits and busts. The collection is separately housed in the Pybus Room, and contains numerous valuable manuscripts, incunabula, medical classics and first editions. A catalogue was compiled by Joan S. Emmerson.[97]

One other private collection must be mentioned as an eclectic accumulation of items acquired mainly as the working collection of an outstanding bibliographer, Sir Geoffrey Langdon Keynes (1887–1982). Furthermore it is notable on account of the fact that the published catalogue of part of the library is happily not a sale catalogue, but was compiled by the collector, and published during his lifetime. Entitled *Bibliotheca bibliographici. A catalogue of the library formed by Geoffrey Keynes* (London, 1964), it lists some 4300 items in a handsomely produced volume, beautifully illustrated, printed and bound. It contains 'Religio bibliographici', Sir Geoffrey's presidential address to the Bibliographical Society, and includes remarkable author collections devoted to Jane Austen, William Blake, Timothy Bright, Rupert Brooke, Sir Thomas Browne, John Donne, John Evelyn, Edward Gibbon, William Harvey, Robert Hooke and many others of whose writings Sir Geoffrey compiled bibliographies, or edited literary studies. It represents but a section of an admirably selected working library, one notable for the fine condition of its contents. The seventeenth-century items might have come straight from the press, and the entire collection is now housed in the library of Cambridge University.[98]

Notes

1. Malcolm, L. W. G., 'The medical man as a collector in the seventeenth and eighteenth centuries', *Med. Life*, 42 (1935) pp. 566–620.

2. Eales, Nellie B., 'On the provenance of some early medical and biological books', *J. Hist. Med.*, 24 (1969) pp.183–92. The catalogue of the library, compiled by Dr Eales, was published as *The Cole Library of early medicine and zoology*, 2 vols (Reading, 1969 and 1975).

3. Peachey, George C., 'Book-plates of medical men', *Proc. Roy. Soc. Med.*, 23 (1930) pp.493–5. See also Fishbein, Morris, 'Medical bookplates', *Bull. Soc. Med. Hist. Chicago*, 11 (1922) pp.303–20; Radbill, Samuel X., *Bibliography of medical ex libris literature* (Los Angeles, 1951); Radbill, Samuel X., 'The symbolism of the staff of Aesculapius as illustrated by medical bookplates', *J. Albert Einstein Med. Center*, 10 (1962) pp.108–19; Cosgrave, MacDowel, 'Book-plates of Irish medical men', *Dublin J. Med. Sci.*, 146 (1918) pp.274–83; Curtin, Roland G., 'The book-plates of physicians, with remarks on the physician's leisure-hour "hobbies"', *Internat. Clin.*, 20th ser., 11 (1910) pp.222–53; Poole, M. E. M., 'Bookplates', *Bull. Med. Lib. Assn*, 24 (1936) pp.145–8.

4. Weimerskirch, Philip J., 'Libraries of physicians: a review of the literature', *AB Bookman's Weekly* (20 April 1987) pp.1705–7.

5. Wells, Ellen B., 'Scientists' libraries: a handlist of printed sources', *Ann. Sci.*, 40 (1983) pp.317–89.

6. Bishop, W. J., 'Some medical bibliophiles and their libraries', *J. Hist. Med.*, 3 (1948) pp.229–62; Herrlinger, Robert, 'Über die Bibliophilie der Ärzte', *Librarium*, 2, (1959) pp.68–74; Henkle, Herman H., 'The physician as book collector. Notes on famous libraries', *J. Internat. Coll. Surg.*, 34 (1960) pp.107–17; Keys, Thomas E., *Applied medical library practice* (Springfield, Ill., 1958) chapter 12, pp.148–89; the following books also contain material on some of the medical collectors mentioned in this chapter: Elton, Charles Isaac and Mary Augusta Elton, *The great book collectors*, 1893; Fletcher, William Younger, *English book collectors*, 1902; Lawler, John, *Book auctions in England in the seventeenth century (1676–1700)* (1906) and De Ricci, Seymour, *English collectors of books and manuscripts (1530–1930), and their marks of ownership* (1930).

7. Sangwine, Eric, 'The private libraries of Tudor doctors', *J. Hist. Med.*, 33 (1978) pp.167–84.

8. Thornton, John L., 'St Bartholomew's Hospital, London, and its connection with eminent book collectors', *J. Hist Med.*, 6 (1951) pp.481–90.

9. Keys, Thomas E., 'Bookmen in biology and medicine I have known', *J. Hist. Med.*, 30 (1975) pp.326–48; Keys, Thomas E., 'Libraries of some twentieth-century American bibliophilic physicians', *Lib. Quart.*, 24 (1954) pp.21–34.

10. Lorenz, Bernd, 'Notizen zu Privatbibliotheken deutscher Ärzte des 15.–17. Jahrhunderts', *Sudhoffs Archiv*, 67 (1983) pp.190–8; and his 'Notizen zu Privatbibliotheken deutscher Ärzte des 18.–19. Jahrhunderts', ibid., 69 (1985) pp.50–61.

11. Rose, Paul Lawrence, *The Italian renaissance of mathematics* (Geneva, 1975) pp.7–8.

12. Cordella, Romano, 'La biblioteca di un medico Nursino del sec. XV', *Spoletium*, 25 (1983) pp.89–90; Caroti, Stefano, 'La biblioteca di un medico fiorentino: Simone di Cinozzo di Giovanni Cini', *La Bibliofilia*, 80 (1978) pp.123–38.

13. Stauber, Richard, *Die Schedelsche Bibliothek* (Freiburg im Breisgau, 1908) (reprinted Nieuwkoop, 1969).

14. Goldschmidt, Ernst Philip, 'Hieronymus Muenzer and other fifteenth-century bibliophiles', *Bull. N.Y. Acad. Med.*, 14 (1938) pp.496–508.

15. Fisch, Max H., *Nicolaus Pol Doctor 1494. With a critical text of his guiac tract, edited with a translation by Dorothy M. Schullian* (New York, 1947).

16. Palmer, W. M., 'Cambridgeshire doctors in the olden times', *Proc. Cambridge Antiquarian Soc.*, 15 (1911) pp.200–79.

17. Leedham-Green, E. S., *Books in Cambridge inventories: book-lists from Vice-Chancellor's Court probate inventories in the Tudor and Stuart periods*, 2 vols (Cambridge, 1986).
18. Sayle, C., 'The library of Thomas Lorkin', *Ann. Med. Hist.*, 3 (1921) pp.310–23.
19. Grierson, P. 'John Caius' library', In *Biographical history of Gonville and Caius College*, 7 (1978) pp.509–25.
20. Emden, Alfred B., *A biographical register of the University of Oxford, A.D. 1501 to 1540* (Oxford, 1974).
21. Gunther, R. T., 'The row of books of Nicholas Gibbard of Oxford', *Ann. Med. Hist.*, 3 (1921) pp.324–6.
22. Reed, A. W., 'John Clement and his books', *The Library*, 4th ser., 6 (1926) pp.329–39.
23. Baker, Donald C., and John L. Murphy, 'The books of Myles Blomefylde', *The Library*, 5th ser., 31 (1976) pp.377–85; Baker, Donald C. and John L. Murphy, 'Myles Blomefylde, Elizabethan physician, alchemist and book collector', *Bodleian Lib. Rec.*, 11 (1982) pp.35–46.
24. James, Montague Rhodes, 'Lists of manuscripts formerly owned by Dr. John Dee. With preface and identifications', *Trans. Bib. Soc., Supplement* (1921).
25. Watson, A. G., 'An identification of some manuscripts owned by Dr. John Dee and Sir Simonds D'Ewes', *The Library*, 5th ser., 13 (1958) pp.194–8.
26. Kiessling, Nicolas K., *The library of Robert Burton* (Oxford, 1988) (Oxford Bibliographical Society Publications, N.S.2). Burton's donations had been previously listed by S. Gibson and F.R.D. Needham. 'Lists of Burton's library', *Oxford Bibliog. Soc. Proc. Papers*, 1, 1922–6, pp.222–46.)
27. Thornton, John L., 'The two catalogues of Jean Riolan's library, Paris, 1654 and London, 1655', *J. Hist. Med.*, 23 (1968) pp.287–9.
28. Finch, S. Jeremiah, *A catalogue of the libraries of Sir Thomas Browne and Dr Edward Browne, his son: a facsimile reproduction with an introduction, notes and index* (Leiden, 1986).
29. See Keynes, Sir Geoffrey, *A bibliography of Sir Thomas Browne, Kt., M.D.* (Cambridge, 1924) pp.182–3.
30. Bib. Osler., 4532.
31. British Library, Sloane MS. 1906. See 'Journal of a visit to Paris in the year 1664, By Edward Browne. Edited by Geoffrey Keynes', *St Bart's Hosp. Rep.*, 56, i (1923) pp.1–34.
32. See Thornton, John L., 'Dr. Edward Browne (1642–1708) as a bibliophile', *Lib. World*, 54 (1952–3) pp.69–73; and Thornton, John L., 'Medicine as recorded in Edward Browne's travels in Europe', *St Bart's Hosp. J.*, 58 (1954) pp.207–10.
33. See Rhodes, Philip, 'The Bartholin family', *J. Obstet. Gynaec. Brit. Emp.*, 64 (1957) pp.741–3.
34. *Thomas Bartholin. On the burning of his library and On medical travel, translated by Charles D. O'Malley* (Lawrence, Kansas, 1961).
35. See Hanford, James H., 'Dr. Paget's library', *Bull. Med. Lib. Assn*, 33 (1945) pp.90–9.
36. *Bibliotheca Scarburghiana; or, a catalogue of the incomparable library of Sir C. Scarburgh* (London, [1695]). See also Newman, Charles, 'Sir Charles Scarburgh', *Br. Med. J.*, 3 (1975) pp.429–30.
37. *A catalogue of the library of the late learned Dr. Francis Bernard ... Which will be sold by auction at the doctor's late dwelling house in Little Britain; the sale to begin on Tuesday, Oct. 4, 1698.*
38. *Bibliotheca Bernardiana: or, a catalogue of the library of the late Charles Bernard, Esq., Serjeant Surgeon to Her Majesty ... With several MSS. ancient and modern which will begin to be sold by auction on Thursday, the 22nd of March, 1710/11. At the Black-Boy Coffee-House in Ave-Mary-Lane, near Ludgate-Street ...* The copy in the Library of the Royal College of Surgeons is priced in ink throughout.
39. See Harrison, John R. and Peter Laslett, *The library of John Locke*, 2nd edn (London, 1971); Harrison, John R., and Peter Laslett, 'The library of John Locke', *Times Literary Supplement*, 27 December 1957; and Laslett, Peter, 'John Locke's books and papers for his own university', *Times Literary Supplement*, 11 March 1960.

40. See Payne, Leonard M., Leonard G. Wilson and Sir Harold Hartley, 'William Croone, F.R.S. (1633–1684)', *Notes Roy. Soc. Lond.*, 15 (1960) pp.211–19.
41. *Bibliotheca Hookiana; sive catalogus diversorum librorum ... quos Doct. R. Hooke ... sibi congessit*, Londin., 1703. Facsimile reproduction in Feisenberger, H. A., *Sale catalogues of libraries of eminent persons. Volume II: scientists* (London, 1975).
42. See Bishop, W. J., 'Le Dr. William Salmon (1644–1713) et sa bibliothèque', *Librarium*, 1 (1959) pp.79–83.
43. See Brooks, E. St John, *Sir Hans Sloane. The great collector and his circle*, (1954); Francis, Sir Frank, 'Sir Hans Sloane, 1660–1753, as a collector', *Lib. Assn Rec.*, 63 (1961) pp.1–5; Thomson, W. W. D., 'Some aspects of the life and times of Sir Hans Sloane', *Ulster Med. J.*, 7 (1938) pp.1–17; and Chance, Burton, 'Sketches of the life and interests of Sir Hans Sloane, naturalist, physician, collector and benefactor', *Ann. Med. Hist.*, N.S.10 (1938) pp.390–404.
44. Nickson, M. A. E., 'Hans Sloane, book collector and cataloguer, 1682–1698', *Br. Lib. J.*, 14 (1988) pp.52–89.
45. Eyles, V. A., 'John Woodward, F.R.S., F.R.C.P., M.D. (1665–1728): a bio-bibliographical account of his life and work', *J. Soc. Bibl. Nat. Hist.*, 5 (1971) pp.399–427.
46. Appleby, John H., and Andrew Cunningham, 'Robert Erskine and Archibald Pitcairne – two Scottish physicians' outstanding libraries', *The Bibliotheck*, 11 (1982) pp.3–16.
47. *Catalogue de la bibliothèque de feu M. Falconet, doyen des médecins*, 2 vols (Paris, 1763).
48. Russell, K. F., 'The anatomical library of Dr. Richard Mead (1673–1754)', *J. Hist. Med.*, 2 (1947) pp.97–109; see also Dobson, Austin, 'The Bibliotheca Meadiana', *Bibliographica*, 1 (1895) pp.404–18; Carter, H. S., 'Richard Mead', *Scot. Med. J.*, 3 (1958) pp.320–4.
49. McCarthy, Muriel, 'Dr Edward Worth's library in Dr Steevens' Hospital', *J. Irish Coll. Phys. Surg.*, 6 (1977) pp.141–5.
50. See Watson, Richard F., 'Angelica to candy. Dr. Shepherd's Library, Preston', *North Western Newsletter*, No. 60 (May, 1960) pp.1–3.
51. Tait, Haldane P., and Archibald T. Wallace, 'Dr. William Smellie and his library at Lanark, Scotland', *Bull. Hist. Med.*, 26 (1952) pp.403–21 (Appendix, Medical books in William Smellie Library, Lanark, pp.415–21).
52. See Barnes, Henry, 'On Anthony Askew, M.D., F.R.S., and his library', *Proc. Roy. Soc. Med.*, 9 (1916) Section of Hist. of Med., pp.23–7.
53. *A catalogue of the manuscripts in the Library of the Hunterian Museum in the University of Glasgow. Planned and begun by the late John Young; continued and completed under the direction of the Young Memorial Committee by P. Henderson Aitken* (Glasgow, 1908).
54. Ferguson, Mungo, *The printed books in the Hunterian Museum in the University of Glasgow ... With a topographical index by David Baird Smith* (Glasgow, 1930).
55. Illingworth, Sir Charles, 'Some old books and ancient coins from the Hunter collection', *Med. Hist.*, 17 (1973) pp.168–73; MacKenna, R. Ogilvie, 'William Hunter as book collector', *Scottish Soc. Hist. Med., Report of Proceedings*, (1953–4) pp.5–7, 9–10.
56. Abraham, James Johnston, *Lettsom, his life, times, friends and descendants* (1933) p.304.
57. Wilson, Julia E., 'An early Baltimore physician and his library (Dr. John Crawford, 1746–1813)', *Ann. Med. Hist.*, 3rd ser., 4 (1942) pp.63–80 (list of books, pp.75–9).
58. Wright-St Clair, Rex E., 'History of surgery and introduction to surgical lectures, by Monro Primus', *Med. Hist.*, 5 (1961) pp.286–90; and Wright-St Clair, Rex E., *Doctors Monro: a medical saga* (1964). This contains a chronology, a bibliography of their writings, and lists of portraits.
59. See Erlam, Harry D., 'Alexander Monro, primus', *Univ. Edinburgh J.* (Summer, 1954) pp.77–105; and Mullin, W. J., 'The Monro family and the Monro collection of books and MSS', *N.Z. Med. J.*, 35 (1936) pp.221–9.
60. See Sharp, J. A., 'Alexander Monro Secundus and the interventricular foramen', *Med. Hist.*, 5 (1961) pp.83–9; see also Guthrie, Douglas, 'The three Alexander

Monros and the foundation of the Edinburgh medical school', *J. Roy. Coll. Surg. Edinb.*, 2 (1956) pp.24–34.

61. 'Blumenbach's library', *J. Hist. Med.*, 10 (1955) pp.123–4.
62. Wright, Reginald W. M., 'Bath Hospital Medical Library', *The Record: Bulletin of the Victoria Art Gallery and Municipal Library, Bath*, 1 (1948) pp.225–34.
63. 'Catalogue of the medical library of the late Matthew Baillie, M.D., and left by him to the Royal College of Physicians of London, 1823' (Royal College of Physicians manuscript). See also Payne, L. M. and C. E. Newman, 'The history of the College Library: the last thirty years in Warwick Lane', *J. Roy. Coll. Phycns Lond.*, 9 (1974) p.98.
64. Viets, Henry R., 'Doctors afield – Georg Kloss (1787–1854)', *New England J. Med.*, 257 (1957) pp.34–6.
65. Emblen, D. L., 'The library of Peter Mark Roget', *Book Collector*, 18 (1969) pp.449–69.
66. Op. cit. in note 9 above.
67. See Viets, Henry R., 'Oliver Wendell Holmes: his books', *Bull. Hist. Med.*, 38 (1964) pp.530–3.
68. Viets, Henry R., 'William Read and his books: a bibliographic research pattern in 1861', *New England J. Med.*, 269 (1963) pp.562–5.
69. Keys, Thomas E., 'The medical books of William Worrall Mayo, pioneer surgeon of the American Northwest', *Bull. Med. Lib. Assn*, 31 (1943) pp.119–27; Keys, Thomas E., 'The medical books of Dr. Charles N. Hewitt', *Proc. Staff Mtgs Mayo Clinic*, 16 (1941) pp.732–6.
70. See Forfar, J. A., 'The library of Professor J. M. Charcot at the Salpêtrière Hospital, Paris', *Bull. Med. Lib. Assn*, N.S.27 (1939) pp.237–41.
71. Wangensteen, O. H., and S. D. Wangensteen, 'Lister, his books, and evolvement of his antiseptic wound practices', *Bull. Hist. Med.*, 48 (1974) pp.100–28.
72. Details of his life and activities are available in the Sir John Williams Centenary Number of the *National Library of Wales Journal*, 1, iv (1940).
73. See Abbott, Maude E. (ed.), *Classified and annotated bibliography of Sir William Osler's publications (based on the Chronological bibliography by Minnie Wright Blogg) ... Second edition, revised and indexed* (Montreal, 1939).
74. Kingsbury, M. E., 'Book collector, bibliographer, and benefactor of libraries: Sir William Osler', *J. Lib. Hist.*, 16 (1981) pp.187–98; Keys, Thomas E., 'Sir William Osler and the medical library', *Bull. Med. Lib. Assn*, 49 (1961) pp.24–41, 127–48; Ruhräh, John, 'Osler's influence on the medical libraries in the United States', *Ann. Med. Hist.*, 1st ser., 2 (1919) pp.170–83.
75. Gwyn, N. B., 'Sir William Osler's contributions to Library of Academy of Medicine, Toronto', *Bull. Acad. Med. Toronto*, 11 (1938) pp.154–8; Packard, Francis R., 'Sir William Osler and the Library of the College of Physicians of Philadelphia', *Trans. Coll. Phycns Philad.*, 3rd ser., 42 (1920) pp.147–50; Noyes, Marcia C., 'Osler influences on the Library of the Medical and Chirurgical Faculty of the State of Maryland', *Bull. Johns Hopkins Hosp.*, 30 (1919) pp.212–13.
76. Cushing, Harvey, *The life of Sir William Osler*, 2 vols (Oxford, 1925); one volume edition (London, 1940). See also Bett, W. R., *Osler: the man and the legend* (1951); MacNalty, Sir Arthur Salusbury, 'Osler, the medical historian', *Proc. Roy. Soc. Med.*, 56 (1963) Suppl., pp.3–9; Packard, Francis R., 'William Osler; the men and institutions with which he was associated in Philadelphia', *Canadian Med. Assn J.*, 27 (1932) pp.117–25; Atcheson, Donald, 'Willie Osler, William Osler, E. Y. Davis, Doctor Osler, Sir William Osler and their libraries', *McGill Med. Undergrad. J.* (February 1938) pp.36–43; Malloch, Archibald, 'William Osler', *Acad. of Med. Bull. Toronto* (May 1932); *Bull. Johns Hopkins Hosp.*, 30 (July 1919) contains articles on various aspects of Osler's life and association, completed by a bibliography of his writings by Minnie Wright Blogg.
77. See Francis, W. W., 'At Osler's shrine', *Bull. Med. Lib. Assn*, 26 (1937) pp.1–8.
78. See *W. W. Francis: Tributes from his friends on the occasion of the thirty-fifth anniversary of the Osler Society of McGill University* (Montreal, 1956); and Stevenson, Lloyd G., 'W. W. Francis, 1878–1959', *Bull. Hist. Med.*, 34 (1960) pp.373–8.

79. Hollender, M. H., 'The Albert Moll hypnosis collection'. *Int. J. Clin. Exp. Hypn.*, 35 (1987) pp.1–7. See also Shelley, Harry S., and Mary H. Teloh, 'The Moll Collection on hypnotism at Vanderbilt', *Bull. Med. Lib. Assn*, 65 (1977) pp.65–6.

80. See LeFanu, W. R., 'Sir D'Arcy Power', *Proc. Roy. Soc. Med.*, 56 (1963) Suppl., pp.24–5.

81. See Beaman, A. Gaylord, *A doctor's odyssey; a sentimental record of LeRoy Crummer, physician, author, bibliophile, artist in living, 1872–1934* (Baltimore, 1935) (bibliography, pp.311–31).

82. See Kleberg, Tönnes, 'Erick Waller', *Libri*, 6 (1955) pp.76–85; Lindroth, Sten, 'Erik Waller, M.D., PhD., November 29, 1875–January 28, 1955', *Bull. Hist. Med.*, 30 (1956) pp.88–90; and Fulton, John Farquhar, 'Axel Erik Waller, 1875–1955', *J. Hist. Med.*, 10 (1955) pp.226–7.

83. See Koch, Sumner L., 'Dr. H. Winnett Orr, 1877–1956', *Bull. Amer. Coll. Surg.*, 42 (1957) pp.118–21.

84. See Cavanagh, G. S. T., 'The Clendening Collection', *Bull. Med. Lib. Assn*, 48 (1960) pp.190–4.

85. Durling, Richard J. and Phoebe Peck, 'Some highlights from the collection', *News to the Friends of the Library of the History of Medicine ... University of Kansas Medical Center, Kansas City, Kansas*, 10th anniversary number (Nov. 1961) 9 pp.

86. See Holman, Emile, 'Sir William Osler and Harvey Cushing: two great personalities and medical bibliophiles', *Stanford Medical Bulletin*, 19 (1961) pp.173–85.

87. See *A bibliography of the writings of Harvey Cushing, prepared on the occasion of his seventieth birthday, April 8, 1939, by the Harvey Cushing Society, 1939* [Compiled by John Fulton]; see also Baumgartner, Leona, 'Harvey Cushing as book collector and litterateur', *Bull. Hist. Med.*, 8 (1940) pp.1055–66.

88. Fulton, John Farquhar, *Harvey Cushing, a biography* (Oxford, 1946); Thomson, Elizabeth H., *Harvey Cushing, surgeon, author, artist* (New York, 1950). See also, for example: Fulton, John F., 'Harvey Cushing and his books', *St Bart's Hosp. J.*, 52 (1948) pp.62–4, 80–2; Reeves, David L., 'The Harvey Cushing Library', *J. Neuro-surg.*, 20 (1963) pp.545–56; Ross, Sir James Paterson, 'Harvey Cushing, 1869–1939', *St Bart's Hosp. J.*, 51 (1947–8) pp.162–7; and Stanton, Madeline E., 'Harvey Cushing: book collector', *J. Amer. Med. Assn*, 192 (1965) pp.149–52.

89. *The making of a library: extracts from letters 1934–1941 of Harvey Cushing, Arnold C. Klebs, John F. Fulton. Presented to John Fulton by his friends on his sixtieth birthday, 1 November, 1959* (New Haven, Conn., 1959); See also Thomson, Elizabeth H., 'Early manifestations of bibliomania in three collectors: Harvey Cushing, Arnold Klebs, and John Fulton', *J. Albert Einstein Med. Cent.*, 10 (1962) pp.98–107.

90. 'Incunabula scientifica et medica. Short title list', *Osiris*, 4 (1938) pp.1–359; for details of his other writings see Lang, Annie, 'Bibliography of the writings of Arnold C. Klebs', *Bull. Hist. Med.*, 8 (1940) pp.523–32. See also Baumgartner, Leona, 'Arnold C. Klebs, 1870–1943', *Bull. Hist. Med.*, 14 (1943) pp.201–16; Baumgartner, Leona, 'Arnold Klebs as humanistic scholar', *Bull. Med. Lib. Assn*, 32 (1944) pp.85–95; and Fulton, John Farquhar, 'The library of a scholar: Arnold C. Klebs', *Yale Univ. Lib. Gaz.*, 22 (July 1947) pp.1–6.

91. Stanton, Madeline E. and Elizabeth H. Thomson, 'Bibliography of John Farquhar Fulton, 1921–1962, *J. Hist. Med.*, 17 (1962) pp.51–71; LeFanu, William Richard, 'John Fulton's historical and bibliographical work', *J. Hist. Med.*, 17 (1962) pp.38–50.

92. See also Muirhead, Arnold, 'John Fulton – book collector, humanist and friend', *J. Hist. Med.*, 17 (1962) pp.2–15; Muirhead, Arnold, 'Portrait of a bibliophile. IX. John Farquhar Fulton, 1899–1960', *Book Collector*, 11 (1962) pp.427–36; and Stevenson, Lloyd G., 'John Farquhar Fulton, 1899–1960', *Bull. Hist. Med.*, 35 (1961) pp.81–6. *J. Hist. Med.*, Vol. 17, Jan. 1962 is a special John Fulton Number.

93. Schuman, Henry, 'The Josiah C. Trent Collection in the history of medicine', *Bull. Med. Lib. Assn*, 46 (1958) pp.352–66; Schuman, Henry and Martha Alexander, *Fifty English medical books, 1525–1640, from the Josiah C. Trent Collection in the history of medicine. An annotated catalogue* (Durham, N. Carolina, 1956).

94. Royal College of Physicians of London, *The Evan Bedford Library of Cardiology* (1977).
95. Bedford, Evan, 'On collecting a cardiologic library', *J. Roy. Coll. Phycns Lond.*, 6 (1972) pp.227–34.
96. Hellman, Alfred M., *A collection of early obstetrical books. An historical essay with bibliographical descriptions of 37 items, including 25 editions of Roesslin's Rosengarten* (New Haven, Conn., 1952); Hellman, C. Doris (Mrs Morton Pepper), 'Additions to the Alfred M. Hellman collection of early obstetrical books', *Academy Bookman*, 11 (1958) pp.2–11.
97. Emmerson, Joan S., *Catalogue of the Pybus Collection of medical books, letters and engravings, 15th to 20th centuries, held in the University Library, Newcastle upon Tyne* [Manchester] (1981). See also her 'F. C. Pybus: the man and his books', *Health Lib. Rev.*, 4 (1987) pp.141–50.
98. See *To Geoffrey Keynes: articles contributed to "The Book Collector" to commemorate his eighty-fifth birthday* (London, 1972); LeFanu, W., 'Sir Geoffrey Keynes (1887–1982)', *Bull. Hist. Med.*, 56 (1982) pp.571–73.

10 Medical libraries of today

Roy B. Tabor

Quality, not quantity, measures the effectiveness of any library.
(Gertrude L. Annan)

The field of medicine is particularly well documented and its secondary literature of indexes, abstracts and bibliographies is the envy of other scientific disciplines. Much of this material is located in national libraries and institutions or in university medical school libraries. But during the past twenty years there have been significant changes in the world of medical libraries. Since the mid-sixties there has been a considerable development of libraries for practitioners and these have been based in hospitals, although often open to other health care staff. Because of this multidisciplinary approach the term 'health care library' has tended to be used increasingly to describe this trend. Similarly university collections have extended their role and allowed access from a much wider public.

The wealth of medical literature is increasing at an exponential rate and this is associated with an obsolescence factor of around 10 per cent each year. Together these contribute to a significant change in the nature and role of medical and health care libraries. Medical libraries are no longer the sole province of the medical profession. There is also an increasing emphasis on the information service aspects of libraries particularly as these serve the wide range of practitioners. Further influences on such changes include the sophistication of information technology and the rapid rate of its application in health care libraries. It is now possible to search on-line databases and catalogues and retrieve information rapidly from the medical literature, which could only have been done with laborious difficulty a few years ago. Communications technology has played a large part in this development and major libraries and their collections have become accessible in a way not previously possible. The now ubiquitous personal computer on the desk of the end-user has ushered in the age of the 'virtual library', that is the world's collections of health sciences literature are brought to the individual at his place of work.

In this chapter some of the principal medical libraries of the world are described and, as in previous editions, some note is made of the size and nature of their collections. It is not easy to measure the activity and value of a library and where stock figures are quoted this is only intended as a guide. The value of a library as a source of information may be inversely proportionate to its size. Some libraries are destined to function as repositories of historical material; some concentrate on providing the latest research material by means of current journals and monographs while others cater for specific user populations such as undergraduates. Most combine some of these functions and cooperate with other libraries to share the total resources. Cooperation has always been a strong feature of medical libraries but, under the influences of information technology and financial constraints, which during the eighties have been seriously affecting library collections, there have been positive moves to create formal networks. A prime mover and leader in this type of development has been the National Library of Medicine in Bethesda, Md, and that example is echoed in many different ways across the world. In the United Kingdom regional medical library networks have been developed within the National Health Service (NHS) and the network concept has been introduced in India (HELLIS) and in the Philippines (HERDIN). It is this networking aspect which becomes so apparent in these descriptions of modern medical libraries.

Biomedical library and information services in Great Britain need to be understood within the contexts of the British Library network and the network of health care libraries operating within the NHS. The British Library (BL) itself provides the principal reference and lending library service on a national scale, and these are complemented by a range of libraries of the Royal Colleges, pharmaceutical companies and university medical school libraries. Supplementing these major libraries is a large network of smaller medical and nursing libraries distributed throughout the NHS in all parts of the country. For the past twenty years NHS libraries have been developing their own special role, especially in providing information services for patient care. These changes are having significant influence on information provision in the biomedical field.

In 1973 the BL was created by amalgamating a number of existing libraries including the British Museum Library, the Science Reference Library and the National Lending Library of Science and Technology (NLL). The NLL was renamed the British Library-Lending Division – now, Document Supply Centre (BLDSC) – and is now one of the largest collections of medical and scientific literature in the United Kingdom. BLDSC has a very large stock of periodicals – about 56 000 are received – in all subjects and languages. The library also collects all important English and foreign language report literature, conference proceedings and monographs. To supplement its collections there are a number of back-up libraries and these include the Royal Society of Medicine and the Department of Health and Social Security (DHSS). Together this national library resource offers a formidable array of medical and scientific literature services including loans and photocopying. The existence of this library service has influenced the pattern of interlibrary loans in the smaller libraries in the United Kingdom. Previously a librarian might spend a considerable amount of time approaching several other libraries for specific loans, but most frequently the BLDSC is now the first choice for a loan application. For the field of health care the back-up of the DHSS Library means that the subject area of clinical medicine is now greatly extended to in 'ide a range of health care management topics and social welfare informa 1.

There are, in addition to BLDSC, a number of medical libraries serving specific user groups. London is particularly well served and an account of the medical libraries was provided by W. R. LeFanu.[1] Certain of the older examining bodies, such as the Royal Colleges, and medical societies and institutions, contain libraries with lengthy histories, and are rich in historical material, in addition to maintaining current collections. The Royal College of Physicians of London Library was founded in 1518, being based on the collection of Thomas Linacre, and houses several significant benefactions. It received 680 volumes from Dr Holsbosch, and in 1632 William Harvey drew up rules for the use of the library, later paying for the erection of a new building which was opened in February 1653, and establishing a trust in 1656 providing for the upkeep of the collection. Dr Christopher Merrett (1614–95) became the first librarian in 1653, and compiled a catalogue, printed in 1660, which lists 1300 volumes. In 1666 the building was completely destroyed, and although Merrett managed to save some of the books, a partial list of which has been compiled by Eleanore Boswell[2] his own library was destroyed. He was expelled from the College in 1681, officially for non-attendance, but there had been trouble with other officials of the College, and the only reliable information available is that contributed by Sir Charles Dodds[3] in an interesting article on the first Harveian Librarian. On the death of the Marquis of Dorchester in 1680 he bequeathed over 3000 books to the College, and these were housed in a new building in 1687. John F. Fulton[4] has written a paper on the Dorchester Collection, based on an exhibition held at the College in 1958, and a catalogue of the Collection inscribed on vellum is in the library. The library of D. Lloyd Roberts was acquired in 1921, consisting of about 1800 volumes, including 50 incunabula. The Royal College of Physicians houses a total of about 100 incunabula, of which there is a typescript catalogue, 40 000 volumes, 600 manuscripts, 10 000 pamphlets, 5000 autograph letters, 5000 portraits, and 2000 bookplates. A printed catalogue of the books was published in 1912, and is still very useful, and catalogues of oriental manuscripts (1951) and of prints (1952) have also appeared. Exhibitions are frequently held in the library, and the catalogues of these are most informative. This library concentrates on historical and biographical material, and is housed in spacious premises in Regents Park. The history of the College library has been well documented by Payne and Newman.[5]

The Royal College of Surgeons was founded in 1800 as successor to the

Company of Surgeons (1745) which was itself an offshoot from the Barber Surgeons Company founded in 1540. The Library of the Royal College of Surgeons of England was founded in 1800, and Robert Willis was appointed as the first librarian in 1828. W. R. LeFanu[6] has described the development of the collection, which includes numerous manuscripts, of which a catalogue was prepared by Victor G. Plarr in 1928,[7] and a collection of 56 incunabula which W. R. LeFanu and A. C. Klebs described in 1931.[8] The library now stocks 160000 volumes, 50000 pamphlets, 3000 portraits and 2000 bookplates. It is particularly rich in the literature of surgery, dentistry, anaesthesia, anatomy, physiology and pathology, and the historical collection is of special value. It includes manuscripts of John Hunter, Edward Jenner, Lord Lister, and many other eminent medical men. W. R. LeFanu[9] has prepared a catalogue of portraits, busts and drawings, and of English books printed before 1701 housed in the College. This is a reference library open only to Fellows or other diplomats of the College but active cooperation is fostered with other libraries.

The Royal College of Obstetricians and Gynaecologists was founded in 1929, and the library was started three years later with the gift of books by William Blair Bell. For some years the collection was mainly historical, a large proportion of the books coming from the collection of Roy Samuel Dobbin (1873–1939), but in 1961 a grant was received from the Wellcome Trustees to bring the collection up to date. A catalogue of the library up to 1850, compiled by W. J. Bishop, was printed in 1956 but the stock has increased considerably since then, and the library offers a useful service to its Fellows and Members.[10] The College of General Practitioners was founded in 1957, and is building up a useful library within its limited field, but is also providing a photocopying service to members by means of cooperation with other medical libraries.

The Royal Society of Medicine was formed in 1907 by the amalgamation of 18 medical societies. The success of this enterprise was largely due to Sir John Young Walker MacAlister, for several efforts had previously been attempted at amalgamation, but without success. The larger societies absorbed by the Royal Medico-Chirurgical Society of London (1805) included the Pathological Society of London (1846), The Epidemiological Society (1850), the Odontological Society of Great Britain (1856), and the Obstetrical Society of London (1858). These societies brought with them extensive libraries, money and members, and their combination resulted in a central building, administered to the benefit of all concerned. The collections brought together in 1907, later bequests and subsequent acquisition policy ensured the development of a broadly based postgraduate medical collection covering the biomedical sciences, clinical practice and clinical research. The Royal Society of Medicine is divided into Sections, so that specialists are well catered for, the transactions of meetings being published in the *Proceedings of the Royal Society of Medicine* issued monthly. While primarily a library of current research and practice it also houses a large collection of historical material, the oldest book being dated 1474, and largely complete runs of most nineteenth-century and many major twentieth-century medical journals. Over 2000 journals are currently taken, covering all aspects of medicine, with particular emphasis on biochemistry, immunology and brain sciences. Over 10000 non-current journal sets are held and retained indefinitely and the library has an extensive collection of pamphlets of the eighteenth and nineteenth centuries. Holdings are listed in the British Union Catalogue of Periodicals and in the World List of Scientific Periodicals. Access to the library for reference purposes is available to all members of the Society; borrowing facilities are restricted to some categories of members. Non-members may use the library in person only on the introduction of a Fellow. Institutional membership is available for some corporate bodies such as pharmaceutical research companies. The library's photocopy service is available worldwide to non-members and interlending services are provided through the British Library Document Supply Centre. The library, which had been extended in 1953, was again enlarged and extensively refurbished in 1985–6 to enable it to manage the growth of the literature beyond the end of the century. The RSM library has a cooperative working arrangement with the Wellcome Institute for the History of Medicine which includes the transfer of stock from the RSM to the Wellcome Institute to ensure that material is housed in the library most appropriate to research needs. The history and development of the library has been described by Philip Wade.[11]

The year 1832 saw the beginning of one of the most important medical societies when the Provincial Medical and Surgical Society was formed at Worcester by Charles Hastings. It was established for the advancement of medical science, and to promote intercourse among members. Branches and divisions were formed all over the world, and some of these have eventually become separate associations. The Society published *Transactions* annually until 1853, when their place was taken by the *Association Medical Journal*, which in 1857 became the *British Medical Journal*. The title of the Society had been changed the previous year to the British Medical Association. It interests itself in everything connected with the profession, including medical reform, public health, and professional ethics. The biography of the founder, Sir Charles Hastings (1794–1866) by William H. McMenemey[12] contains much information on the early days of the Society.

The Nuffield Library[13] of the British Medical Association (named after Lord Nuffield, an honorary member of the BMA), was founded in 1887 and houses the collection formed by Sir Charles Hastings, founder of the BMA. The stock consists of 30000 books, about 2000 sets of periodicals of which over 1100 are current, 3000 Government reports and 3500 pamphlets. The library was moved to the refurbished Great Hall of BMA House in 1986, and has readers' desks fitted with computer terminals and telephone lines. Microfilm and microfiche readers are available. It is available to Members and Associate Members of the BMA, and others at the discretion of the librarian. Enquirers can contact the library by telephone, telex or telefax. The Nuffield Library provides a fast photocopying service to other libraries as well as to individual enquirers.

The nucleus of the library of the Wellcome Institute for the History of Medicine consists of books collected by and for Sir Henry Wellcome between 1898 and 1936. Today it is the largest and most comprehensive European collection in the history of medicine. It contains some 400000 printed books dating from the fifteenth to the twentieth centuries and ranks internationally in size and quality among the finest three libraries serving this field. The collection comprises much more than medical literature in the narrow sense. In addition to extensive holdings of material on clinical medicine and therapeutics there are large collections relating to the history of the biological sciences in general – particularly physiology, botany and chemistry, whose histories are closely intertwined with that of the healing arts. Important holdings relate to travel, ethnography, alchemy, tobacco, smallpox and vaccination, venereal diseases and veterinary medicine, as well as hospitals, case histories and nursing. Acquisitions from other institutions have been made recently, including part of the library of the Medical Society of London, and a large collection (*c.*24000 volumes) of mostly eighteenth- and nineteenth-century books belonging to the Royal Society of Medicine and the library of the Royal Society of Health (*c.*30000 volumes). The collection from the Medical Society of London (*c.*11000 volumes) includes some 200 manuscript volumes dating from the twelfth century onwards. The library holds over 600 incunabula representing most of the great names in the history of medicine from antiquity, the European Middle Ages and the Renaissance.

A *Catalogue of Incunabula* and three volumes of the *Catalogue of Printed Books* in the Wellcome Institute Library have already been published and further volumes are in preparation.[14] The development of a machine-readable bibliographic record of all printed holdings published after 1850 is in progress. Noteworthy are the American collection, including Latin-America and the Caribbean, Oriental books and manuscripts (*c.*10000) and Iconographics, including paintings, prints, photographs and illustrated books. There is also a significant Contemporary Medical Archives Centre (established 1979) which encourages the preservation of twentieth-century archive materials.

In addition to being one of the earliest London medical societies to be founded, The Medical Society of London is also the oldest existing medical society in the metropolis (founded 1773). The ninth President, James

Sims, possessed an extensive library, and in 1802 he sold a large proportion of it to the Society for £500 and an annuity. Lettsom also gave several hundred books to the Society and its library was one of the richest historical medical libraries in Great Britain. A catalogue of incunabula and manuscripts was compiled by Warren R. Dawson,[15] and John Leaney[16] has described some of the most outstanding items. In the seventies the Wellcome Historical Library purchased the larger proportion of this library and the remainder was purchased by a Canadian philanthropist and now is housed in the rare books collection of the University of Toronto. (It should be noted that an error in the STC indicates that these books are in the library of Kingston University, Ontario.)

The Hunterian Society was established on 3 February 1819, as the London Medical and Physical Society, the title being changed at the second meeting. The Society possesses a remarkable collection of books and relics relating to John Hunter, and published its *Transactions* from 1831 to 1914, from 1936 to 1939, and from 1945. It instituted the Hunterian Society Medal, which is awarded annually for an essay. In 1831 the Harveian Society of London was founded as the Western London Medical Society, and instituted the Harveian Lectures, which have been delivered by many prominent professional men. This Society also houses a small collection of books and reprints by or relating to William Harvey.

The amalgamation of the Belfast Medical Society (1806) and the Belfast Clinical and Pathological Society (1853) in 1862 heralded the birth of the Ulster Medical Society, which has an extensive library. The Society published its *Transactions* in the *Quarterly Journal of Medical Science* from 1873 to 1892 but printed its own *Transactions* from 1892 to 1931 and then founded the *Ulster Medical Journal*. The Society is housed in the Whitla Medical Institute, which was presented by Sir William Whitla.

Government Departmental libraries include that of the Department of Health and Social Security which, though it does not specialize in clinical medicine, has one of the largest national collections on health and social services. It is particularly rich in material on the history of public health services from the middle of the nineteenth century, and holds large collections of Government publications including Parliamentary Papers and Debates, reports of Government medical officers and publications of international bodies such as the World Health Organization (WHO). The stock consists of some 200 000 volumes and over 2000 sets of journals, and there are branch libraries with specialized collections covering the safety of medicine, the literature of health building and design, and NHS equipment and supplies. The library produces several abstracting and indexing bulletins including *Health Service Abstracts* (successor to *Hospital Abstracts*), *Nursing Research Abstracts* and *Quality Assurance Abstracts* (in conjunction with the Kings Fund Quality Assurance Project). From the end of 1983 all data has been entered on the library's computerized information system, and as DHSS-DATA is available for on-line search-ing by outside users using the commercial systems of Data-Star and Scicon.[17]

The Medical Research Council maintains two large institutes and many smaller research units throughout the country. The oldest library is that of the National Institute for Medical Research at Mill Hill[18] which originated at Hampstead in 1920, moving to its present premises in 1950. This library covers the basic sciences, while clinical sciences are covered by the library of the Clinical Research Centre (CRC), opened in 1970, at Harrow.[19] The CRC Library also provides a multidisciplinary service to the staff of Northwick Park Hospital and Harrow Health District. Both of these large collections are available at all times to the staff of their institutes. Together with two other, smaller, professionally staffed unit libraries, those of the Radiobiology Unit at Didcot and the Clinical and Population Cytogene-tics Unit at Edinburgh, they provide a back-up service to all staff of the MRC and coordinate union catalogues of serials and books. Other signifi-cant collections exist at the Laboratory for Molecular Biology and the Dunn Nutrition Unit, both at Cambridge, and the MRC Laboratories at Carshalton.

Library services to the armed forces are now organized on a tri-service basis, coordinated through the library of the Ministry of Defence (MOD) and focussed on the central library at the Royal Army Medical College, Millbank. Multidisciplinary library services are provided to the Army, Navy and Royal Air Force and the MOD union catalogue of periodicals is heavily used for inter-library loans purposes. Early naval medical libraries have been described by Lattimore.[20]

The Library of the Royal College of Nursing (established in 1921) houses the finest collection of nursing literature in Europe (over 40 000 volumes), and takes over 200 current periodicals. Services are provided primarily for members of the College and to students and staff of the Institute of Advanced Nursing Education (IANE). There are two specia-list collections, the Steinberg collection of nursing research theses, and the Historical collection demonstrating the development of nursing. This library also acts as a back-up service to the British Library Document Supply Centre.

The Pharmaceutical Society of Great Britain possesses an outstanding collection of modern and historical books devoted to pharmacy and cognate subjects.

The 12 medical schools in London, all affiliated to the University of London, are undergoing change with various mergers and reorganiza-tions. Final decisions are still being taken and it is uncertain what impli-cations these changes will have for the libraries concerned (see Table 10.1). Several of the schools possess libraries dating from the early nineteenth century and some house special collections of writings by their alumni.[21]

Individually they cannot cater for all the requirements of their staff and students, but they cooperate in inter-lending, and their members can use the University of London library. Some of these libraries have begun to introduce automated systems, while others are still in the planning stage. Charing Cross and Westminster Medical School have already merged and there is an important teaching development using fibre-optic cable to link students with teaching staff on the different sites. This could have considerable potential for library services eventually.

Table 10.1   London medical school libraries

	(Est.)	*Current periodicals*	*Total bookstock*
St Bartholomew's	(1800)	250	17000
King's College	(1831)	368	7000
Charing Cross	(1834)	350	8000
Middlesex	(1835)	240	4000
St George's	(1836)	500	20000
Westminster	(1938)	190	5000
St Thomas's	(1842)	207	12000
London	(1854)	300	9000
St Mary's	(1854)	275	5000
Royal Free	(1874)	370	4000
Guy's	(1903)	460	14000
University College	(1907)	300	15000

There are numerous postgraduate medical institutes in London financed by the British Postgraduate Medical Federation, most of which have been established since the war. Older ones include the London School of Hygiene and Tropical Medicine, founded in 1899 as the London School of Tropical Medicine, which in 1921 amalgamated with the Tropical Diseases Bureau (1908–20) to form the Tropical Diseases Library, and becoming the London School of Hygiene and Tropical Medicine in 1928. This now houses 47000 volumes, 45000 pamphlets, and contains several outstanding collections. Comprehensively covering hygiene, tropical medicine, parasitology and related topics, its printed card catalogue represents about 40000 separate items, and is useful to other libraries as representing the contents of the largest library devoted to these subjects.[22] The Postgraduate Medical School of London, Hammersmith was founded in 1935, and houses 14 200 volumes, 10000 pamphlets, and takes 360 current journals. An index of the contents of these is prepared and circulated to subscribers, who find it a most useful guide to current literature. The Institute of Cancer Research (1951) 14000 volumes; Institute of Cardiology (1948–9) 1300 volumes; Institute of Child Health (1946) 3000 volumes; Institute of Dermatology 2500 volumes; Institute of Diseases of the Chest (1946) 7000 volumes; Institute of Laryngology and

Otology (1946) 1500 volumes; Institute of Neurology (1938) 5000 volumes; Institute of Ophthalmology (1948) 9000 volumes; Institute of Orthopaedics (1946) 5000 volumes; Institute of Psychiatry (1924) 18000 volumes; Institute of Urology (1950) 500 volumes. Although these collections may appear very small, they are highly specialized, and in certain instances well organized to serve their readers.

The Barnes Library occupied new premises in 1959, having previously functioned as the Medical School Library of Birmingham University. Originally established in 1875, it now carries a stock of 135000 volumes. It is the largest medical library in the West Midlands and covers both clinical and pre-clinical sciences. It also acts in a coordinating role to the West Midlands Regional Health Libraries network of 140 member libraries. There is a large collection of older medical literature including the Birmingham Medical Institute's historical collection and a special collection on the plague. A separate branch serves the General and Dental hospitals.

The Medical Library of the University of Bristol moved into new premises in 1965 and was further extended in 1977. It was founded in 1893 as the joint library of the Medical School (1833) and the Bristol Medico-Chirurgical Society (1890) and incorporates collections from the Bristol Royal Infirmary (1894) and individual nineteenth-century gifts. The stock now totals around 105000 bound volumes, including 3000 pre-nineteenth-century and about 19000 nineteenth-century items. A total of 1100 serials are received currently and there is an automated issue and cataloguing system. This library also serves doctors and many health professionals in the NHS South West region.[23]

Cambridge University has numerous medical departmental libraries. Provision is divided between the pre-clinical departments and clinical medicine. The former includes Anatomy (17 200 volumes), Biochemistry (13000 volumes), Genetics (10100 volumes), Pathology (11000 volumes), Pharmacology (3100 volumes) and Physiology (13 800 volumes). Clinical medicine is served by the Medical Library at Addenbrookes Hospital which was formed in 1973 by the amalgamation of several departmental libraries and now contains around 62000 volumes. Since 1976 the Medical Library has also acted as the Regional Medical Library for the NHS East Anglia region. It is a branch of the University Library which benefits from copyright deposit and itself has notable collections in medical science and the history of medicine. The Whipple Library, in the Department of the History and Philosophy of Science, contains 17 500 volumes on the history of science and medicine.

The University of Leeds Medical and Dental Library was formed in 1977 by the amalgamation of Medical Library (1831) and the Dental Library.[24] It includes the library of the Old Infirmary (about 1767), and of the Leeds and West Riding Medico-Chirurgical Society (1875), and stocks 95000 volumes. The University of Leeds Oncology Information Service

founded in 1974 forms part of the library and provides a current awareness service publishing 23 bulletins, covering specific sites or regions,
drawn from 1300 major biomedical journals. An AIDS bulletin was first
issued in 1985.

The Manchester Medical Library was founded in 1834, and the first
catalogue issued the following year lists 1075 volumes and pamphlets. In
1931 the books were transferred to the University, and among them are
numbered a dozen incunabula and about 600 books printed before 1600.
Holdings of books printed before 1700[25] (a 1972 printed catalogue lists
2685 items) were augmented by a further 300 very fine items (108 incunabula among them) when the University Library merged with the John
Rylands University Library in 1970.[26] Particularly rich in nineteenth-
century texts, the bookstock numbered 170000 volumes in 1981 when the
Medical Library moved into the new University Library building. A
thousand periodicals are currently taken. The Manchester Medical
Collection includes archives of the Manchester Medical Society and its
members and an extensive collection of publications by Manchester
doctors.[27] A separate Faculty Library serves the staff and the 1400 medical
undergraduates of the Medical School.

The Medical Library of Newcastle University (31000 volumes) includes
the libraries of the University of Durham College of Medicine, the Royal
Victoria Infirmary and Newcastle Medical Society. It contains the Pybus
collection of historical medical books (2300 books, 1100 engravings).[28]
The main library of the University of Sheffield houses over 1000 pre-1850
medical works, the majority donated in 1901 from the Sheffield Royal
Infirmary, and the medical and dental library holds some 40000 volumes.
At Leicester there is a new medical school library (1978) and its collection
is a merger from the University and the postgraduate medical library at
Leicester Royal Infirmary; this houses an historical collection originally
associated with the Leicester Medical Society.[29] Nottingham is another
new medical school (1973) and its medical library in the Queens Medical
Centre holds a total of some 73000 volumes and serves the School of
Nursing and Nottingham hospitals.

Liverpool University houses the former medical departmental libraries
and has a stock of 40000 books, some of these coming from the Royal
Infirmary Medical School (1834) and from the Liverpool University
College Faculty of Medicine (1884).[30] The older Liverpool Medical Institution Library dates from about 1773, and was founded by practitioners
as a reading club. It was rehoused in 1837 and now contains over 40000
volumes.[31]

The University of Southampton created its new medical school in 1971
and was designed to be integrated in the NHS regional health system of
the Wessex Regional Hospital Board (now the Regional Health Authority). This integration was emphasized in the title used for the medical

school library – the Wessex Medical Library – which serves also as the hospital library for the Southampton General Hospital and also acts in a focal role for the NHS Wessex Regional Library Information Service (WRLIS). The library holds around 35 000 books and takes 1250 periodicals.

Several important medical collections are housed in Scotland,[32] where some of the universities date from an early period. Aberdeen University Library dates from 1475, but the Medical School was founded as recently as 1937, and stocks 5000 volumes. The Medico-Chirurgical Society of Aberdeen was founded in 1789, and the library came into existence two years later. It contains over 10 000 books and some of the more important have been described by Mabel D. Allardyce.[33] Dundee University, founded in 1881 as University College, Dundee in affiliation with St Andrew's University, houses 27 000 medical volumes. St Andrew's University, founded 1411 with the formation of a library beginning in 1456, contains 25 000 medical items, including many historical books.

The Library of the Royal College of Physicians of Edinburgh was founded in 1681 by the gift of about 100 books from Sir Robert Sibbald. The first printed catalogue was published in 1767 and had 2346 entries; it was followed by several others, the last being printed in 1898. The library houses over 600 volumes of manuscripts, 16 incunabula and over 200 000 printed books. It is maintained as a modern medical library, but with a very valuable historical collection.[34] The Royal College of Surgeons of Edinburgh dates back to 1505, but was chartered under its present title in 1778, and the library probably dates from 1696. It contains 23 000 volumes. The Royal Medical Society, Edinburgh,[35] founded 1737, has a stock of about 30 000 volumes, mainly of historic interest. A Faculty of Medicine was instituted in Edinburgh University in 1726, and the Erskine Medical Library was established in 1931. This houses 26 500 volumes and a large collection of engraved medical portraits.

Glasgow also houses several large medical collections, the University, founded in 1451, being the home of the remarkable Ferguson Collection devoted to alchemy and chemistry (8000 volumes) and the Hunterian Collection. This latter was bequeathed to the University by William Hunter and handed over by Matthew Baillie in 1807. It consists of about 600 manuscripts, a catalogue of which was printed in 1908, 534 incunabula, and over 10 000 printed books, of which a catalogue was printed in 1930.[36] The Royal College (formerly Faculty) of Physicians and Surgeons of Glasgow dates from 1599, and the library was opened in 1698. It stocks 150 000 volumes, including several special collections, together with portraits, medals, instruments and diplomas.[37]

In Wales, the University of Wales College of Medicine (UWCM) received its first Charter as a School of the University of Wales in 1931 and its second as a College of the University in 1984. The Library comprises a

Main Library, located at the University Hospital of Wales, Cardiff, and 3 branch libraries located in other local hospitals. The UWCM network of libraries holds about 30000 books and receives 800 current periodicals; it is gradually being extended to cover libraries in other Cardiff hospitals. The UWCM Main Library provides certain facilities for all medical libraries in Wales and functions as a coordinating centre for these libraries. An historical collection of some 2000 volumes includes a complete set of Sydenham Society publications donated by the Cardiff Medical Society.

The medical library arrangements in Northern Ireland are particularly noteworthy; they are centred on the Northern Ireland Health and Social Services Library, Queens University Medical Library and provide resources and services to the hospitals throughout the country. This is a joint service between the University and Department of Health and Social Security Service (Northern Ireland).[38] The central library holds around 100000 volumes and about 1300 current periodicals. The Republic of Ireland has several medical collections in Dublin, including the rich medical collection at Trinity College, founded in 1591, which has had copyright privilege since 1801. The Royal College of Physicians of Ireland has a large historical collection based on the library of Sir Patrick Dun (1642–1713), printed catalogues of which were issued in 1794 and 1828.[39] The Royal College of Surgeons in Ireland, Dublin was founded in 1784 and in 1816 acquired the library of the Physico-Chirurgical Society. It also houses the Arthur Jacob Library (1876) and the Butcher-Wheeler Library (1943); a new library is now being built, to be opened in 1990.[40] Steevens' Hospital, Dublin contains the library collected by Edward Worth (1678–1733). University College, Cork, founded in 1845 as Queen's College, Cork, became a constituent college of the National University of Ireland in 1909.

No description of medical and health care libraries in the United Kingdom would be complete without mentioning the development of regional library services within the National Health Service. Most of the 15 Regions in England and Wales have cooperative library services and many are focussed on a major library which is usually the university medical school library. But in five regions other arrangements apply. In the four Thames regions of London a regional librarian has been appointed as part of the university postgraduate medical education system and these librarians coordinate and direct a network of medical and nursing libraries and, to varying degrees, enable library provision to be made available to all categories of NHS staff, including managers. The Wessex region has pioneered the development of NHS libraries since 1967 when the first regional librarian was appointed. This multidisciplinary library service has undertaken many research studies to ascertain the information needs of practitioners and managers and is developing a unique information system for health care – Health Compass; this aims to put a guide to sources of health information at an electronic terminal on the desk of end-users to be accessed when and where the information is required. Another unique feature of the Wessex Regional Library Information Services is its emphasis on the information needs of patients and relatives.

France's medical libraries are among the most successful and forward-looking of the country's libraries, incorporating advanced technology into their services. Mostly government-funded, they are either academic librar-ies in universities and teaching hospitals, or libraries of important national institutions such as the Centre National de la Recherche Scientifique (CNRS) or the Institut National de la Santé et de la Recherche Médicale (INSERM).

The old Faculty of Medicine of Paris Library is now called the Biblioth-èque Interuniversitaire de Médecine (BIUM) and is a focal library of the French library network. Based on the German pattern, this is essentially a controlled-acquisition network and 15 Centres d'Acquisition et de Diffu-sion de l'Information Scientifique et Technique (CADIST) have been designated covering 15 specialized fields. BIUM houses a valuable stock[41] which in 1395 consisted of 13 manuscripts and has grown to over 800 000 volumes. There are around 1100 manuscripts and some 90 medical incu-nabula.[42] A further 113 incunabula are held at the Académie de Médecine in Paris.[43]

Locating literature has been made easier by the creation of a 'Periodi-cals in French libraries' database called the *Catalogue Collectif National des publications en série (CCN)*; this collates details of the collections of libraries and documentation centres from all over France. France is also participating in the European Community electronic document delivery system (DOCDEL) with its own project, TRANSDOC. This will allow electronic delivery of information stored on microfiche or on optical disk using advanced techniques of digitalization of text and pictures.

In recent years a complete reform of medical documentation has been undertaken which will link and facilitate access to medical information in the universities, hospital libraries and other institutions. SITS is a special videotex medical host and the largest French host is Télésystèmes-Questel which offers a number of important medical databases, including PAS-CAL, a multidisciplinary base half of which is devoted to the life sciences and medicine with bilingual indexing and searching.

A large amount of information is also available through the French videotex system, Minitel. It is possible to search every database offered, either by ESA-IRS or by Télésystèmes-Questel. Medical documentation is thus being made accessible on a wide scale from local terminals and is backed up by the national document delivery system.

In the Federal Republic of Germany medical libraries are integrated into the national library system and are not organized separately. Three levels of medical libraries can be distinguished, the Central Library of

Medicine in Cologne, university libraries, and hospital libraries. The last group vary considerably in size and are not connected with the lending network of research libraries neither do they possess data terminal equipment to access databases, as automation is still at an early stage. Generally to obtain literature they turn to the nearest general scientific library or directly to the Central Library of Medicine in Cologne. The latter represents the national library for the medical sciences and collects in its field as comprehensively as it can. In 1984 it held about 600 000 bound volumes and subscribed to more than 6500 periodicals.

There is close cooperation with the Deutsches Institut für Medizinische Dokumentation und Information (DIMDI) in Cologne which has mounted numerous foreign and domestic databases for information retrieval. The Central Library tries to obtain all literature recorded on DIMDI's databases and users' literature requests are transmitted on-line from DIMDI to the Central Library. A central periodicals database is maintained at the Deutsches Bibliotheksinstitut in Berlin, consisting of some 360 000 titles in all subjects; on-line consultation is possible and this forms a strong basis for interlending activities. It is expected that the introduction of Bildschirmtext, an interactive videotex technique, will have considerable effect on the retrieval of literature and inter-library lending by small libraries as well as individuals. This is leading to a future interconnection of the various on-line catalogues to open them for common use.

There are 430 libraries and information centres at universities, research institutes and hospitals within the medical scientific information system of the German Democratic Republic. There is no central medical library but a degree of coordination is provided by the Institute for Scientific Information in Medicine (IWIM) which acts as a central register of library resources. In addition the German State Library in Berlin holds a central catalogue of monographs and periodicals. There is a regional medical library in each of the 15 regions which organizes and coordinates the activities of the libraries in its own region.

The medical libraries in Belgium are located principally in the universities, although there is a movement now to network hospital libraries at least in the French-speaking region. Notable university medical libraries include Louvain (46 000 volumes, 950 periodicals), Antwerp (60 000 volumes), Brussels Free University (35 000 volumes) and Liège (founded 1983). There are specialist libraries at the Institute for Hygiene and Epidemiology, Brussels and the Central Library of Medical Services (military and aviation medicine).

In the Netherlands, the Universities of Leyden, Utrecht, Groningen and Amsterdam have extensive medical collections, and the Royal College of Physicians, Amsterdam contains over 100 000 volumes. A survey of medical libraries in this country was published by F. P. Koumans.[44]

Norway, until 1948, had only one university – in Oslo – but in recent years three more have been founded and all have medical schools. The University of Oslo's Biomedical Library has functioned as the central medical library in Norway since 1947 (175 000 volumes, 1000 periodicals), Bergen (founded 1956) has a stock of 12 000 volumes and 795 periodicals, Trondheim has 14 300 volumes and 717 periodicals, while Tromsø (founded 1973) has around 50 000 volumes and 980 periodicals. There are just over 100 general hospitals and almost half have a medical library with one or more fully trained librarians. The National Hospital, Oslo has around 50 000 volumes and 500 periodicals, while Oslo City Hospital has 46 800 volumes and 471 periodicals.

An initiative by the University of Oslo to produce a union list of foreign periodicals and union catalogue of foreign books has resulted in a printed version for biology and medicine being produced in 1982. The microfiche version is updated three times a year and since 1983 it has been searchable on-line. Co-operation between medical libraries is good but there is also cooperation on a Scandinavian scale with a union list of scientific periodicals within all fields (NOSP) which is shortly to be accessible on-line.

The central medical libraries in Norway are able to search MEDLINE which is based at the Karolinska Institute in Stockholm (KIBIC). This is the Swedish National Resource Library of Medicine and holds 3300 medical periodicals and receives 250 000 requests for loans and photocopies each year. In addition to MEDLINE it hosts SWEMED which covers medical articles, reports and dissertations from Sweden. The university libraries of Göteborg, Linköping, Lund, Umea and Uppsala also have large medical collections. At Uppsala the university medical school contains the remarkable medico-historical collection donated by Erik Waller.

The University Library, Scientific and Medical Department, Copenhagen, acts as the central library in Denmark and holds a collection of about 1.2 million books and some 6000 biomedical periodical titles. There are other medical collections at the State and University library of Arhus (founded 1902), Odense University Library (founded 1965) and the library of the Medical Historical Museum, University of Copenhagen (founded 1910). There are libraries in most of the big county hospitals, staffed with trained librarians, and these cooperate through inter-library lending networks using the local university library as a first resort. Books may be located through the Danish National Acquisitions Catalogue of Foreign Language Materials (ALBA) and periodicals are located through the Scandinavian on-line database NOSP or the newly established Danish on-line base DASP.

The Republic of Iceland is a small country of almost 250 000 people, over half of whom live in the Reykjavik area. There are 50 hospitals and some 79 Health Centres. The National Library (founded 1818) conserves

Icelandic medical publications, but there is no medical school library. The largest library, in the National Hospital, has some 320 current periodical titles and altogether there are around 700 unique foreign medical periodicals held in the country. There is an active inter-library cooperation with a strong dependence also on Sweden and Denmark. A MEDLARS service has been established since 1973 and there are now 12 libraries accessing the MEDLINE database hosted at the Karolinska Medical Institute in Sweden (KIBIC).[45]

In Finland there are some 75 medical libraries, but most of these are small and without trained staff. The largest and most important is the Central Medical Library in Helsinki (founded 1966) which is an independent institution affiliated with the University. It was formed from the collections of several medical societies, taking some 2396 periodicals. It is the national resource library in medicine and has an active inter-library loan programme. There are other very active libraries in the medical industry, research institutes and the medical faculties of the universities of Turku, Oulu, Knopio and Tampere. The Central Medical Library has compiled a bibliography of Finnish medical materials, FINMED, and a database MEDIC since 1978. It has also pioneered the use of automated information systems in Finland with access to MEDLARS in Sweden.

There are around 300 medical libraries in Switzerland, in the universities, pharmaceutical industry and in hospitals, but there is no central medical library nor is there any structured system. In contrast the public library system is well organized, with a focus on the Swiss National Library in Berne. The inter-library lending service is based on five regional medical libraries and there are good links with the United Kingdom (British Library Document Supply Centre) and with the Federal Republic of Germany. The Commission for Biomedical Libraries of the Department of the Interior compiles BIOMED, a union list of biomedical periodicals; the second edition (1983) lists 12000 biomedical periodicals in 300 libraries. DOKDI, the documentation service of the Swiss Academy of Medical Sciences in Berne used to be exclusively connected with the NLM but, since 1982, 80 per cent of searches are now undertaken on Data-Star. There are no national biomedical databases.

The World Health Organization library at Geneva currently receives over 2500 periodicals and annuals in addition to numerous governmental public health reports, and houses a working collection of over 35000 volumes, as well as a small historical collection on international health. Services are provided to WHO staff members throughout the world, to delegates to the World Health Assembly, members of the Executive Board and participants at WHO meetings. The WHO Library also promotes the strengthening of health libraries, documentation centres and other literature services at country level.

The tradition of medical libraries in Italy dates back to the foundation of the oldest university institutions in the main cultural centres of the country (Bologna, Florence, Genoa, Milan, Naples and Rome). Precious incunabula and rare books are preserved in these libraries, as for example the Medical Central Library of the University in Florence which contains the manuscripts of Lorenzo Bellini (1643–1704), Marcello Malpighi and others,[46] and the Library of History of Medicine, University 'La Sapienza', in Rome (over 1500 medical monographs of historical interest and herbaria, among others). The Library of Medicine and Surgery of the Catholic University in Rome, established only in 1961, now has a collection of 176000 monographs and 5800 periodicals, 80 per cent of which are in foreign languages. There are many other important medical libraries, belonging to research institutions, which were founded between 1920 and 1935, such as in Rome, the Central Library of the Italian National Research Council (whose global collections amount to 500000 monographs and 3000 periodicals), the State Medical Library, located in the 'Policlinico Umberto I' (one of the main Roman hospitals), and the Library of the Italian National Health Institute (whose total collection amounts to 160000 monographs and 3000 current periodicals covering all subjects related to public health). The Documentation Service of the latter Institute is the Italian reference centre for MEDLARS and other on-line systems. Medical libraries in Italy, attached to universities, medical schools, hospitals, medical societies and research institutions, have developed considerably in recent years. The lack of a consolidated medical librarianship policy is being overcome by several cooperative projects carried out by librarians of national scientific organizations and local institutions. In addition, the creation of the Group of Biomedical Libraries inside the Italian Library Association and the introduction of new technologies in library procedures is helping to improve access to the medical literature.

The main historical collections of biomedical literature in Spain are located in Barcelona (School of Medicine Library, Universidad Central de Barcelona; Academy of Medical Sciences Library) and Madrid (School of Medicine Library, Universidad Computense; the library of the Instituto Nacional de las Salud; and the library of the Royal Academy of Medicine). Current Spanish biomedical literature is indexed in the *Indice Medico Español*, edited and published by the Instituto de Informacion y Documentacion en Biomedicina de Valencia. Library networking is at an early stage. A union list of serials (*Catalogo colectivo de publicacions periodicas en bibliotecas espanolas: 2: Medicina*) has been available since 1971 and a third edition is in preparation. Since 1980 the 'Coordinadora de Documentacion Biomedica de Catalunya' has been in operation, building the *Catalogo colectivo*; its second edition will be available for on-line searching. Similar professional organizations, such as the Biomedical Group of the Asociación Andaluza de Bibliotecarios, are working towards networking activities. A significant challenge facing Spanish biomedical librarianship was introduced by the Ley 14/1986, General de Sanidad, which entitles patients and relatives to a thorough and continued, oral/written information in plain terms, about the diagnosis, prognosis and alternative treatments. Health information systems will be initiated by the Health Authorities and all levels of medical education will be integrated with the total health care system. Both universities and health authorities now need to develop imaginative answers to these new problems through networking and resource sharing. The next few years promise to be a testing time for health care library and information professionals in Spain.

Medical libraries in Portugal fall into two categories – government (universities, research institutes, hospitals) or private (pharmaceutical companies, chemical industry and medical associations). There are more than 50 medical collections across the country but those providing the more regular services are located in the principal urban centres of Lisbon, Porto and Coimbra. Some important institutions are concerned to merely maintain their collections and lack any dynamic development of modern library information services. The smaller hospital libraries are keen to develop information services but lack the money to develop adequate document collections. Important library collections exist at the Faculty of Medicine, University of Lisbon (founded 1815) which contains the collection of the Royal Surgery School and has works from the sixteenth century; Faculty of Medicine, University of Porto (founded 1825) with some 3000 historical works from the fifteenth to eighteenth centuries; Lisbon City Hospital (founded 1918) which holds the Archives of the Capital's Hospitals, 1504–1755; Faculty of Medicine, University of Coimbra (founded 1853) with 2267 manuscripts, 8 incunabula and some 350 books from the sixteenth century. A National Information System is still in process of development and inter-library loans operate at a low level without any automation. Library development is constrained by lack of policy and funding, difficulties in professional training of library staff, and passiveness of users.

The most extensive medical library collections in Greece can be found in the Evangelismos Hospital, Athens General Hospital, the National Institute for Research, Agia Sophia Paediatric Hospital, the Democritus Nuclear Research Centre and the 251 General Air Force Hospital. Most hospital libraries are small and some are specialized: such as the Eginition Hospital which holds mainly neurology and psychiatry. The only official medical library catalogue in Greece was published in 1977.

The medical libraries in Turkey are based primarily in the university medical schools. Before 1963 there were only four medical schools but there are now 22. The universities may be located on a single campus where a central library serves all users; alternatively in the traditional

Turkish universities there are separate faculty or departmental libraries. Istanbul University Medical Faculty Library was the first to be established in the early years of the new Turkish Republic (1933). The most recent one is the Marmara University Medical Faculty Library (1985). These library collections vary between 3000–115000 volumes and between 20–600 current periodicals. The largest and most important libraries are in the universities of Hacettepe, Ankara, Ege and Istanbul. The Medical Centre Library at Hacettepe acts as a focus for inter-library loans both nationally and internationally and has pioneered library automation in the country. Most of the state hospitals have their own medical library but few are able to provide adequate services. Major constraints on effective library development include the lack of library funding and lack of qualified librarians.

There are about 4000 medical libraries in the USSR, which operate within a nationwide network system. The primary focus is the All-Union Scientific Institute for Medical and Medico-technical Information (VNIIMI) which coordinates the hierarchical structure of the system according to geographical location and professional specialty. There is a second focus in the Central Medical Scientific State Library (GCNMB) which governs the activities of libraries. VNIIMI is concerned with the information centres of the republic and main research institutes, whereas GCNMB governs the medical libraries of the republic, medical research institutes, medical universities, and the medical libraries of districts, hospitals and polyclinics. The GCNMB is one of the world's largest libraries, with a stock of over 3 million items and around 2000 current periodicals. It also provides extensive information services including translations and serves as a bibliographical centre with a particular emphasis on grey literature. Documentation on medical literature forms part of the National System of Scientific-Technical Information (GSNTI) which includes ten all-union institutes in specific fields, 86 central branch information centres, several hundred local information centres and some 11000 information centres in institutions. GSANTI organizes the regular flow of foreign medical literature down to the users and gathers information on the national literature at local levels to be aggregated at the all-union institutes. A feature of the Soviet system is the high qualifications of the staff – around 20 per cent of the staff in the medical information centres are physicians. Automated information systems have been progressively introduced during the past ten years and databases such as ASSISTENT (from VNIIMI) are used for current awareness purposes. 75 per cent of the sources are written in English and only 14 per cent in Russian. But international databases from MEDLARS and Excerpta Medica are also used for on-line searches. Other important medical library collections are held at the Fundamental Library of the USSR Academy of Medical

Sciences, Moscow and the Kharkov State Scientific Medical Library, which now has a stock of over 1 million items.

There are six republics in Yugoslavia and two autonomous provinces, all with a high degree of autonomy; there are also five official languages, in all of which medical literature is published and medicine is taught. The largest libraries are in the medical schools; two of these have collections of more than 100 000 volumes, 25 have between 5000 and 50 000 volumes but the majority of individual libraries have fewer than 5000 volumes. Only one medical library takes more than 1000 current periodicals, while more than half the libraries subscribe to fewer than 100 titles. The two most significant medical libraries in Serbia are at the Medical Faculty, University of Belgrade – 500 foreign periodicals and 60 Yugoslav periodicals – and at the Medical Faculty, Nis – 300 foreign periodicals and 40 Yugoslav periodicals. Regional medical library networks are still developing and union catalogues and periodical lists have been compiled; there is a union list of medical periodicals in medical school libraries produced at irregular intervals. Library automation is not highly developed but there has been access to on-line databases through DIMDI since 1979.

In Poland, the Central Medical Library, Warsaw was founded in 1945 and forms the centre of medical bibliographical services in Poland; it publishes Polska Bibliografia Lekarska, which constitutes a national index of Polish medical writings.

A survey of medical libraries in the United States of America (1979) indicated a total of some 2775 health sciences libraries, although the National Library of Medicine (NLM) records some 4000 'basic unit' libraries (mostly in hospitals), 125 resource libraries (at medical schools), seven Regional Medical Libraries (covering all geographic regions of the United States) and the National Library of Medicine itself in Washington DC. The greatest concentration of these libraries lies in the North Eastern part of the country in the States of New York, Pennsylvania, Illinois, Ohio, Massachusetts and Michigan. The surveys carried out by the American Medical Association, Division of Library and Archival Services in 1969, 1973 and 1979 have shown a gradual overall decline in the number of medical libraries by 5–7 per cent every three years. These changes include an increase in medical school and hospital libraries with the decrease in medical society and other types of libraries. The decrease may be associated with the closing of certain special hospitals (for example, chronic disease and tuberculosis (TB) hospitals) and changes in medical practice, such as the closing of long-term state psychiatric hospitals.

Overall, the aggregate resources of health sciences libraries are increasing with an associated increase in inter-library cooperation. In all this Federal support has been an important factor; between 1964 and 1980 Federal support for the NLM grew from approximately $4 055 000 to over $46 350 000. This high level of support has contributed to the growth of individual libraries and the development of networking, and undoubtedly American libraries have been very well resourced.

In 1960–1 Bloomquist estimated that 1200–1500 current journals would be required 'to meet the needs of a medical school community of good quality';[47] at that time only 25 per cent of the libraries surveyed met such standards. By 1980–1, 126 medical school libraries indicated an average number of current serial titles of 2415. By comparison the average number of periodicals in hospital libraries (1979) in 1739 hospitals was 130, although libraries in hospitals with more than 500 beds had an average of 230 current periodicals.[48]

During the period 1960–80 medical schools in the USA grew at a faster rate than the general economy. Consequently the medical school libraries have grown to a position of leadership among American health sciences libraries and together have the greatest aggregate of resources. This is certainly owing to the unprecedented amount of Federal support. But in recent years Federal and State funding has diminished and this trend is likely to continue. This is leading to new coalitions being formed and the introduction of new technology to ensure that these libraries can continue as active agents in medical information processing. In the 1979 survey hospital libraries received an average of 569 items on inter-library loan and loaned 616 items. For larger hospitals, of more than 500 beds, an average of 1864 items were received and an average of 20 items were loaned. This survey indicated a total of 1949 hospital libraries, an overall increase of 12.8 per cent since 1969; this may be partly explained by the revision and raising of the requirements by the Joint Commission on Accreditation of Hospitals which have clarified and made more stringent the condition of libraries as prerequisite for hospital approval.[49] Today hospital librarians form 40 per cent of the membership of the Medical Library Association.

Hospital libraries have greatly expanded their roles and have become more involved in both undergraduate and postgraduate medical education. They have also responded to the need for continuing education of other staff, both in their own hospital and in their region. In some cases there is a new commitment to research.

The most significant medical library in the world is the National Library of Medicine at Bethesda. Founded in the Surgeon General's Office, Washington in 1836, a catalogue prepared in 1840 lists 228 volumes. In 1865 John Shaw Billings was appointed assistant to the Surgeon General, and by the time he left the collection had grown to 300 000 volumes, and now is around 3.7 million items. Billings was responsible for launching the *Index Medicus* and the *Index-Catalogue*,[50] and for initiating the development of an institution which has had a profound effect on medical research throughout the civilized world. Medical librarians rely heavily upon the catalogues, bibliographies, lending facilities and general cooperation of the National Library of Medicine. About 1868 there were two plans for a national medical library in America, one sponsored by the American Medical Association (founded 1847) and housed in the Smithsonian Building. This project was abandoned in 1895 and the 7500 books collected were handed over to the Newberry Library in Chicago, and later transferred to the John Crerar Library in 1907.[51] The second scheme was based on the Surgeon General's Library, and not only survived, but reached fruition in the rehousing of the Library in new, adequate premises in 1962. This ensured the full development of MEDLARS, and the promotion of other centres to cooperate in its exploitation to the full.

The Library collects exhaustively in all major areas of the health sciences and the current total is now 3.7 million items. Housed within the Library is one of the world's finest medical history collections of old (pre-1871) and rare medical texts, manuscripts and incunabula. A catalogue of the latter was published in 1950.[52] The Library may be used by all health professionals and health science students, either in the reading rooms or by inter-library loan. NLM serves as the national resource for all US health science libraries and lending and other services are provided through a Regional Medical Library Network. Some 2 million inter-library loan requests are filled each year within this Network.

In 1965 the Medical Library Assistance Act (MLAA) enabled the National Library of Medicine to initiate many programmes to assist American health sciences libraries, including the establishment of the Regional Medical Library Network (RMLN). The primary goal was to 'improve the flow of medical information from the point of generation to the ultimate user for the purposes of research, education and medical practice'.[53] By 1972 an NLM policy statement described a four-level hierarchical network model; these included base units (mainly hospital libraries), resource libraries (mainly medical school libraries), Regional Medical Libraries and the NLM. Each level was responsible for providing back-up information resources for the lower level. Faced by the need to provide a more cost-effective grouping a new configuration for the RML was approved in 1981, reducing the network from 11 regions to seven. A revised mission statement was also issued: 'The mission of the RML Program is to provide health science practitioners, investigators, educators and administrators in the United States with timely, convenient access to health care and biomedical information resources.'

The revised RML Program goals emphasized the provision of a basic level of information services to health professionals, development of optimal efficiency and performance at each health science library, sharing of resources and expertise among network institutions, especially for document delivery, and the use of modern technology to promote the transfer of biomedical and other health science information.[54] Two factors had emerged in this revision which altered the structure and emphasis of the network: improved computer capabilities at NLM made it possible to automate several of the RML services[55] and health care professionals were changing their information-seeking patterns from dependence upon libraries to a direct interaction with databases through personal computers. By 1982 a third generation of NLM's Medical Literature Analysis and Retrieval Systems (MEDLARS) was being implemented and access to the databases was being made easier by new software developments.

In 1982 the seven RMLs joined with NLM to create a new file of serials holdings – SERHOLD; this, together with SERLINE (Serials Online) now serves as the national, machine-readable database of periodicals and includes some 550000 holdings statements from over 1000 health science libraries. This serves as a basis of NLM's automated inter-library loan request and referral system DOCLINE (Documents Online). A prototype has been tested by the Mid-Continental RML Program in Nebraska and essentially will allow any request to be entered via any ASCII terminal. Requests check the serial holdings listed in SERHOLD and are then automatically routed to libraries reporting holdings until the request is filled. During 1983–4 the RML Network has allowed direct inter-library access, with each participant responsible for locating and requesting materials directly from any holding library. A common electronic mail system (ONTYMELL) has been adopted for interlibrary loan and this will serve as an interim measure until DOCLINE is fully operational.

The MEDLARS system had been established (1964) to achieve rapid bibliographic access to NLM's vast store of biomedical information. Today MEDLARS search facilities are available on-line to individuals and institutions throughout the world. The MEDLINE database, essentially the Index Medicus on-line, currently contains over 5 million references going back to 1966. Since it became operational in 1971 a further 20 databases have been developed – for cataloguing and serials information, toxicological and chemical data, cancer and other specialized areas of health and disease. A further development of great significance occurred in mid-1987, with the issue of the MEDLINE database on CD-ROM (Compact Disk) using optical technology. One compact disk holds at least a full year's records of the Index Medicus and is frequently updated. This will certainly influence end-user searching of the database but it remains to be seen what effect it will have on on-line database-searching through the mainframe hosts.

An important development in US medical school libraries has been the introduction of local Integrated Library Systems (ILS). The purpose is to facilitate the library's internal functions and at the same time to enhance the user's ability to exploit the total resources by direct access to on-line catalogues and other data files. A significant feature in the development of

ILS is that the master bibliographic files have been derived from one of the major bibliographic cataloguing services, such as OCLC, using the MARC format. The standardization imposed by MARC has contributed to the economic conversion of these data. ILS systems have been implemented at Georgetown University, Washington University School of Medicine Library and as L8/2000 by OCLC as their local turnkey system.

A further significant development in health science libraries has been the concept of the Integrated Academic Information Management System (IAIMS). In 1979 the NLM contracted with the Association of American Medical Colleges (AAMC) to study the health science libraries role in the transfer of information during the next decade.[56] The resultant report is a landmark for all health science libraries, emphasizing that library automation is a necessity and should not be delayed. Three distinct types of networking are described in which the library must engage: system-to-library networks (e.g. MEDLINE, OCLC), library-to-library networks (the RML Network) and library-to-user networks. A particularly significant factor is that the library should be actively involved in the integration of all internal and external information databases needed by medical personnel. The NLM continues to support IAIMS aggressively with funding for a number of research and development programmes. 'The IAIMS concept has introduced an enormous challenge in the application of technology to achieve more effective management and dissemination of information in medical centres ... The health science library never again will be able to limit its concerns to the information resources available within its physical walls.'[57]

It would be impractical to mention all the larger medical libraries in the United States, although a number were included in the previous edition. The following libraries are particularly noteworthy. The library of the University of California Medical Center, San Francisco dates from 1915, and the collection has grown to 628 000 volumes (1986). It includes several historical collections, including sections devoted to anaesthetics, medicine in California, Osleriana, and the Crummer Medical History Room which contains eleven incunabula. The Biomedical Library of the University of California, Los Angeles was established in 1947, and has grown rapidly since that date, having 437 000 volumes in 1986. This combination of medical and biological material offers tremendous scope for the development of a comprehensive library devoted to the life sciences. This library is now the designated Regional Medical Library for the Pacific Southwest Regional Medical Library Service.

The second largest medical collection in the United States is the Francis A. Countway Library of Medicine, opened in 1965, with over 527 000 volumes, 775 incunabula, and over 5000 current periodicals, formed by the fusion of the Boston Medical Library and Harvard Medical Library. This serves an extensive area, and has cooperative facilities with libraries in New Haven, New York, Philadelphia, Baltimore and Bethesda. The Boston Medical Library was founded in 1805, with John Fleet as its first librarian[58] but it moved several times until 1900, when it became settled until its amalgamation with Harvard. It includes several special collections, and James F. Ballard[59] prepared a catalogue of its manuscripts and 654 incunabula. Harvard University School of Medicine and Public Health Library, dating from 1783, also contains valuable special collections and the joint libraries, while retaining their identities, have combined their resources to provide a central medical library in Boston that will form a focal point for medical research.[60]

Colombia University Medical Library, New York was formed in 1929 by the amalgamation of the libraries of the College of Physicians and Surgeons (1807) which in 1814 had merged with the Columbia (Kings) College School of Medicine (1767). It has access to other extensive collections, and serves several other institutions. In 1986 Columbia stocked 406000 volumes, and it possesses a particularly notable collection on plastic surgery.

Yale's first separate collection of medical books was formed in 1814 by the Medical Institution of Yale College and a history of this has been contributed by Frederick G. Kilgour.[61] A catalogue issued in 1865 listed only 1204 volumes, and these were transferred to Yale University Library about 1880. The present Yale Medical Library was opened in 1941, and it contains some 349000 volumes of periodicals, books and monographs. This library houses large collections of manuscripts, incunabula, and material connected with Boyle, Browne, Galen, Harvey, Hippocrates, Jenner, Paré and Vesalius. It is also the home of the outstanding libraries collected together by Harvey Cushing, Arnold C. Klebs, John F. Fulton and smaller donations by George Milton Smith, Clements C. Fry and Samuel C. Harvey. These have made Yale one of the main centres for the study of medical history, and several useful publications have been issued by the Historical Library.

The Library of Medical Sciences, University of Maryland originated in 1813, and it contains the John Crawford Collection, on which it was founded, the Cordell Collection, devoted to the history of medicine, and the Grieves Collection on the history of dentistry. It stocked almost 278000 volumes in 1986. This library is designated as the Regional Medical Library for the Southeastern/Atlantic Regional Medical Library Services.

The University of Nebraska College of Medicine Library originated in Omaha Medical College (1881), and the University of Nebraska College of Medicine (1883), these being amalgamated in 1903. The books belonging to the Omaha-Douglas County Medical Society were added in 1916, and journals belonging to the Nebraska State Medical Association were deposited a year later. The library housed over 210000 volumes in 1986, and possesses the ophthalmology collection of Harold Gifford, and the Charles F. and Olga C. Moon collection on obstetrics and gynaecology.[62] This library serves as the Regional Medical Library for the Mid-continental Regional Medical Library Program.

An early survey of medical libraries in the New York State by Wesley Draper[63] reveals that at that time there were over a hundred medical libraries in the State, including four libraries belonging to county medical societies. New York itself houses a number of prominent medical libraries, including the New York University–Bellevue Medical Center Library, centrally situated in a new building. It has a capacity for 200000 volumes, and contains a collection of rare books, in addition to a comprehensive modern stock. The New York Academy of Medicine dates from 1847, but it did not have a library for some years. A building to house the Academy was erected in 1874, and Samuel S. Purple donated 2000 books. Five years later it absorbed the Medical Library and Journal Association of New York (1864). The Library was opened to the public in 1878, and a new building was opened in 1926, when the collection numbered 133000 volumes. In 1927 the collection of medical classics belonging to E. C. Streeter was purchased, and a new Rare Book and History Room was opened to readers in 1933, and named after Archibald Malloch.[64] The Fenwick Beekman Collection[65] was donated to the Academy, and contains outstanding series of the writings of John Hunter, Jenner, Beaumont, Cowper, Cheselden and others. The New York Academy of Medicine Library functions as an up-to-date collection, but with rich historical material in most branches of medicine, and also outstanding collections of manuscripts, letters, medals, postage stamps and medical instruments.[66] This library is designated as the Regional Medical Library for the Greater Northeastern Regional Medical Library Program.

The University of Texas Medical Branch Library (established 1893) now holds some 240000 volumes and is the designated Regional Medical Library for the South Central Regional Medical Library Program. The University of Washington Health Services Library, Washington was opened in 1949 and now holds some 327000 volumes; it is the designated Regional Medical Library for the Pacific Northwest Regional Health Sciences Library Services.

Among other notable libraries is that of the American College of Surgeons Library in Chicago formed in 1921, being based on the library of John B. Murphy, to which collections from Albert J. Ochsner, William McDowell Mastin and others have been added. The orthopaedic collection assembled by H. Winnett Orr is of particular significance, and a catalogue of this, edited by L. Marguerite Prime and Kathleen Worst, has been published.[67] In addition to housing a valuable historical collection, this library performs an extensive service to readers in search of modern literature, and bibliographies, abstracts and translations are prepared.

The American Medical Association in Chicago first had a collection of books in 1869 but it was housed in several locations until it was eventually absorbed by the John Crerar Library. Premises for a library were acquired in 1903, and a modern collection of journals and reprints has been built up, providing a service to members and to subscribers to the Journal and other specialist periodicals published by the Association. The Association also cooperated with the National Library of Medicine in the production of the Cumulated Index Medicus up to 1965.

The John Crerar Library, Chicago, founded in 1894, houses the DuBois Reymond Collection on comparative physiology, the Meissner Collection devoted to physiology, the Baum Collection on medical history, the Martin Collection on gynaecology, the Grulee Collection devoted to paediatrics, and the Robert Sonnenshein Collection of medical portraits. This library is responsible for the preparation and publication of Leukemia Abstracts.[68]

The Johns Hopkins Hospital, Baltimore, was opened in 1889, the School of Medicine Library was started in 1893, and the School of Hygiene and Public Health was established in 1916. Their libraries were amalgamated in the William H. Welch Medical Library, opened in 1929.[69] The Institute of the History of Medicine is housed in the same building. Special collections include the Morison Dermatological Collection, the Howard A. Kelly Collection, the Hugh H. Young Urological Collection, the Henry J. Berkely Collection on Psychiatry, the William Osler Collection, the William Stewart Halsted Collection, the Leonard L. Mackall Collection, the Ahlfield Teratological Collection and the Henry Barton Jacobs Collections.

The first medical library in the United States was that of the Pennsylvania Hospital founded in 1762, John Fothergill (1712–80) giving the first books to the Hospital in that year. The following year it was decided to found the library, and Fothergill further assisted in the project, John Coakley Lettsom, another benefactor, acting as their agent for the acquisition of books. In 1787 the library of Benjamin G. Barton was purchased and the collection rapidly grew, several catalogues being issued. The library is rich in historical matter, and in herbals.[70] The Library of the College of Physicians of Philadelphia was founded in 1788, and it has continued to grow, housing 224 000 volumes, including several special collections. Among these are the Samuel Lewis Library (13 900 volumes), a collection on tuberculosis, de Schweinitz's collection on ophthalmology, J. P. Crozer Griffith's collection on paediatrics, a large number of manuscripts, autographs and engravings of portraits of physicians, and also 416 incunabula.[71] Jefferson Medical College Library originated in 1894, and was housed in a new building in 1929.

In Canada the population increased between 1961 and 1986 from 14 million to 26 million and the commitment to the provision of health care services increased similarly. There are now 16 medical schools and their library collections have increased in size. A particularly significant development has been the creation of the Health Sciences Resource Centre (HSRC) which functions as part of the Canada Institute for Scientific and Technical Information (CISTI). HSRC is not a 'national library of medicine' but serves as an access point to the medical and health related literature. Although CISTI has only a modest stock (450 000 volumes and 45 000 serial titles) it is one of the most active lenders in North America. HSRC also provides some unique services, including administration of the national MEDLARS network, and acts as the primary access point for the biomedical community into the extensive services and expertise available at CISTI. HSRC also provides a biomedical information service for institutions without such facilities and undertakes MEDLINE searches for users without access to a terminal. CISTI plays an important role in the development of information technology in Canadian libraries.

Of the 12 university medical libraries serving medical schools and other health professionals the average intake of current periodical titles is around 1700. There are a number of other active medical libraries of which two merit special mention: in British Columbia the BC Medical Library Service is maintained by the College of Physicians and Surgeons and is an active partner with the Woodward Library at the University of British Columbia in serving the information needs of the medical profession and the hospitals throughout the Province; in Ontario the Academy of Medicine (Toronto) maintains a library for its Fellows but also has a reciprocal arrangement with the Science and Medical Library at the University of Toronto to serve the medical community in the Greater Metropolitan area.

Two topics are actively being developed in Canadian health science libraries – automation of library services and patient education services. The language problem in Canada is prominent in that there is an overwhelming emphasis on English language texts, serials and reference works and the Francophone community experiences difficulties similar to those in other bilingual countries.

Most of the South American countries house medical schools, produce numerous medical journals, and have an extensive medical literature dating back several centuries. A survey of early Mexican medical books, and of medical libraries has been made by Francisco Guerra.[72] (In this connection it is worth noting that the Mexican collection in the Wellcome Institute for the History of Medicine in London is the most complete collection of original texts of 1557–1833 in existence. That library also holds useful material for Argentina and Brazil.) In Argentina the University of Buenos Aires' Faculty of Medicine Library was founded in 1863, and has grown considerably since 1895, when it was housed in a new building.[73] A detailed description of the rare books in the Bibliotheca de la

Sociedad de Obstetricia y Ginecología de Venezuela has been published by M. A. Sanchez Carvajal.[74] This library also houses up-to-date books on obstetrics and gynaecology.

An interesting history of early Australian medical libraries has been written by Bryan Gandevia and Ann Tovell,[75] indicating their sudden development in the middle of the nineteenth century. They were usually housed by medical societies, such as the Port Philip Medical Association (1846), the Victoria Medical Association (1852), and the Medical Society of Victoria, formed in 1855 by the amalgamation of the Victoria Medical Association and the Medico-Chirurgical Society of Victoria (1854). The Australian Medical Subscription Library was formed in Sydney in 1846, and the Medical Association of South Australia was founded in 1851, but its books were dispersed five years later. Most of these libraries did not function for long, and the books have disappeared, with the exception of a few which have been identified in other collections. The medical schools house libraries, Melbourne Medical School (1862) in particular being noteworthy, and Melbourne is also the home of the Central Medical Library Organization formed in 1953 by the key medical libraries in the city.[76] This maintains union lists of periodicals, and facilitates cooperation in other ways. The Royal Australasian College of Surgeons, Melbourne, founded in 1927, houses the Gordon Craig Library, of which a catalogue was issued in 1941, and has also acquired the historical library of Leslie Cowlishaw (died 1943), which is particularly rich in the history of medicine in Australia. Medical libraries are also maintained in the University of Sydney (40 000 volumes), the Department of Public Health, New South Wales (25 000 volumes), the Medical Library of Western Australia, formed by the amalgamation of the University medical library and that of the British Medical Association; and the University of Adelaide Medical School Library, which in 1949 incorporated the medical section of the University and the South Australian branch of the British Medical Association (BMA). The psychiatric material in these collections was surveyed by Iris Gunner,[77] and Sheila R. Simpson[78] has surveyed medical libraries in New South Wales. The historical material in these libraries has inspired several Australian medical authors to contribute invaluable studies to the literature, and the writings of K. F. Russell, Ann Tovell and Bryan Gandevia, for example,[79] are useful to medical historians in general, and to those interested in Australian medical history in particular. Judith Lloyd has written an excellent account of the early history of the Adelaide Hospital Medical Library 1870–90, which updates earlier accounts.[80]

The National Library of Australia, Canberra, in 1981 inaugurated the Australian Bibliographic Network (ABN) which is based on similar principles to the American regional medical library system. The National Library is also the focus and host to the Australian MEDLARS service and offers services throughout the continent as well as to New Zealand

and to other countries in the Western Pacific and South East Asia. In addition to the MEDLINE database it provides a National Drug Information Service for hospital pharmacists, an Australian Medical Index to periodicals and a HEALTHNET national on-line union catalogue of State health department libraries and certain public hospitals and medical institutes. Some State health departments have appointed librarians with responsibility to develop hospital libraries. Inter-library loans operate primarily within each metropolitan area; some inter-state traffic exists but the vast distances involved cause inevitable delays in document delivery.

The Faculty of Medicine at the University of Tasmania was established in 1963 and its medical library in 1964. The preclinical requirements are supported by the university's Biomedical Branch Library and the clinical library is located at the Royal Hobart Hospital. The latter holds some 12 000 books and takes around 750 current periodicals; library services are provided also to the professional hospital staff, and, by special arrangement, to medical and dental practitioners in the State of Tasmania.

New Zealand's medical and health literature resources are not centralized in any national collection. Five substantial collections are based in the four University Medical or Clinical School libraries and the Department of Health library. There are also a number of small to medium-size hospital libraries and a few special libraries. The Universities of Auckland and Otago (Dunedin) have medical schools and the latter also has two Clinical Schools (Christchurch and Dunedin). When the Otago Medical School was founded in 1875 the books belonged to the New Zealand Medical Association of Dunedin. Despite initial slow development the library has received several donations of great value, including the Monro Collection, and now contains a fine collection of early printed books and manuscripts.[81]

The Department of Health Library in Wellington has a substantial collection in public health and health services administration with numerous other special interests, including food and nutrition, occupational health and toxicology. There are 29 branch libraries in other centres throughout the country. The Country's public hospitals are organized into 29 hospital boards, but 16 of these are large enough to join the national inter-library loans network. This interloan system, administered jointly by the New Zealand Library Association and the National Library of New Zealand is currently undergoing change and a New Zealand Bibliographic Network (NZBN) (1984) is emerging which will be available on-line. Until recently the National Library collected little medical literature, but it is envisaged that this policy will change and in future is likely to support the health sciences more actively.

Since 1981, New Zealand has had access to the Australian MEDLINE network and there are now 13 New Zealand members. The New Zealand MEDLINE Co-ordinator is based at Wellington Medical Library.

Because MEDLINE coverage of Australian and New Zealand medical periodicals is poor the National Library of Australia and the Australian Department of Health developed a national database, the Australian Medical Index (AMI). New Zealand material is now added to AMI, making it the Australasian Medical Index; this went on-line in 1985.[82]

In South Africa the largest medical libraries are based on the medical schools and there is a substantial library at the Department of National Health. In the Cape Province there are medical libraries at the University of Cape Town (69000 volumes and 1087 current periodicals) and at the University of Stellenbosch, established 1957 (38000 volumes). Major libraries in the Transvaal are located at Witwatersrand University (Johannesburg) founded 1926 (50000 volumes and 950 current periodicals), University of Pretoria's clinical library at the H. F. Verwoerd Hospital, and the most recently established (1976) Medical University of Southern Africa (MEDUNSA). There are significant collections at the South African Institute for Medical Research, the National Institute for Occupational Diseases and at the National Research Institute for Virology. In Natal the focus is on the University of Natal Medical Library (40000 volumes and 838 current periodicals) but the province is unusual in its multiplicity of hospital libraries (26) all administered by the Natal Provincial Library Service. The Natal Medical Libraries Interest Group, formed in 1980, has stimulated a greatly improved service in the Natal Hospital libraries.

An important contribution to medical documentation in South Africa occurred when the South African Medical Research Council was established in 1969. The Institute for Medical Literature (IML) – now the Institute for Biomedical Communication – was created in 1976 and access to MEDLINE became available the same year, connecting directly to the NLM in Washington. There is also available a South African Medical Literature database (SAMED). Medical libraries may also use SABINET, the South African Bibliographic and Information Network which offers a nationwide, shared-access computerized bibliographic database, which, by providing location data, acts as a valuable union catalogue for South African libraries.[83]

In Nigeria, University College, Ibadan was founded in 1948. The Medical Research Institute, Yaba and the Library of Medical Headquarters, Lagos was combined to form the Central Medical Library at Yaba and there is also a medical library at the West African Institute for Trypanosomiasis Research in Kaduna.[84]

In India there are about 400 medical and biomedical libraries throughout the sub-continent. Generally these are attached to medical schools, large teaching hospitals, district hospitals and pharmaceutical, medical and scientific research institutions. Most of these libraries function in isolation and vary widely in their stock and range of services. The National Medical Library in New Delhi is the largest medical library in India and subscribes to over 2000 current periodicals; it also has the national responsibility for biomedical information systems.

Recognizing the fundamental importance of health literature and information in support of health care programmes, the World Health Organization South East Asia Regional Office initiated the development of HELLIS (Health Literature Library and Information Service) in 1976. In 1980 a policy was endorsed to create a structure of a National Medical Library, six regional medical libraries (RML), referral libraries and peripheral libraries. The RMLs will function mainly as regional coordinating centres and will organize mobile libraries for primary health workers in the rural areas. In total the constituent libraries of the HELLIS network in India number more than 500 with a wide range of administrative authorities. There is a concentration of medical libraries in the metropolitan cities but many libraries do not have even a minimum capacity for active participation in the network. Few libraries have Index Medicus or Excerpta Medica and most libraries do not have catalogues or periodical lists. Two directories of health and medical libraries in India were compiled during 1980; there are 106 medical colleges and 18 dental colleges.

In the Western region a small body of librarians have formed the Indian Medical Libraries Association (Western region) and have begun a programme of training and cooperation. A union list of periodicals available in the region has been compiled and inter-library lending has been greatly facilitated.

There are numerous medical libraries in Malaysia; the three largest are the medical faculty libraries of the University of Malaya, founded 1963 (93 000 volumes and 1366 current periodicals), the National University of Malaysia, founded 1974 (50 000 volumes and 1000 current periodicals) and the Science University of Malaysia (28 000 volumes and 700 current periodicals). Their function is to serve their own staff and students. There are several smaller libraries within the Ministry of Health, attached to government hospitals and health centres; the largest of these is at the Institute for Medical Research (IMR). The library at the IMR (founded 1901) in Kuala Lumpur is the oldest library in the country. It is the national focal point for the WHO's Regional Biomedical Information Programme and is responsible for compiling the national medical bibliography and for undertaking on-line searches for the medical and health personnel in the country. All major government hospitals and training schools (such as nursing training schools) have small libraries. There are also small libraries at the administrative headquarters of the Ministry of Health and at the Public Health Institute (PHI). There is close cooperation between all the libraries in the country and most of the country's needs can be met from within the country by means of inter-library loans.

Health and medical information services in Singapore are focussed on the medical library of the University of Malaya, founded in 1905. The library now has over 115000 volumes and around 1100 current periodicals and serves all personnel in the medical and health services, both in Singapore and in neighbouring countries. It is a designated 'WHO National Focal Point' library and cooperates with the medical libraries in five Asian countries (Indonesia, Malaysia, Philippines, Singapore and Thailand). MEDLARS services have been available since 1975 through the National Library of Australia, but since 1983 direct on-line access to DIALOG and MEDLINE (1984) has been available.

In 1973 the Southeast Asian Medical Information Centre (SEAMIC) published BIBLIOMED-SM, the author and subject indexes to the Singapore/Malaysia periodicals, with entries dating back to 1890. A supplement, 1974–9 was published in 1982 and this has now been automated to an on-line service – PERIND.

There is a wealth of biomedical information in the Philippines among medical institutions and health-related agencies. Each of the 27 medical schools has its own library, many of which are associated with private universities or religious institutions. The need for cooperation between all these libraries is acutely recognized and a recent development has been the creation of the HERDIN network (Health Research and Development Information Network) focussed on the Philippines Council for Health Research and Development (PCHRD). Other cooperating agencies are the Ministry of Health and the University of the Philippines, Manila (UPM). The intention is to establish a library-based information network which will serve all health care staff and agencies throughout the twelve Health Regions in the country.

An index to Philippine medical literature has been compiled, the *Philippine Index Medicus*, and volumes 2–8 (1917–79) have already been published. The UPM medical library is the SEAMIC Key Station in the country, coordinating activities and cooperative projects, including the Union list of medical periodicals in South East Asian countries, and provides off-line access to MEDLARS in both Australia and Japan. Throughout the Philippines library funding is extremely limited and few libraries can afford subscriptions to *Index Medicus, Excerpta Medica* or the *Tropical Diseases Bulletin*. However a new Medical and Health Libraries Association (MAHLAP) is being organized and there are initiatives to improve staff training and to introduce library automation.

The Japan Medical Library Association (JMLA) lists over one hundred cooperating member libraries, mostly university medical libraries. The largest of these are Osaka University (300000 volumes, 6184 periodicals), Tohoku University (296000 volumes, 3338 periodicals), Kyushu University (253000 volumes, 2601 periodicals), Tokyo Medical and Dental University (234000 volumes, 1889 periodicals), University of Tokyo (227000 volumes, 2334 periodicals) and Nigata University (221000 volumes, 1772 periodicals). The average medical library has 58000 volumes and 1443 current periodicals – more than half of these are foreign journals. In the field of medical sciences the total number of periodicals published in Japan is 1779, of which 1640 are in Japanese and 139 in foreign languages.

The JMLA has high affiliation requirements: all members must hold more than 10000 books and subscribe to more than 300 current periodicals. This accounts for the apparently high stock figures listed above. The Association does, however, organize inter-library loan services and publishes a list of some 15000 biomedical periodicals in member libraries.

International cooperation is fostered by SEAMIC, a project implemented in 1979 by a private foundation, the International Medical Foundation of Japan (IMFJ) but funded entirely by the Japanese government. Services include three programmes – data exchange on infectious diseases, compilation of health statistics and health documentation and publications services. For the latter, SEAMIC compiles medical bibliographies and union lists of periodicals for each of its member countries.

There are at least 2300 medical libraries of various categories throughout China, of which 122 are medical college libraries, and these form the core of the medical library system. Noteworthy features are that some 40 per cent of library directors are medically qualified and that the libraries are open not only to their primary users but also to the public community. Since 1977 there has been a very active programme of library development, with funding increasing by some 150 per cent in some libraries.

Since 1982 four multi-provincial medical library and institute of medical information networks have been founded – Central-south, East, Northeast and North China – along with 18 local networks. Many provinces have formed their own networks. Their principal responsibilities include inter-library loans and resources sharing, cooperative acquisition, and compiling union lists of periodicals. Staff training and exchange of experience are also featured. The Chinese Medical University and College Library Association (CMUCLA) was formed in 1985 and promotes and coordinates programmes of continuing education and collection development.

Information services receive particular attention with 55 medical college libraries setting up information departments, and 35 of these have specific subject services. Cooperation between the Chinese Academy of Medical Sciences Institute of Medical Information (CAMS) and the National Library of Australia has provided a MEDLARS service to some 15 libraries. In June 1987 CAMS in Beijing became a full MEDLARS Centre for China. The Health Sciences Library of CAMS has been designated as the National Medical Library of China and has some 5700 periodical titles in 10 languages, although most of them are in English. This library has a special collection of traditional Chinese medicine, some of them rare books from the thirteenth century. A union catalogue of books and serials on Chinese traditional medicine in foreign languages is currently under compilation.

The medical libraries mentioned above, and others throughout the world, function as repositories of medical literature for the benefit of research, education and above all for ensuring a high quality of patient care. This last function has become specially prominent during the past 20 years. The number of new journals continues to increase and these serve as important vehicles for the communication of new knowledge in medicine and across the whole field of health. A significant development has been the opening up of the traditionally exclusive medical libraries to other health care-related staff and this has been coupled with rising standards for nursing and paramedical education. In some countries, notably the USA, the United Kingdom and Sweden, there is a realization that the patient is an equal partner with the doctor and his health care team in collaborating with an effective diagnosis and treatment. This has led to a number of initiatives to provide appropriate libraries or information services for the non-medically trained public. Such developments illustrate the changing nature of the health care library world.

At the heart of these changes lie the rapidly developing information and communications technologies which are influencing the design and future role of medical library networks. One example is the ADONIS trial document delivery service which supplies 219 biomedical periodicals published in 1987–8 on CD-ROM. Weekly texts are available in this laser disk format which can be searched (with individual articles printed out) on demand; each article is given a unique identification number. Because the text is in a standard ASCII form it can be transmitted by telefacsimile and, in future, by satellite communication to any part of the world. This technology holds significant implications for networks and for health care libraries throughout the world.

Although the great medical library collections continue to grow and provide the basis for medical education and a source of medical knowledge, the demand for medical literature is producing new solutions in different parts of the world. There is an increasing emphasis on cooperation, and library networks are changing character and becoming potentially more effective as new technology is introduced. Library services are reaching out to the practitioners beyond the library building and new services are being provided. Library information services are adapting to changes in health care practice in both the Western world and the developing countries. But marked contrasts remain, with the Third World unable to obtain basic medical literature and the industrialized West having large library resources and well-developed inter-library loans systems. There is a worldwide crisis in health care provision resulting from increased demand, a rising population, and restricted resources. Medical and health care libraries of the future can be expected to continue to play an important role in providing information support to practitioners in the field of medicine and health.

Notes

1. LeFanu, W. R., 'Medical libraries', in Raymond Irwin and Ronald Staveley (eds), *The libraries of London*, 2nd rev. edn (1961) pp.302–7.

2. Boswell, Eleanore, 'The Library of the Royal College of Physicians in the Great Fire', *Lib. Trans. Bib. Soc.*, N.S.10 (1929–30) pp.313–26.

3. Dodds, Sir Charles, 'Christopher Merrett, F.R.C.P. (1614–1695), first Harveian Librarian', *Proc. Roy. Soc. Med.*, 47 (1954) pp.1053–6.

4. Fulton, John, 'The library of Henry Pierrepont, first Marquis of Dorchester (1606–1680), F.R.C.P., F.R.S.,' *J. Hist. Med.*, 14 (1959) pp.89–90; see also Payne, L. M. and C. E. Newman, 'The history of the College Library: the Dorchester Library', *J. Roy. Coll. Phycns Lond.*, 4 (1970) pp.234–46.

5. Payne, L. M., and C. E. Newman, 'The history of the College Library', *J. Roy. Coll. Phycns Lond.*, 4 (1970) pp.234–46; 5 (1971) pp.385–96; 7 (1973) pp.145–53; 8 (1974) pp.283–93; 9 (1974) pp.87–98; 11 (1977) pp.163–70; 12 (1978) pp.189–95; 18 (1984) pp.66–73, 198–202.

6. LeFanu, W. R., 'The history of the library of the College', *Ann. Roy. Coll. Surg. Engl.*, 9 (1951) pp.366–82; LeFanu, W. R., 'The Library', in Sir Zachary Cope, *The Royal College of Surgeons of England: a history* (1959) pp.257–73.

7. Plarr, Victor G., *Catalogue of manuscripts in the library of the Royal College of Surgeons* (1928).

8. LeFanu, W. R. and A. C. Klebs, 'Incunabula in the library of the Royal College of Surgeons of England', *Ann. Med. Hist.*, N.S.3 (1931) pp.674–6.

9. LeFanu, W. R., *A catalogue of the portraits and other paintings, drawings and sculpture in the Royal College of Surgeons of England* (1960); LeFanu, W. R., *English books printed before 1701 in the library of the Royal College of Surgeons of England* (1963).

10. Shaw, Sir William Fletcher, *Twenty-five years: the story of the Royal College of Obstetricians and Gynaecologists, 1929–1954* (1954); Thornton, John L. and Patricia C. Want, 'Roy Samuel Dobbin (1873–1939), book collector and benefactor of the Royal College of Obstetricians and Gynaecologists', in *Proceedings of the XXIII International Congress of the History of Medicine* (London, 1974), pp.1087–98; Royal College of Obstetricians and Gynaecologists, *Short-title catalogue of books printed before 1851 in the Library ...*, 2nd edn (1968).

11. Wade, Philip, 'The history and development of the library of the Royal Society of Medicine', *Proc. Roy. Soc. Med.*, 55 (1962) pp.627–36; Godbolt, Shane, *The incomparable Mac* (1983); Davidson, M., *The Royal Society of Medicine. The realization of an ideal (1805–1955)* (1955); Power, Sir D'Arcy, *The foundations of medical history* (Baltimore, 1931); Moore, Sir Norman and S. Paget, *The Royal Medical and Chirurgical Society of London: centenary 1805–1905* (1905); Wade, P., 'After forty years: the library of the RSM in retrospect and prospect', *Proc. Roy. Soc. Lond. (Biol.)*, 69 (1976) pp.751–4.

12. McMenemey, W. H., *The life and times of Sir Charles Hastings, founder of the British Medical Association* (1959).

13. Wright, D., 'The new Nuffield Library at the British Medical Association', *Health Libraries Review*, 3 (1986) pp.164–6.

14. *A catalogue of printed books in the Wellcome Historical Medical Library*, I. Books printed before 1641 (1962); II. Books printed from 1641–1850 A–E (1966); III. Books printed from 1641–1850 F–L (1976); IV. Books printed from 1641–1850 M–R (in preparation); Poynter, F. N. L., *A catalogue of incunabula in the Wellcome Historical Medical Library* (London, 1954).

15. Dawson, W. R., *Manuscripta medica: a descriptive catalogue of the manuscripts in the library of the Medical Society of London* (1932).

16. Leaney, J., 'Treasures of a medical library', *Books*, No.332 (Nov.–Dec. 1960) pp.217–

21; see also Freeman, E. J., 'Some of the rarer books in the collection of the Medical Society of London', *Trans. Med. Soc. Lond.*, 90 (1974) pp.43 8.

17. Kahn, Ann, 'The Department of Health and Social Security Library in context', *Medical, Health and Welfare Libraries Group Newsletter*, No.19 (March 1983) pp.5 26; Cotton, Joanna, 'The DHSS integrated library system', *Health Libraries Review*, 2 (1985) pp.170 6.

18. Morton, Leslie T., 'The library of the National Institute for Medical Research', *Library World*, 62 (1960 1) pp.249 51.

19. Wade, Jenny, 'The library services of the Clinical Research Centre and Northwick Park Hospital, Harrow', *Library Association Medical Section Bull.*, 103 (1975) pp.1 4.

20. Lattimore, M. I., 'Early naval medical libraries, personal and corporate', *J. Roy. Nav. Med. Service*, 69 (1983) pp.107 11.

21. See, for example, Hibbott, Y., 'The collection of early printed books in the Medical School Library', *St Thomas' Hosp. Gaz.*, 79 (1981) pp.64 72; Thornton, John L., 'Books [in the College Library]', in Victor Cornelius Medvei and John L. Thornton (eds), *The Royal Hospital of Saint Bartholomew 1123 1973* (1974) pp.308 31.

22. *Dictionary catalogue of the London School of Hygiene and Tropical Medicine*, 7 vols (1965); Barnard, Cyril C., *London School of Hygiene and Tropical Medicine. History of the Library ...* (1947).

23. Roberts, A. E. S., 'The medical library of the University of Bristol', *Med. J. South-West*, 73 (1958) pp.12 14; Roberts, A. E. S., 'An exhibition of important anatomical books [in the Medical Library, University of Bristol]', ibid., pp.104 7.

24. Collins, Anne M. and J. A. Sharp, 'Some books in the Historical Collection of the Medical and Dental Library', *University of Leeds Review*, 22 (1979) pp.172 90; Wood, P. B. and J. V. Golinsk, 'Library and archive resources in the history of science and medicine at the University of Leeds', *Br. J. Hist. Sci.*, 14 (1981) pp.263 81.

25. Parkinson, E. M. and A. E. Lumb, *Catalogue of medical books in Manchester University Library, 1480 1700* (1972); 'John Rylands Library Manchester: pre-1700 medical books in the Rylands Library', *Bull. John Rylands Lib.*, 54 (1971) pp.2 5.

26. 'Notes and News', *Bull. John Rylands Lib.*, 54 (1971 2) pp.2 5.

27. Elwood, W. J. and A. F. Tuxford, *Some Manchester doctors: a biographical collection to mark the 150th anniversary of the Manchester Medical Society, 1834 1984*, Manchester, 1984.

28. Emmerson, J. S. (ed.), *Catalogue of the Pybus collection of medical books, letters and engravings, 15th 20th centuries, held in the University Library, Newcastle-upon-Tyne* (Manchester University Press for the University Library, 1981).

29. Frizelle, E. R., *A history of the library of Leicester Medical Society*, Leicester, 1973.

30. Jones, I. B., 'Symposium on three types of medical libraries. I. A university medical library', *Bull. Med. Lib. Assn*, 41 (1953) pp.220 4.

31. 'Liverpool Medical Institution', *Br. Med. J.* (1963) i, pp.179 80; and Lee, W. A., 'Symposium on three types of medical libraries. II, Medical Society libraries', *Bull. Med. Lib. Assn*, 41 (1953) pp.224 9.

32. Jolley, Leonard, 'Medical libraries of Great Britain. II. Medical libraries of Scotland', *Br. Med. Bull.*, 8 (1952) pp.256 61; Jolley, Leonard and Margaret D. Bell, 'Medical libraries of Scotland', *Bull. Med. Lib. Assn*, 43 (1955) pp.356 65; Hargreaves, G. D. (ed.), *A catalogue of medical incunabula in Edinburgh libraries* (Edinburgh, 1976); Bird, D. T., *A catalogue of sixteenth-century medical books in Edinburgh libraries* (Edinburgh, 1982); Dewey, N., 'The early medical libraries of Edinburgh and Glasgow', *AB Bookman's Weekly*, 28 April 1986, pp.1946 8.

33. Allardyce, Mabel D., *The library of the Medico-Chirurgical Society of Aberdeen*, (1934).

34. Pendrill, Geoffrey R., 'The Royal College of Physicians of Edinburgh, its origin and functions', *Scot. Med. J.*, 6 (1961) pp.526 31.

35. Cormack, J. J. C., 'The Society's Library', *Bull. Med. Lib. Assn*, 48 (1960) pp.125 41.

36. Young, John and P. Henderson Aitken, *A catalogue of the manuscripts in the library of the Hunterian Museum in the University of Glasgow* (1908); *The printed books in the Library of the Hunterian Museum in the University of Glasgow. A catalogue prepared by Mungo Ferguson. With a topographical index by David Baird Smith* (1930); see also

Ferguson, Mungo, 'Note on some medical MSS and books in the Hunterian Library', *Glasgow Med. J.*, 108 (1922) pp.51–4.

37. Goodall, Archibald L., 'The Royal Faculty of Physicians and Surgeons', *J. Hist. Med.*, 10 (1955) pp.207–25; Goodall, Archibald L., 'The history of the Royal Faculty of Physicians and Surgeons', *Glasgow Med. J.*, 30 (1949) pp.89–100; Alstead, Stanley, 'Origins of the Royal Faculty of Physicians and Surgeons of Glasgow', *Br. Med. J.* (1949) II, pp.1223–4; Bowman, A. K., 'The Royal Faculty of Physicians and Surgeons of Glasgow, 1599–1949', *Lancet*, 1949, II, pp.1002–4.

38. Linton, W. D., 'The Ulster way: a regional health care library service', *Bibliotheca Medica Canadiana* (1981) pp.178–80.

39. Kirkpatrick, T. Percy C. 'Dun's Library in the Royal College of Physicians of Ireland', *Bull. Med. Lib. Assn*, 26 (1938) pp.201–10; Widdess, J. D. H., *A history of the Royal College of Physicians of Ireland, 1654–1963* (1963); and Widdess, J. D. H., 'Medical libraries in the Republic of Ireland', *Libri*, 3 (1954) pp.81–7.

40. Widdess, J. D. H., *A Dublin school of medicine and surgery. An account of the Schools of Surgery, Royal College of Surgeons, Dublin, 1789–1948* (1949).

41. Hahn, André *et al.*, *L'Histoire de la médecine et du livre médical à la lumière des collections de la Bibliothèque de la Faculté de Médecine de Paris* (1962); see also Hahn, André, 'History of the Library of the Faculté de Médecine, Paris', *Histoire de la Médecine*, 4 (1954) pp.8–20.

42. Hahn, André and Paule Dumaître, 'Les manuscrits à la bibliothèque de la Faculté de Médecine de Paris', *Sem. Hôp. Paris*, 30 (1954) pp.4447–54. Hahn, André and Paule Dumaître, 'Les incunabules médicaux de la bibliothèque de la Faculté de Médecine de Paris', *Sem. Hôp. Paris*, 25 (1949) pp.4001–9.

43. Genty, Maurice and Geneviève Nicole-Genty, 'Les incunabules de l'Académie de Médecine', *Presse Méd.*, 63 (1955) pp.1316–18; and *Libri*, 3 (1954) pp.420–2.

44. Koumans, F. P., 'Medical libraries in the Netherlands', *Bull. Med. Lib. Assn*, 42 (1954) pp.155–7.

45. Olafsson, Helen A., 'Medical libraries in Iceland', *Health Libraries Review*, 5 (1988) pp.11–15.

46. Mannelli, Maria Assunta, 'History of the library of the Faculty of Medicine and Surgery of Universita degli Studi in Florence', *Bull. Med. Lib. Assn*, 52 (1964) pp.575–8.

47. Bloomquist, H., 'The status and needs of medical school libraries in the United States', *J. Med. Educ.*, 38 (1963) pp.145–163.

48. Lyders, R. (ed.), *Annual statistics of medical school libraries in the United States and Canada 1980–81* (Houston, Assoc. of Academic Health Sciences Library Directors and Houston Academy of Medicine – Texas Medical Center Library, 1981).

49. Topper, J. M. *et al.*, 'JCAH accreditation and the hospital library: a guide for librarians', *Bull. Med. Lib. Assn*, 68 (1980) pp.212–19.

50. Titley, Joan, 'Printed catalogues of American medical libraries before 1850: a check list', *J. Hist. Med.*, 19 (1964) pp.252–3.

51. Wilson, William Jerome, 'Early plans for a national medical library', *Bull. Med. Lib. Assn*, 42 (1954) pp.426–34.

52. Schullian, D. M. and F. E. Sommer, *A catalogue of incunabula and manuscripts in the Army Medical Library* (New York [1950]).

53. Wilson, M. P. 'Implications of planning for regional libraries; our underlying philosophy', *Bull. Med. Lib. Assn*, 56 (1968) pp.46–8.

54. Department of Health & Human Services, 'Public Health Services. National Institutes of Health, National Library of Medicine. Request for Proposal NLM-82-104/JPS. Statement of Work Section IV.'

55. Walker, W. D. and K. M. Due, 'The United States', in *Medical librarianship in the eighties and beyond: a world perspective*, ed. by F. M. Picken and A. M. C. Kahn (Mansell, 1986).

56. Walker, W. D. and K. M. Due, op. cit. in note no. 55 above, p.243.

57. Walker, W. D. and K. M. Due, op. cit. in note no. 55 above, p.244.

58. Viets, Henry R. 'John Fleet and the first Boston Medical Library', *New Engl. J. Med.*, 268 (1963) pp.1254–5.

59. Ballard, James F., *A catalogue of the medieval and Renaissance manuscripts and incunabula in the Boston Medical Library*, Boston [privately printed] (1944).
60. Colby, Charles C. and Ralph T. Esterquest, 'The Francis A. Countway Library of Medicine, Harvard Medical Library–Boston Medical Library', *Bull. Med. Lib. Assn*, 48 (1960) pp.121–4.
61. Kilgour, Frederick G., *The Library of the Medical Institution of Yale College and its catalogue of 1865* (1960). See also Fulton, John F., Frederick G. Kilgour and Madeline E. Stanton, *Yale Medical Library: the formation and growth of its historical library* (New Haven, 1962) (this is a translation of 'Die medizinische Bibliothek der Universität Yale', *Librarium*, 2 (1959) pp.87–102); Kilgour, Frederick G., 'The first century of medical books in the Yale College Library', *Yale Univ. Lib. Gaz.*, 35 (1961) pp.101–5.
62. Farris, Betty R., 'The Charles F. and Olga C. Moon collection on obstetrics and gynaecology in the University of Nebraska College of Medicine Library. Introduction by C. F. Moon', *Bull. Med. Lib. Assn*, 48 (1960) pp.243–77.
63. Draper, Wesley, 'Medical libraries of New York State', *New York State Journal of Medicine*, 57 (1957) pp.584–94.
64. Doe, Janet, 'The Mallach Room', *Bull. N.Y. Acad. Med.*, 30 (1954) pp.221–22.
65. Annan, Gertrude L., 'The Fenwick Beekman Collection', *Bull. N.Y. Acad. Med.*, 37 (1961) pp.277–80.
66. Galdston, Iago, 'The New York Academy of Medicine 1847–1947', *J. Hist. Med.*, 2 (1947) pp.147–62.
67. *A catalogue of the H. Winnett Orr Historical Collection and other rare books in the Library of the American College of Surgeons* (Chicago, 1960).
68. Henkle, Herman H., 'The Medical Department of Crerar Library', *Centaur of Alpha Kappa Kappa* (1956) pp.7–12.
69. *The William H. Welch Medical Library of the Johns Hopkins University. An account of its origin and development, together with a description of the building* (Baltimore, 1930), (reprinted from the *Bulletin of the Johns Hopkins Hospital*, 46, 1930).
70. Thompson, Kathryn S., 'America's oldest medical library: the Pennsylvania Hospital', *Bull. Med. Lib. Assn*, 44 (1956) pp.428–30; Packard, Francis R., *Some accounts of the Pennsylvania Hospital from its first rise to the beginning of the year 1938* (Philadelphia, 1938) Chapter IV, pp.63–70; and Packard, Francis R., 'Early medical libraries in America, being an account of the origin and growth of the libraries of the Pennsylvania Hospital and of the College of Physicians of Philadelphia', *Med. Lib. and Hist. J.*, 5 (1907) pp.96–108.
71. A list of 409 of these is contained in: 'Census of incunabula in Library of College of Physicians of Philadelphia', *Trans. Stud. Coll. Phycns Philad.*, 6 (1938) pp.159–93.
72. Guerra, Francisco, 'The bibliography and medical libraries of Mexico', *Libri*, 3 (1954) pp.191–5.
73. Risolia, Vicente A., 'Medical libraries in the Republic of Argentina', ibid., pp.130–3.
74. Sanchez Carvajal, M. A., 'Los libros viejos y raros de la Bibliotheca de la Sociedad de Obstetricia y Ginecologia de Venezuela', *Rev. Obstet. Ginec. (Caracas)*, 14 (1954) pp.495–574; *Rev. Obstet. Ginec. de Venezuela*, 22 (1962) pp.11–68.
75. Gandevia, Bryan and Ann Tovell, 'The first Australian medical libraries', *Med. J. Australia* (1964) I, pp.314–320; Tovell, Ann, 'The first Australian medical libraries', (Corres.). *Med. J. Australia*, 52 (1965) p.947.
76. Brown, A. J., 'Medical library cooperation in Melbourne, Australia. The Central Medical Library Organization', *Bull. Med. Lib. Assn*, 44 (1956) pp.110–14.
77. Gunner, Iris, 'Psychiatric library resources in Australia: a brief survey', *Australian Lib. J.*, 9 (1960) pp.171–6.
78. Simpson, Sheila R., 'Medical libraries in New South Wales', *Australian Lib. J.*, 13 (1964) pp.199–208.
79. Russell, K. F., *British anatomy, 1525–1900. A bibliography* (1963); Tovell, Ann and Bryan Gandevia, 'Early Australian medical associations', *Med. J. Australia* (1962) I, pp.756–9.
80. Lloyd, Judith, 'Medical libraries in S. Australia', *Australian Lib. J.*, 18 (1969) pp.175–8.
81. Erlam, H. D., 'University of Otago Medical School Library', *New Zealand Libraries*, 19

(1956) pp.120–5; Erlam, H. D., 'The history of medical librarianship in New Zealand', *Libri*, 3 (1954) pp.196–203.

82. Mosley, Isobel, *Medical and health library resources and services in New Zealand, in medical and biological libraries in Asia/Oceania* (Tokyo, IFLA Section of Biological and Medical Sciences Libraries, 1986).

83. Musiker, R., *Medical libraries in comparison to South African libraries* (1986).

84. Cannon, D. A., 'The development of medical library facilities in Nigeria', *Libri*, 3 (1954) pp.184–7.

Bibliography

The bibliography below is not intended to be comprehensive but is restricted to the general histories consulted. Only a selection of the bibliographies and catalogues mentioned in the book are included here. Books are published in London unless otherwise indicated. The arrangement is based on the order adopted in the book and is as follows:

General information sources
Biography
Medical history – general
Ancient and medieval
Incunabula and other early printed books
Sixteenth to nineteenth centuries
Herbals and medical botany
Book illustration
Periodicals
Private libraries
Institutional libraries
Medical societies

General information sources
Bibliotheca Osleriana: a catalogue of books illustrating the history of medicine and science (1929).
Brodman, E., *The development of medical bibliography*, [n.p.] (1954) (Medical Library Association Publication, No. 1; reprinted 1981).
Corsi, P. and P. Weindling (eds), *Information sources in the history of science and medicine* (1983).
Dannatt, R. J., 'Primary sources of information', in L. T. Morton and S. Godbolt (eds), *Information sources in the medical sciences*, 3rd edn (1984) pp. 17–43.
Fulton, J. F., *The great medical bibliographers: a study in humanism* (Philadelphia, 1951).
Garrison, F. H., *An introduction to the history of medicine: with a medical chronology, suggestions for study and bibliographic data ...*, 4th edn (Philadelphia and London, 1929, reprinted 1960).
Guerra, F., 'Some bibliographers of early medical Americana', *J.Hist.Med.*, 17 (1962) pp. 94–115.
McGrew, R. E., *Encyclopedia of medical history* (1985).

Malclès, L. N., *Les sources du travail bibliographique*, 3 vols in 4 (Geneva and Paris, 1950–8) (vol. 3, Sciences exactes et techniques).

Monfalcon, J. B., *Précis de l'histoire de la médecine et de bibliographie médicale* (Paris, 1826).

Morton, L. T. (comp.), *Garrison and Morton's Medical bibliography: an annotated check-list of texts illustrating the history of medicine*, 4th edn (1983).

Power, Sir D'Arcy, *The foundations of medical history* (Baltimore, 1931).

Power, Sir D'Arcy and C. J. S. Thompson, *Chronologia medica: a handlist of persons, periods and events in the history of medicine* (1923).

Sheehy, E. P., *Guide to reference books*, 9th edn. (Chicago, 1976) (Supplement, 1980).

Thornton, J. L. and R. I. J. Tully, *Scientific books, libraries and collectors*, 3rd rev. edn (1971) (Supplement, 1976).

Viets, H. R., 'The bibliography of medicine', *Bull.Med.Lib.Assn*, 27 (1958) pp. 105–17.

Walford, A. J., *Walford's guide to reference material*, 4th edn. 3 vols, (1980–6) (Vol. 1, Science and technology).

Biography

Bailey, H. and W. J. Bishop, *Notable names in medicine and surgery*, 3rd edn (1959).

Dictionary of scientific biography, ed. C. C. Gillispie, 16 vols (New York, 1970–80).

Gascoigne, R. M., *A historical catalogue of scientists and scientific books, from the earliest times to the close of the nineteenth century* (New York, 1984).

Greenwood, M., *Some British pioneers of social medicine* (1948).

Hirsch, A. (ed.), *Biographisches Lexikon der hervorragenden Ärzte aller Zeiten und Völker*, 2nd edn. 5 vols (Berlin, 1929–35, reprinted, with additions, 1970).

Jacquart, D., *Dictionnaire biographique* ... (see Wickersheimer, E., below).

McMichael, W., *The gold-headed cane*, 2nd edn (1828).

Morton, L. T. and R. J. Moore (comps), *A bibliography of medical and biomedical biography*, Aldershot, 1989.

Osler, Sir William (ed.), *Great men of Guy's* (Metuchen, NJ, 1973).

Power, Sir D'Arcy (ed.), *British masters of medicine* (1936).

Sigerist, H. E., *Great doctors: a biographical history of medicine* (1933).

Talbot, C. H. and E. A. Hammond, *The medical practitioners of mediaeval England* (1965).

Wickersheimer, E., *Dictionnaire biographique des médecins en France au moven âge*, 2 vols (Paris, 1936) (Supplement by D. Jacquart, Geneva, 1979).

Medical history – general

Ackerknecht, E. H., *A short history of medicine* (New York, 1955).

Brock, T. D. (translator and ed.), *Milestones in microbiology* (1961).

Brown, A., *Old masterpieces in surgery: being a collection of thoughts and observations engendered by a perusal of some of the works of our forbears in surgery* (Omaha, NE, 1928, based on articles published in *Surg.Gynec.Obstet.*).

Bynum, W. F., R. Porter and M. Shepherd (eds), *The anatomy of madness* ..., 3 vols (1985–8).

Castiglione, A., *A history of medicine. Translated from the Italian and edited by E. B. Krumbhaar* (New York, 1946).

Cole, F. J., *A history of comparative anatomy, from Aristotle to the eighteenth century* (1944).

Elgood, C., *A medical history of Persia and the Eastern Caliphate from the earliest times until the year A.D. 1932* (Cambridge, 1951).

Friedenwald, H., *The Jews and medicine*, 2 vols (Baltimore, 1944).

Grainger, T. H., *A guide to the history of bacteriology* (New York, 1958).

Guthrie, D., *A history of medicine* ... (1958).

Hall, T. S., *Ideas of life and matter: studies in the history of general physiology*, 2 vols (Chicago, 1969).

Hoeppli, R., *Parasites and parasitic infections in early medicine and science* (Singapore, 1959).

Howard-Jones, N., 'Our medical literature – then and now', *Br.J.Med. Educ.*, 7 (1973) pp. 70–85.

Huard, P. and M. Wong, *La médecine chinoise au cours des siècles* (Paris, 1959).

Keys, T. E., *The history of surgical anaesthesia* ... (New York, 1945, revised reprint, 1963).

Krumbhaar, E. B., 'The early history of anatomy in the United States', *Ann.Med.Hist.*, 4 (1922) pp. 271–86.

Major, R. H., *Classic descriptions of disease, with biographical sketches of the authors*, 3rd edn (1945, frequently reprinted).

Major, R. H., *A history of medicine*, 2 vols (Springfield, Ill., 1954).

Needham, J., *A history of embryology*, 2nd edn rev. (Cambridge, 1959).

Osler, Sir William, *The evolution of modern medicine: a series of lectures delivered at Yale University in April 1913* (New Haven, Conn. and London, 1921).

Parker, G., *The early history of surgery in Great Britain: its organization and development* (1920).

Power, Sir D'Arcy, 'The beginnings of the literary renaissance of surgery in England', *Proc.Roy.Soc.Med.*, 22 (1929) pp. 77–82.

Power, Sir D'Arcy, *A short history of surgery* (1933).

Power, Sir D'Arcy, *A mirror for surgeons: selected readings in surgery* (Boston, 1939).

Ricci, J. V., *The genealogy of gynaecology: history of the development of gynaecology throughout the ages, 2000 B.C. – 1800 A.D.*, 2nd edn, enlarged and revised (Philadelphia and Toronto, 1950).

Science, medicine and history, see Underwood, E. A. below.

Sigerist, H. E., *American medicine* (New York, 1934).

Sigerist, H. E., *A history of medicine*, 2 vols (New York, 1951–61).

Singer, C., *The evolution of anatomy: a short history of anatomical and physiological discovery to Harvey* (1925).

Singer, C. and E. A. Underwood, *A short history of medicine*, 2nd edn (Oxford, 1962).

South, J. F., *Memorials of the craft of surgery in England … Edited by D'Arcy Power* (1886).

Spencer, H. R., 'Lloyd Roberts Lecture: the renaissance of midwifery', *Trans.Med.Soc.Lond.*, 48 (1925) pp. 71–105 (also published separately).

Still, Sir George Frederic, *The history of paediatrics: the progress of the study of diseases of children up to the end of the XVIIIth century* (1931, reprinted 1965).

Thorndike, L., *A history of magic and experimental science*, 6 vols (New York, 1923–41).

Underwood, E. A. (ed.), *Science, medicine and history: essays on the evolution of scientific thought and medical practice, written in honour of Charles Singer*, 2 vols (1953).

Ancient and medieval

Baader, G. and G. Keil, *Medizin im mittelalterlichen Abendland* (Darmstadt, 1982) (Wege der Forschung, 363).

Ballard, J. F., 'Medieval manuscripts and early printed books illustrating the evolution of the medical book from 1250–1550 A.D.', *Bull.Med.Lib.Assn*, 23 (1935) pp. 173–88.

Ballard, J. F., 'Demonstration of manuscripts and printed books of the late Middle Ages and the early Renaissance', *Bull.Med.Lib.Assn*, 27 (1938) pp. 165–77.

Beccaria, A., *I codici di medicina del periodo presalernitano, secoli IX, X, e XI* (Rome, 1956).

Bonsor, W., *The medical background of Anglo-Saxon England: a study in history, psychology and folklore* (1963), (Publications of the Wellcome Historical Medical Library, N.S.III).

Campbell, D., *Arabian medicine and its influence on the Middle Ages*, 2 vols (1926).

Cockayne, O., *Leechdoms, wort-cunning and starcraft of early England, being a collection of documents, for the most part never before printed, illustrating the history of science in this country before the Norman Conquest*, 3 vols (1864–66, reprinted 1961).

Corbett, J. A., *Catalogue des manuscrits alchimiques latins*, 2 vols (Brussels, 1939, 1951).

Corner, G. W., *Anatomical texts of the earlier middle ages: a study in the transmission of culture* (Washington, 1927).

Diels, H., *Die Handschriften der antiken Ärzte*, 2 vols (Leipzig, 1905–7, reprinted 1970).

Dunlop, D. M., 'Arabic medicine in England', *J.Hist.Med.*, 11 (1956) pp. 166–82.

Durling, R. J., 'Medico-historical research in medieval and renaissance manuscripts', in P. M. Teigen (ed.), *Books, manuscripts and the history of medicine: essays on the fiftieth anniversary of the Osler Library* (New York, 1982) pp. 31–43.

Durling, R. J., 'A guide to the medical manuscripts mentioned in Kristeller's "Iter Italicum" III', *Traditio*, 41 (1985) pp. 341–65.

Gratton, J. H. G. and C. Singer, *Anglo-Saxon magic and medicine: illustrated specially from the semi-pagan text 'Lacnunga' ...* (1952).

Grmek, M. D., *Recueil d'anciens manuscrits relatifs à la médecine, aux mathématiques, à la physique, à l'astronomie, à la chimie et aux sciences naturelles, conservés en Croatie et en Slovénie* (Zagreb, 1963).

Halleux, R., *Les textes alchimiques* (Turnhout, 1979) (Typologie des sources du moyen âge occidental, 32).

Haskins, C. H., *Studies in the history of mediaeval science* (Cambridge, Mass., 1927, reprinted New York, 1960).

Jones, W. H. S., 'Philosophy and medicine in ancient Greece', *Bull. Hist.Med.*, Supplement No. 8 (1946) (whole issue).

Kollesch, J., 'Papyri mit medizinischen, naturwissenschaftlichen und mathematischen Texten', *Archiv für Papyrusforschung*, 26 (1978) pp. 141–8.

Kristeller, P.O., *Iter Italicum: a finding list of uncatalogued or incompletely catalogued humanistic manuscripts of the renaissance in Italian and other libraries*, 3 vols so far (London and Leiden, 1963–83).

Lawn, B., *The Salernitan questions: an introduction to the history of medieval and renaissance problem literature* (Oxford, 1963).

Lindberg, D. C. (ed.), *Science in the middle ages* (Chicago, 1978).

MacKinney, L. C. and T. Herndon, 'American manuscript collections of medieval medical miniatures and texts', *J.Hist.Med.*, 17 (1962) pp. 284–307.

Marganne, M. H., *Inventaire analytique des papyrus grecs de médecine* (Geneva, 1981).

Moore, Sir Norman, 'The Schola Salernitana: its history and the date of its introduction into the British Isles', *Glasgow Med.J.*, 69 (1908) pp. 241–68.

Payne, J. F., *The Fitz-Patrick Lectures for 1903: English medicine in the Anglo-Saxon times ...* (Oxford, 1904).

Riesman, D., *The story of medicine in the middle ages* (New York, 1935).

Robbins, R. H., 'Medical manuscripts in Middle English', *Speculum*, 45 (1970) pp. 393–415.

Russell, J. C., 'Medical writers of thirteenth-century England', *Ann.Med. Hist.*, N.S.7 (1935) pp. 327–40.

Sarton, G., *Introduction to the history of sciences*, 3 vols (Washington, 1927–48).

Schumacher, J., *Antike Medizin: die naturphilosophischen Grundlagen der Medizin in der grieschen Antike*, 2nd edn. (Berlin, 1963).

Sigerist, H. E., *Studien und Texte zur frühmittelalterlichen Rezeptliteratur* (Leipzig, 1923) (Studien zur Geschichte der Medizin, 13, reprinted Liechtenstein, 1977).

Sigerist, H. E., 'The Latin medical literature of the early middle ages', *J.Hist.Med.*, 13 (1958) pp. 127–46.

Singer, D. W., 'A review of the literature of the Dark Ages, with a text of about 1110', *Proc.Roy.Soc.Med.*, 10 (1917) Section of Hist. of Med., pp. 107–60.

Singer, D. W., 'Survey of medical manuscripts in the British Isles dating before the sixteenth century', *Proc.Roy.Soc.Med.*, 12 (1918–19) Section of the Hist. of Med., pp. 96–107.

Singer, D. W. and A. Anderson, *Catalogue of Latin and vernacular alchemical manuscripts in Great Britain and Ireland dating from before the XVIth century*, 3 vols (Brussels, 1928–31).

Singer, D. W. and A. Anderson, *Catalogue of Latin and vernacular plague tracts in Great Britain and Eire in manuscripts written before the sixteenth century* (Paris and London, 1950).

Sudhoff, K., 'Pestschriften aus den ersten 150 Jahren nach der Epidemie des "schwartzen Todes" 1348', *Archiv für Geschichte der Medizin*, 5 (1911) pp. 36–87.

Voigts, L. E., 'Editing Middle English medical texts: needs and issues', in T. H. Levere (ed.), *Editing texts in the history of science and medicine* (New York, 1982), pp. 39–68.

Voigts, L. E., 'Scientific and medical books', in J. Griffiths (ed.), *Book production and publishing in Britain, 1375–1475* (Cambridge, 1989).

Wickersheimer, E., *Les manuscrits latins de médecine du haut moyen âge dans les bibliothèques de France* (Paris, 1966).

Wilson, W. J., 'Catalogue of Latin and vernacular alchemical manuscripts in the United States and Canada', *Osiris*, 6 (1939) pp. 1–836.

Incunabula and other early printed books

Ballard, J. F., 'Medical incunabula in the William Norton Bullard Collection', *Boston Med.Surg.J.*, 196 (1927) pp. 865–75.

Ballard, J. F., 'Medieval manuscripts and early printed books illustrating the evolution of the medical book from 1250–1550 A.D.', *Bull.Med.Lib.Assn*, 23 (1935) pp. 173–88.

Ballard, J. F., 'Demonstration of manuscripts and printed books of the late Middle Ages and the early Renaissance', *Bull.Med.Lib.Assn*, 27 (1938) pp. 165–77.

Buhler, C. F., 'Scientific and medical incunabula in American libraries', *Isis*, 35 (1944) pp. 173–5.

Buhler, C. F., *The fifteenth century book. The scribes, the printers, the decorators* (Philadelphia, 1960).

Chance, B., 'Early printing of medical books and some of the printers who printed them', *Bull.Hist.Med.*, 22 (1948) pp. 647–63.

Cowlishaw, L., 'Some early printed books: their authors and printers', *Med.J.Australia* (1926) II, pp. 77–81.

Dox, I., 'Medical incunabula', *Med. Heritage*, 1 (1985) pp. 121–6.

Duff., E. G., *Fifteenth-century English books: a bibliography of books and documents printed in England, and of books for the English market printed abroad* (Oxford, 1917) (Bibliographical Society, Illustrated Monographs, No. 18).

Goff, F. R. (ed.), *Incunabula in American libraries: third census* (New York, 1964, reprinted Millwood, N.Y., 1973. Supplement, New York, 1972).

Haebler, K., *Hundert Kalendar–Inkunabeln* (Strasbourg, 1905).

Heitz, P. and W. S. Schreiber, *Pestblätter des XV. Jahrhunderts* (Strasbourg, 1901).

Keys, T. E., 'The earliest medical books printed with movable type: a review', *Lib.Quart.*, 10 (1940) pp. 220–30.

Klebs, A. C., 'Incunabula scientifica et medica: short title list', *Osiris*, 4 (1938) pp. 1–359 (reprinted Hildesheim, 1963).

Osler, Sir William, *Incunabula medica* (1923).

Peddie, R. A., *Fifteenth-century books: a guide to their identification. With a list of the Latin names of towns, and an extensive bibliography of the subject* (1913).

Singer, D. W., 'Some plague tractates (fourteenth and fifteenth centuries)', *Proc.Roy.Soc.Med.*, 9 (1916) Section of Hist. of Med., pp. 159–212.

'Some early printed books: their authors and printers', *Med.J.Australia* (1926) II, pp. 77–81.

Stillwell, M. B. (ed.), *Incunabula in American libraries: second census of fifteenth-century books owned in the United States, Mexico and Canada* (New York, 1940).

Stillwell, M. B., *The awakening interest in science during the first century of printing, 1450–1550: an annotated checklist of first editions viewed from the angle of their subject content* (New York, 1970).

Sudhoff, K., *The earliest printed literature on syphilis; being ten tractates from the years 1495–1498. In complete facsimile, with an introduction and other accessory material by Karl Sudhoff, adapted by Charles Singer* (Florence, 1925) (Monumenta Medica, 3).

Sixteenth to nineteenth centuries

Abraham, J. J., 'The early history of syphilis', *Br.J.Surg.*, 32 (1944–5) pp. 225–37.

Annan, G. L., 'Medical Americana', *J.Amer.Med.Assn*, 192 (1965) pp. 139–44.

Austin, R. B., *Early American imprints: a guide to works published in the United States, 1668–1820* (Washington, 1961).

Bennett, H. S., *English books and readers, 1475–1557: being a study in the history of the book trade from Caxton to the incorporation of the Stationers' Company*, 2nd rev. edn (Cambridge, 1969).

Billings, J. S., 'Literature and institutions', in E. H. Clarke *et al.*, *A century of American medicine, 1776–1876* (Philadelphia, 1876) pp. 291–366.

Boas, M., *The scientific renaissance, 1450–1630* (1962).

Brown, J. R. and J. L. Thornton, 'Physiology before William Harvey', *St Bart's Hosp.J.*, 63 (1959) pp. 116–24.

Colebrook, L., 'The story of puerperal fever, 1800–1950', *Br.Med.J.*, (1956) I, pp. 247–52.

Cope, Sir Vincent Zachary, 'The evolution of anatomy and surgery under the Tudors. Thomas Vicary Lecture delivered at the Royal College of Surgeons of England on 25th October, 1962', *Ann.Roy.Coll.Surg. Engl.*, 32 (1963) pp. 1–21.

Copeman, P. W. M. and W. S. C. Copeman, 'Dermatology in Tudor and early Stuart England', *Br.J.Derm.*, 82 (1970) pp. 78–88, 182–91.

Coury, C., 'La méthode anatomo-clinique et ses promoteurs en France: Corvisart, Bayle et Laënnec', *Méd. de France*, 224 (1971) pp. 13–22.

Debus, A. G., 'The Paracelsians and the Chemists: the chemical dilemma in Renaissance medicine', *Clio Med.*, 7, (1972) pp. 185–99.

Debus, A. G. (ed.), *Science, medicine and society in the Renaissance: essays to honor Walter Pagel*, 2 vols (1972).

Debus, A. G., 'The chemical philosophers: chemical medicine from Paracelsus to Van Helmont', *Hist.Sci.*, 12 (1974) pp. 235–59.

Doetsch, R. N. (ed.), *Microbiology: historical contributions from 1776 to 1908 by Spallanzani, Schwann, Pasteur, Cohn, Tyndall, Koch, Lister, Schloesing, Burrill, Ehrlich, Winogradsky, Warington, Beijerinck, Smith, Orla-Jensen* (New Brunswick, NJ, 1960).

Durling, R., 'Some unrecorded English versions of foreign seventeenth–eighteenth-century works', *Med.Hist.*, 5 (1961) pp. 396–401.

Eamon, W., 'Arcana disclosed: the advent of printing, the books of secrets tradition and the development of experimental science in the sixteenth century', *Hist.Sci.*, 22 (1984) pp. 111–50.

Eccles, A., 'The reading public, the medical profession and the use of

English for medical books in the 16th and 17th centuries', *New-philol.-Mitt.*, 75 (1974) pp. 143–56.

Eisenstein, E., *The printing press as an agent of change*, 2 vols (Cambridge, 1979).

Fye, W. B., 'The literature of American internal medicine: a historical review', *Ann.Intern.Med.*, 106 (1987) pp. 451–60.

Hall, A. R., *From Galileo to Newton, 1630–1720* (1963).

Hunter, M., *Science and society in Restoration England* (Cambridge, 1981).

Keevil, J. J., 'The seventeenth-century English medical background', *Bull.Hist.Med.*, 31 (1957) pp. 408–24.

Keys, T. E., 'Some American medical imprints of the nineteenth century', *Bull.Med.Lib.Assn*, 45 (1957) pp. 309–18.

Lesch, J. E., *Science and medicine in France: the emergence of experimental physiology, 1790–1855* (Cambridge, Mass. and London, 1984).

Lind, L. R., *Studies in pre-Vesalian anatomy. Biography, translations, documents* (Philadelphia, 1975) (Memoirs of the American Philosophical Society, 104).

Malloch, A., 'Certain old American medical works', *Bull.N.Y. Acad.Med.*, 2nd ser. (1936) pp. 545–65.

Olmsted, J. M. D., 'French contributions to physiology in the XIX century', *Texas Rep.Biol.Med.*, 13 (1955) pp. 306–16.

O'Malley, C. D., 'Tudor medicine and biology', *Huntington Lib.Quart.*, 32 (1968) pp. 1–27.

Pelling, M., *Cholera, fever and English medicine, 1825–1865* (Oxford, 1978).

Rath, G., 'Pre-Vesalian anatomy in the light of modern research', *Bull.-Hist.Med.*, 35 (1961) pp. 142–8.

Reiser, S. J., *Medicine and the reign of technology* (Cambridge, 1978).

Russell, K. F., *British anatomy, 1525–1800*, revised and enlarged edn., (Winchester, 1986).

Shaftel, N., 'The evolution of American medical literature', *Int.Rec.Med.*, 71 (1958) pp. 431–54.

Shirley, J. W. and F. D. Hoeniger (eds), *Science and the arts in the Renaissance* (Cranbury, NJ, 1985).

Singer, C., *The evolution of anatomy: a short history of anatomy and physiological discovery to Harvey. Being the substance of the Fitzpatrick Lectures delivered at the Royal College of Physicians of London in the years 1923 and 1924* (1925).

Slack, P., 'Mirrors of health and treasures of poor men: the uses of the vernacular medical literature of Tudor England', in C. Webster (ed.), *Health, medicine and mortality in the sixteenth century* (Cambridge, 1979), pp. 237–73.

Spencer, H. R., *The history of British midwifery from 1650–1800. The Fitz-*

Patrick Lectures for 1927 delivered before the Royal College of Physicians of London (1927).

Thornton, J. L., 'British medical publishers, 1868–1968', *Practitioner*, 201 (1968) pp. 231–7.

Viets, H. R., 'The first American medical publications', *New England J.Med.*, 268 (1963) pp. 600–1.

Walsh, M. N., 'Medical printers of the Renaissance', *Prof.Staff Mtgs Mayo Clin.*, 14 (1939) pp. 582–7.

Wear, A., R. K. French and M. Lonie, *The medical Renaissance of the sixteenth century* (Cambridge, 1985).

Webster, C. (ed.), *The intellectual revolution of the seventeenth century* (1974).

Webster, C., *The Great Instauration: science, medicine and reform, 1626–1660* (New York, 1976).

Webster, C. (ed.), *Health, medicine and mortality in the sixteenth century* (Cambridge, 1979).

Webster, C., *From Paracelsus to Newton: magic and the making of modern science* (Cambridge, 1982).

Wightman, W. P. D., *Science in a Renaissance society* (London, 1972).

Herbals and medical botany

Anderson, F. J., *An illustrated history of the herbals* (New York, 1977).

Arber, A., *Herbals, their origin and evolution in the history of botany, 1470–1670*, new edn (Cambridge, 1938).

Arber, A., 'From medieval herbalism to the birth of modern botany', *Science, medicine and history*, 1 (1953) pp. 317–36.

Barlow, H. M., 'Old English herbals, 1525–1640', *Proc.Roy.Soc.Med.*, 6 (1913) Section of Hist. of Med., pp. 108–49.

Palmer, R., 'Medical botany in northern Italy in the Renaissance', *J.Roy.-Soc.Med.*, 78 (1985) pp. 149–57.

Payne, J. F., 'English herbals', *Trans.Bib.Soc.*, 9 (1906–8) pp. 120–3; 11 (1909–11) pp. 299–310.

Rohde, E. S., *The old English herbals* (New York, 1922).

Singer, C., 'The herbal in antiquity', *J.Hellenic Studies*, 47 (1927) pp. 1–52.

Stannard, J., 'Medieval herbals and their development', *Clio Med.*, 9 (1974) pp. 23–33.

Book illustration

Audette, L. G., 'Stylism in anatomical illustration from the sixteenth to the twentieth centuries', *J.Biocommunication*, 6 (1979) pp. 24–9, 34–7.

Blunt, W., *The art of botanical illustration* ... (1950).

Choulant, L., *History and bibliography of anatomic illustration in its rela-*

tion to anatomic science and the graphic arts ..., rev. edn (New York and London, 1945, reprinted 1962).

Coleman, R. B., 'Illustration of human anatomy before Vesalius', *Surg. Gynec.Obstet.*, 90 (1950) pp. 500–7.

Garrison, F. H., *The principles of anatomic illustration before Vesalius: an inquiry into the rationale of artistic anatomy* (New York, 1926).

Herrlinger, R., *History of medical illustration from antiquity to A.D. 1600* (1970).

Hind, A. M., *A history of engraving and etching*, 3rd rev. edn (New York, 1923).

Hind, A. M., *Engraving in England in the sixteenth and seventeenth centuries* (Cambridge, 1952).

Jones, T. S., 'The story of medical illustration', *J.Internat.Coll.Surg.*, 32 (1959) pp. 697–707.

LeFanu, W. R., 'Some English illustrated medical books', *Book Collector*, 21 (1972) pp. 19–28.

Loechel, W. E., 'The history of medical illustration', *Bull.Med.Lib.Assn*, 48 (1960) pp. 168–71.

MacKinney, L. C., 'Medical illustration, ancient and medieval', *CIBA Symposium*, 10 (1949) pp. 1062–71.

MacKinney, L. C., *Medical illustrations in medieval manuscripts* ... (1965).

Putscher, M., *Geschichte der medizinischen Abbildung, von 1600 bis zur Gegenwart* (Munich, 1972).

Reeves, C., 'Illustrations of medicine in ancient Egypt', *J.Audiovisual Media in Med.*, 3 (1980) pp. 4–13.

Rollins, C. P., 'Illustration in printed medical books', *CIBA Symposium*, 10 (1949) pp. 1072–86.

Thornton, J. L. and C. Reeves, *Medical book illustration: a short history* (Cambridge, 1983).

Weindler, F., *Geschichte der gynäkologisch-anatomischen Abbildungen* (Dresden, 1908).

Wells, E. B., 'Medical illustration and book decoration in the 18th century', *Med.Biol.Ill.*, 20 (1970) pp. 78–84.

Wells, E. B., 'Graphic techniques of medical illustration in the 18th century', *J.Biocommunication*, 3 (1976) pp. 24–7.

Periodicals

Armstrong, J. M., 'The first American journals', in *Lectures on the history of medicine: a series of lectures at the Mayo Foundation* (Philadelphia, 1933) pp. 357–69.

Baird, V. M., 'Nineteenth-century medical journalism in Texas; with a journal checklist', *Bull.Med.Lib.Assn*, 60 (1972) pp. 375–81.

Berry, E. M., 'The evolution of scientific and medical journals', *New Eng.J.Med.*, 305 (1981) pp. 400–2.

Booth, C. C., 'Medical communications: the old and the new. The development of medical journals in Britain', *Br.Med.J.*, 285 (1982) pp. 105–8.

Brockbank, W., 'The history and present state of provincial medical journalism', *Lancet* (1953) I, pp. 433–5.

Brodman, E., 'Medical periodicals', *Lib.Trends*, 10 (1961–2) pp. 381–9.

Cassedy, J. H., 'The flourishing and character of early American medical journalism, 1797–1860', *J.Hist.Med.*, 38 (1983) pp. 135–50.

Chernin, E., 'A worm's eye view of biomedical journals', *Fed.Proc.*, 34 (1975) pp. 124–30.

Coggins, C. C., 'Medical articles in eighteenth-century American magazines', *Bull.Med.Lib.Assn*, 53 (1965) pp. 426–37.

Cumpston, J. H. L., 'The history of medical journalism in Australia', *Med.J.Australia* (1939) II, pp. 1–5.

Desjardins, E., 'La petite histoire du journalisme médical au Canada', *Union Médicale du Canada*, 101 (1972) pp. 121–30, 309–14, 511–18, 1190–6.

Ebert, M., 'The rise and development of the American medical periodical, 1797–1850', *Bull.Med.Lib.Assn*, 40 (1952) pp. 243–76.

Gandevia, B., 'A review of Victoria's early medical journals', *Med.J.Australia* (1952) II, pp. 184–8.

Garrison, F. H., 'The medical and scientific periodicals of the 17th and 18th centuries. With a revised catalogue and check-list', *Bull.Inst. Hist.Med.*, 2 (1934) pp. 285–343.

Gascoigne, R. M., *A historical catalogue of scientific periodicals, 1665–1900, with a survey of their development* (New York, 1985).

King, L. S., 'Medical journalism, 1847–1983', *J.Amer.Med.Assn*, 250 (1983) pp. 744–8.

Kronick, D. A., 'The Fielding H. Garrison list of medical and scientific periodicals of the 17th and 18th centuries; addenda and corrigenda', *Bull.Hist.Med.*, 32 (1958) pp. 456–74.

Kronick, D. A., *A history of scientific and technical periodicals: the origins and development of the scientific and technological press, 1665–1790*, 2nd edn (Metuchen, NJ, 1976).

LeFanu, W. R., *British medical periodicals: a chronological list, 1640–1899*, rev. edn (Oxford, 1984) (Wellcome Unit for the History of Medicine, Research Publications, No. 6).

Lévy-Valensi, J., 'Les origines de la presse médicale française', *Presse Méd.* (1936) II, pp. 2124–5.

Lévy-Valensi, J., 'Histoire de la presse médicale française', *Presse Méd.* (1938) II, pp. 1229–30.

Lopez Piñero, J. M. and M. L. Terrada, 'Las etapas históricas del periodismo médico en España: estudio bibliométrico', *Med. Esp.*, 78 (1979) pp. 95–108.

354 *Thornton's medical books, libraries and collectors*

Luketic, V., 'Early medical journals in Alabama', *Alabama J.Med.Sci.*, 6 (1969) pp. 422–4.

Neelameghan, A., *Development of medical societies and medical periodicals in India, 1780 to 1920* (Calcutta, 1963).

Olschner, K., 'Medical journals in Louisiana before the Civil War', *Bull.-Med.Lib.Assn*, 60 (1972) pp. 1–13.

Onodera, S., 'Past and present of Japanese medical journals', *Bull.Med. Lib. Assn*, 46 (1958) pp. 73–81, 320–34.

Pizer, I. H. and H. Steuernagel, 'Medical journals in St. Louis before 1900 ...', *Bull.Missouri Hist.Soc.* (April 1964) pp. 221–56.

Porter, J. R., 'The scientific journal – 300th anniversary', *Bact.Rev.*, 28 (1964) pp. 211–30.

Robinson, V., 'The early medical journals of America founded during the quarter-century 1797–1822', *Med.Life*, 36 (1929) pp. 553–85.

Rogal, S., 'A checklist of medical journals published in England during the seventeenth, eighteenth and nineteenth centuries', *Br.Stud.Monitor*, 9 (1980) pp. 3–25.

Roland, C. G., 'Canadian medical journalism in the 19th century', *Canadian Med.Assn J.*, 128 (1983) pp. 449–51, 454–5, 458–9.

Runge, E., 'Aus dem Anfängen des deutschen medizinischen Zeitschriftenwesens', *Med.Welt* (1937) II, pp. 950–2, 984–6, 1019–22.

Senadhira, M. A. P., 'The development of scientific journalism in Sri Lanka', in Corea, I. (ed.), *Libraries and people: Colombo public libraries, 1925–1975* (Colombo, 1975) pp. 261–70.

Shadrake, A. M., 'British medical periodicals, 1938–1961', *Bull.Med. Lib.Assn*, 51 (1963) pp. 181–96.

Shafer, H. B., 'Early medical magazines in America', *Ann.Med.Hist.*, N.S.7 (1935) pp. 480–91.

Shultz, S. M. and M. S. Wood, 'Medical journals of Pennsylvania before the Civil War', *Trans.Stud.Coll.Phycns Philad.*, ser. 5, 5 (1983) pp. 244–70.

Snorrason, E., 'Danish physicians and the periodicals of the seventeenth and eighteenth centuries', *Danish Med.Bull*, 5 (1958) pp. 200–9.

'South African medical journals', *S.Afr.Med.J.*, 30 (1956) pp. 311–12, 337–8.

Stieg, M. F., *The origin and development of scholarly historical periodicals* (Tuscaloosa, AL, 1986).

Taniguchi, M., 'An analysis of Japanese medical periodicals', *Bull.Med. Lib.Assn*, 53 (1965) pp. 43–51.

Thomas, M. R., 'Early medical journals of North Carolina', *North Carolina Lib.*, 21 (1962) pp. 4–7.

Winton, R., 'Medical journalism in Australia and New Zealand', *Med. J.Australia* (1961) I, pp. 723–6.

Private libraries

Bishop, W. J., 'Some medical bibliophiles and their libraries', *J.Hist.Med.*, 3 (1948) pp. 229–62.

De Ricci, S., *English collectors of books and manuscripts (1530–1930) and their marks of ownership* (Cambridge, 1930).

Eales, N. B., 'On the provenance of some early medical and biological books', *J.Hist.Med.*, 24 (1969) pp. 183–92.

Elton, C. I. and M. A. Elton, *The great book-collectors* (1893).

Emden, A. B., *A biographical register of the University of Oxford, A.D. 1501 to 1540* (Oxford, 1974) (includes transcripts of book-lists of private collectors).

Fletcher, W. Y., *English book collectors* (1902).

Goldschmidt, E. P., 'Hieronymus Muenzer and other fifteenth-century bibliophiles', *Bull.N.Y.Acad.Med.*, 14 (1938) pp. 496–508.

Henkle, H. H., 'The physician as book collector: notes on famous libraries', *J.Internat.Coll.Surg.*, 34 (1960) pp. 107–17.

Herrlinger, R., 'Über die Bibliophilie der Ärzte', *Librarium*, 2 (1959) pp. 68–74.

Keys, T. E., 'Libraries of some twentieth-century American bibliophilic physicians', *Lib.Quart.*, 24 (1954) pp. 21–34.

Keys, T. E., 'Bookmen in biology and medicine I have known', *J.Hist.Med.*, 30 (1975) pp. 326–48.

Lawler, J., *Book auctions in England in the seventeenth century (1676–1700), with a chronological list of the book auctions of the period* (1906) (first edn 1898, reprinted Detroit, 1968).

Leedham-Green, E. S., *Books in Cambridge inventories: book-lists from Vice-Chancellor's Court probate inventories in the Tudor and Stuart periods*, 2 vols (Cambridge, 1986).

Lorenz, B., 'Notizen zu Privatbibliotheken deutscher Ärzte des 15–17. Jahrhunderts', *Sudhoffs Archiv*, 67 (1983) pp. 190–8.

Lorenz, B., 'Notizen zu Privatbibliotheken deutscher Ärzte des 18–19. Jahrhunderts', ibid., 69 (1985) pp. 50–61.

Malcolm, L. W. G., 'The medical man as a collector in the seventeenth and eighteenth centuries', *Med.Life*, 42 (1935) pp. 566–620.

Palmer, W. M., 'Cambridgeshire doctors in the olden times', *Proc.Cambridge Antiquarian Soc.*, 15 (1911) pp. 200–79.

Sangwine, E., 'The private libraries of Tudor doctors', *J.Hist.Med.*, 33 (1978) pp. 167–84.

Thornton, J. L., 'St Bartholomew's Hospital, London, and its connection with eminent book collectors', *J.Hist.Med.*, 6 (1951) pp. 481–90.

Weimerskirch, P. J., 'Libraries of physicians: a review of the literature', *A B Bookman's Weekly*, 20 April 1987, pp. 1705–7.

Wells, E. B., 'Scientists' libraries: a handlist of printed sources', *Ann.Sci.*, 40 (1983) pp. 317–89 (also published separately, 1983).

Institutional libraries

Bunch, A. J., *Hospital and medical libraries in Scotland: an historical and sociological study* (Glasgow, 1975).

Cannon, D. A., 'The development of medical library facilities in Nigeria', *Libri*, 3 (1954) pp. 184–7.

Dewey, N., 'The early medical libraries of Edinburgh and Glasgow', *A B Bookman's Weekly*, 28 April 1986, pp. 1946–8.

Gandevia, B. and A. Tovell, 'The first Australian medical libraries', *Med.- J.Australia* (1964) I, pp. 314–20.

Guerra, F., 'The bibliography and medical libraries of Mexico', *Libri*, 3 (1954) pp. 191–5.

Henkle, H. H., 'The history of medical libraries in Chicago', *J.Internat. Coll.Surg.*, 40 (1963) pp. 611–19.

Humphreys, K. W., 'The medical books of the mediaeval friars', *Libri*, 3 (1954) pp. 95–103.

Koumans, F. P., 'Medical libraries in the Netherlands', *Bull.Med. Lib.Assn*, 42 (1954) pp. 155–7.

Lattimore, M. I., 'Early naval medical libraries, personal and corporate', *J.Roy.Nav.Med.Service*, 69 (1983) pp. 107–11, 156–60.

LeFanu, W. R., 'Medical libraries', in R. Irwin and R. Staveley (eds), *The libraries of London*, 2nd rev. edn (1961) pp. 302–7.

Lloyd, J., 'Medical libraries in S. Australia', *Australian Lib.J.*, 18 (1969) pp. 175–8.

Olafsson, H. A., 'Medical libraries in Iceland', *Health Lib. Rev.*, 5 (1988) pp. 11–15.

Risolia, V. A., 'Medical libraries in the Republic of Argentina', *Health Lib.Rev.*, 5 (1988) pp. 130–3.

Simpson, S. R., 'Medical libraries in New South Wales', *Australian Lib.J.*, 13 (1964) pp. 199–208.

Whitten, N. E., 'Philadelphia's medical libraries', *Bull.Med.Lib.Assn*, 53 (1965) pp. 245–51.

Widdes, J. D. H., 'Medical libraries in the Republic of Ireland', *Libri*, 3 (1954) pp. 81–7.

Medical societies

Artelt, W., 'Die medizinischen Lesegesellschaften in Deutschland', *Sudhoffs Archiv*, 37 (1953) pp. 195–200.

Barnor, M. A., 'A history of medical societies in Ghana', *Med.J.Australia*, 49, I (1962) pp. 781–2.

Batty Shaw, A., 'The oldest medical societies in Great Britain', *Med. Hist.*, 12 (1968) pp. 233–44.

Bell, W. J., 'For mutual improvement in the healing art: Philadelphia medical societies of the 18th century', *J.Amer.Med.Assn*, 216 (1971) pp. 125–9.

Bishop, W. J., 'Medical book societies in England in the eighteenth and nineteenth centuries', *Bull.Med.Lib.Assn*, 45 (1957) pp. 337–50.

Brown, H., *Scientific organizations in seventeenth century France, 1620–1680* (Baltimore, 1934).

Camp, H. M., 'Men of medicine, 1776–1976: early medical societies', *Illinois Med.J.*, 150 (1976) pp. 49–54.

Cassedy, J. H., 'Medicine and the learned society in the United States, 1660–1850', in A. Oleson and S. C. Brown, (eds.), *The pursuit of knowledge in the early American Republic* (Baltimore, 1976) pp. 261–78.

Cohen, J., C. E. M. Hansel and E. F. May, 'Natural history of learned and scientific societies', *Nature*, 173 (1954) pp. 328–33.

Conradi, E., 'Learned societies and academies in early times', *Pedagogical Seminary*, 12 (1905) pp. 384–426.

'County medical societies', *N.Y.St.J.Med.*, 76 (1976) pp. 2053–72.

Dukes, C. E., 'London medical societies in the eighteenth century', *Proc.-Roy.Soc.Med.*, 53 (1960) pp. 699–706.

McDaniel, W. B., 'A brief sketch of the rise of American medical societies', *Internat.Rec.Med.*, 171 (1958) pp. 483–91.

McMenemey, W. H., 'The influence of medical societies on the development of medical practice in nineteenth-century Britain', in F. N. L. Poynter (ed.), *The evolution of medical practice in Britain* (1961) pp. 67–79.

Mann, G., *Die medizinischen Lesegesellschaften in Deutschland* (Cologne, 1956), (Arbeiten aus dem Bibliothekar-Lehrinstitut des Landes Nordrhein-Westfalen, No. 11).

Neelameghan, A., *Development of medical societies and medical periodicals in India, 1780 to 1920* (Calcutta, 1963).

Ornstein, M., *The role of scientific societies in the seventeenth century*, 3rd edn (Chicago, 1938).

Power, Sir D'Arcy (ed.), *British medical societies* (1939).

Rolleston, Sir Humphry Davy, 'Medical friendship, clubs and societies', *Ann.Med.Hist.*, N.S.2 (1930) pp. 249–66.

Tovell, A. and B. Gandevia, 'Early Australian medical associations', *Med.J.Australia* (1962) I, pp. 756–9.

Index

As in the previous edition, the index includes personal names, names of institutions, titles of journals, and subjects. Under the latter are indicated the names of those contributing to these subjects.

Entries are in word-by-word order. Abbreviations are treated as if they were expanded, *e.g.* 'St Aubin' is treated as 'Saint Aubin' and appears before 'Salerno' in the alphabetical sequence. A name such as 'McKay' is treated as if it were spelt 'MacKay', and it therefore precedes 'MacKenna'. Universities are grouped under the heading 'universities and centres of education'.

Specific entries are used for subject headings, usually in direct phrase form, *e.g.* 'ectopic pregnancy' (not 'pregnancy, etopic'). Capital letters are used for proper names only. Cross-references from one entry to another are given selectively, and double entries are used when they do not occupy more space than '*see*' references would.

References are to page numbers, and the following conventions are used:–

bib. = bibliography, *e.g.* 'bib.349' refers to page 349 in the Bibliography section.

loc. = location of items in the possession of libraries, *e.g.* 'loc.291' refers to a special collection mentioned on page 291.

(n) = note, *e.g.* '79(n100)' refers to note 100 on page 79.

Institute of Medical Information, 335
Academy of Medical Sciences (Moscow), Fundamental Library, 321
Academy of Medicine (New York) *see* New York Academy of Medicine
Academy of Medicine (Richmond, Virginia), 205–6; library, 206
Academy of Medicine (Toronto), library, 288, 329
Academy of Medicine in Ireland, 204
Academy of Sciences (Leningrad), library, 278; museum. 109
Accademia del Cimento (Florence), 85
Accademia del Segreti (Naples), 84
Accademia Nazionale dei Lincei (Rome), 84
Achillini, Alessandro, 47–8
Ackerknecht, E. H., 80(n111), 207(n10), 210(n55), 212(n76); bib.344
Acland, *Sir* H. W., 208(n30)
acromegaly, Marie on, 200
Acta Medica et Philosophica Hafniensia, 224, 273
Acta Medicorum Berolinensium, 225
acupressure, Simpson on, 185
Adami, J. G., 153(n57)
Adams, C. E., 111(n13)
Adams, F., 202
Adams, H. M., 44
Adams, T., 55
Adams, W., 113(n27)
Addenbrookes Hospital Library, Cambridge, 310
Addington, A., 142
Addison, T., 178–9, 206
'Addison's disease', 178
Adelaide Hospital Medical Library, 330
Adelmann, H. B., 101, 110(n11)
ADONIS document delivery system, 336
Aeschylus, 280
Aetius of Amida, 4
Agia Sophia Paediatric Hospital (Greece), library, 319
Agrimi, J. 22, 27(n55)
Ahlfield Collection, W. H. Welch Medical Library, Johns Hopkins, 328

Aitken, P. H., 297(n53), 338(n36)
Akenside, M., 90
Alafovanine, T., 112(n18)
Albinus, B. S., 118; correspondence of, 118; editor of Vesalius, 52; students of, 119, 124, 246
Albinus, C. B., 98
Albucasis, 7, 9, 31, 36
Albury, W. R., 206(n2), 214(n99)
alchemy, Paracelsus on, 57; in Middle Ages, 23
Alderotti, T., 8, 9
Aldobrandino da Siena, 7
Aldus Manutius, 46, 57
Alexander, B., 116
Alexander, M., 293
Alexander of Tralles, 5
Alglave, E., 187
'Ali ibn al-'Abbas, 5
All Souls' College, Oxford, 93, 95
Allardyce, M. D., 312
Allbutt, *Sir* T. C., 200
Allegria, C., 110(n10)
Allen, D. G., 154(n80)
Allestrye, J., 85, 94, 272
almanacs and calendars, 3, 30, 38
Alstead, S., 339(n37)
Alvarez, W. C., 188
Alverny, M. T. d', 25(n2)
Amacher, P., 208(n21)
Ambrosiana Library (Milan), 22, 47
America (*see also* Canada; Mexico; USA), first medical book printed in, 72
American College of Surgeons (Chicago), library, 291, 327
American Journal of the Medical Sciences, 227
American Medical Association, 205–6, 255, 257; library, 328; *Transactions* and *Journal*, 206
American Medical Recorder, 227
amputation and excision (*see also* ovariotomy), Bigelow on, 173; Guthrie on, 170; Hunter on, 128; Fabricius on, 71; Pott on, 121; Syme on, 171; White on, 129; Yonge on, 103
amyl nitrite, Brunton on, 193
anaemia (*see also* pernicious anaemia), Ehrlich on, 202
anaesthesia (*see also* spinal

Ballard, T., 276
Balmer, H., 157(n124)
Baltimore Library Company, 283
Bämler, J., 31
Banckes, R., 44–5
Barber, G., 41(n30), 78(n81)
Barber-Lomax, J. W., 81(n135)
Barbers' Company, 64
Barber-Surgeons' Company, 102, 275, 304
Bardeleben, K. H. von, 164–5
Barge, J. A. J., 114(n30)
Bariety, M., 211(n56)
Barigazzi *see* Berengario da Carpi, J.
Barker, L. F., 164
Barlow, C., 216 (n122)
Barlow, G. H., 178
Barlow, H. M., 45; bib.351
Barlow Collection of Bookplates, Royal College of Physicians of London, 303; Plates 1–2
Barlow, P., 216(n122)
Barnard, C. C., 156(n113), 338(n22)
Barnes, H., 297(n52)
Barnes, R., library of, 270
Barnes Library (Birmingham), 310
Barnor, M. A., bib.357
Baron, J., 155(n95)
'Bartholin's duct' and 'glands', 273
Bartholin, C. (1585–1629), 91, 273
Bartholin, C. (1655–1738), 91, 273
Bartholin, T., 91,106,224; library of, 273–4
Bartholomaeus Anglicus, 33,36,37
Bartlett, B., 133
Barton, B. G., library of, 328
'Basedow's disease' *see* exophthalmic goitre
Baskerville Press, 124,125
Basset, T., 225
Bast, T. H., 151(n11), 164,207(n12)
Bate, G., 96
Bates, D. G., 112(n20)
Bath Hospital, 283
baths (mineral), Fabricius on, 72
Battie, W., 148
Batty Shaw, A., 149,114(n37); bib.357
Bauhin, C., 104
Baum Collection, John Crerar Library (Chicago), 328
Bauman, J., 54

Baumgartner, L., 78(n85), 156(n100,112),299(n87, 90)
Bäumler, E., 219(n149)
Bausch, J. L., 85
Baxby, D., 155(n88,95)
Bay, J. C., 247,251
Bayle, A. L. J., 176
Bayle, G. L., 175, 176
Bayon, H. P., 79(n105)
Beaman, A. G., 298(n81)
Beatrix de Savoie, 7
Beau, E., 182
Beaujon Hospital (Paris), 177
Beaujouan, G., 22
Beaumont, S., 188
Beaumont, W., 188–9,194,227; correspondence and papers of, 188–9
Beccaria, A., 3,22; bib.345
Bechet, P. E., 208(n25)
Becker, L. E., 211(n61)
Bedford, D. E., library of, 153(n64),157(n126),263,294
Beekman, F., 113(n25)
beer, Pasteur on,193; Thudichum on,192
Begbie, W., 206
Behr, G., 153(n57)
Belfast Clinical and Pathological Society,307
Belfast Medical Society,307
Belgium, medical libraries in,315
Bell, *Sir* C., 118,166–7
Bell, J., 166,169
Bell, J. W., 208(n21)
Bell, M. D.,338(n32)
Bell, W., 128
Bell, W. B., library of, 304
Bell, W. J., bib.357
Bellini, L., manuscripts of,318
Belloc, H.,177
Belloni, L.,157(n129)
'Bell's nerve',167
'Bell's palsy',167
Belt, E.,47
Benalius, B.,32
Benassi, E.,117
Benedek,I., 213(n86)
Benedetti, E. L., 219(n146)
Bénédictins du Bouveret,20
Benjamin, J. A.,212(n67)
Bennett, G., 138

Salmon, 296(n42); on Scarpa,
151(n9); bib.343,355,357
Bisset, C., 142
Black, D. A. K., 131
Black, J. W., 184
blackwater fever, Koch on, 194
bladder and bladder diseases, Bell on,
167; Gross on, 172; Guthrie on,
170
Blado d'Asola, A., 58
BLAISE-LINE, 35
Blake, J. B.,
155(n90),240,257,266(n28,33)
Blakey, N., 125
Bland-Sutton, *Sir* J., 203
Blasius, G., 94
Blegny, N. de, 225
Blezza, F., 157(n131)
Bloch, G., 147
Bloch, H., 79(n105)
Bloesch, H., 72
Blogg, M. W., 298(n73,76)
Blomefylde, Myles, library of, 270
blood and blood diseases, Boyle on,
106; Ehrlich on, 202; Hunter on,
128; Hewson on, 144; Mitchell
on, 199; Tuffier on, 202
blood cells and corpuscules (*see also*
haemoglobin), Hewson and
Falconar on, 144; Leeuwenhoek
on, 100; Malpighi on, 100
blood circulation (*see also* pulmonary
circulation), Bartholin on, 91;
Brunton on, 193; Cohnheim on,
164; Descartes on, 90–91; Ent on,
272; Flourens on, 182; Glisson
on, 97; Harvey on, 83,86,88–
91,107; Harvey's precursors on,
60–61; Marey on, 191;
Spallanzani on,143; Wale on,91
blood coagulation, Hewson on,144
blood transfusion, Dieffenbach on,
170; first account of, 92
blood pressure, Ludwig on,190
blood-letting and purging, Broussais
on, 176; Louis on, 177; medieval
and early works on, 3,14,30,38;
Vesalius on, 50
Bloomfield, A. L., 259
Bloomquist, H., 322
Blumenbach, J. F., 120,248;

correspondence of, 120; library
of, 283
Blunt, W., 44; bib.352
Boas, M. *see* Hall, M. Boas
Bodington, G., 179
Bodleian Library (Oxford), 288;
incunabula in, 32; manuscripts
in,71,113(n27),275; Digby
Manuscripts, 15
loc.61,62,93,271,272,276,280,284
Boehm, W., 112(n16)
Boenhum, F., 207(n10)
Boerhaave, H., 130–31,246–7;
correspondence of, 131; editor of
Vesalius, 52; library of, 131;
students of, 118,141,246
Bollet, A. J., 211(n56)
Bonamy, C., 182
bones and bone diseases (*see also*
cranium; dislocations; fractures;
hip; humerus; osteitis deformans;
rickets; spine and spinal injuries),
Albinus on,118; Bell on,166–7;
Blumenbach on, 120; Cheselden
on, 117; Douglas on,122;
Fabricius on,88; Gross on, 171;
Scarpa on,119; Soemmerring
on,119; in 16th c. medicine,51
Bonet, T., 225
Bonnette, P., 210(n55)
Bonsor, W., bib. 345
book clubs and societies,150,204
book illustrations *see* illustrations
book production (*see also*
manuscripts)
fifteenth century *see* incunabula
sixteenth century, 43–82;
Americana, 72; bibliographical
sources, 44,73; library holdings
and catalogues, 44; first
medical book printed in
English, 68
seventeenth century, 83–115;
Americana, 84, 105;
bibliographical sources, 83;
publishing in, 83–4,103–6
eighteenth-century, 116–59;
Americana, 137–8,148–9
nineteenth century, 160–220;
Americana, 203
bookplates,268,303,304; Plates 1–2
Boorde, A., 68

USSR, medical libraries in, 320–1
USSR Academy of Medical Sciences, Fundamental Library, 321
USSR Academy of Sciences, library, 278; museum, 109
Usteri, P., 248
uterine diseases, Addison on, 178; Velpeau on, 171
uterine haemorrhage, Denman on, 126
uterine sound, Simpson and, 184
uterine surgery, Sims on, 185
uterine tumours, Spencer Wells on, 185
uterus in pregnancy, Hunter on, 124–5

vaccination and inoculation, Conolly on, 180–1; Crawford and, 283; Heberden on, 132, Jenner on, 138–9, 149, 150; Koch and, 194; Rush on, 138; Willan on, 147
Val de Grâce Hospital and Medical School (Paris), 176
Valdezoccho, B. de, 32
Vallery-Radot, P., 194
Vallery-Radot, R., 216(n121)
Vallois, H.·V., 212(n76)
Valois, C. de, 10
Valsalva, A. M., 116
Valverde de Amusco, J. de, 53
Van Wyck, W., 59
'Vancouver Convention', 235
Vanderbilt Medical Center Library, 289
Vandergucht, G., 117
Vandevelde, A. J. J., 115(n44)
Vareschis, P. de, 38
vasa lactea *see* lacteal vessels
Vasari, G., 51
vascular surgery, Bell and, 166
vascular system and diseases (*see also* arterial diseases and injuries; arteries; blood circulation; capillaries; phlegmasia alba dolens; veins), Corvisart on, 175; Hall on, 181; Haller on, 144
vasomotor system, Bernard on, 187
Vatican Library, 22
Vaughan, R. B., 218(n144)
Vautrollier, T., 70
vectis (obstetrics), Denman on, 126
vein-men (Middle Ages), 13
veins, Albinus on, 118; Eustachius on,

54; Fabricius on valves in, 88; Guthrie on diseases of, 170
Veldener, J., 32
Velpeau, A. A. L. M., 170
Veltheer, W., 219(n147)
Venegas, J. M., 149
venereal diseases (*see also* gonorrhoea; syphilis), Hunter on, 128; Lind on, 142; Morgagni on, 117
Venezuela, medical libraries in, 329–30
Venn, J., 68
ventilation, Pringle on, 142
Verfasserlexikon, 19
vermiform appendix, Berengario da Carpi on, 48
Verso, M. L., 157(n118)
Vesalius A., 49–53, Plate 4; Boerhaave's edition of, 130; precursors of, 8, 46, 47, 48; professional relations, 54, 67; loc.291, 326
Vescovile Seminario Library (Padua), 22
vesica urinaria *see* bladder and bladder diseases
vesico-vaginal fistula, Sims on surgery for, 185
Vesling, J., 106
veterinary medicine, in Middle Ages, 24
Vicary, T., 53, 64–5
Vicq d'Azyr, F., 120
Victoria Art Gallery and Municipal Library (Bath), 283
Victoria Medical Association Library, 330
Victoria Medical Society, 229; library, 330
Victoria Medico-Chirurgical Society, 330
videotex, 314–15
Viets, H. R., on early Americana, 110(n3); on Fleet, 340(n58); on Kloss, 298(n64); on Laënnec, 177; on plague tracts, 30; on Read, 285; on Thacher, 110(n3); on Wendell Holmes, 298(n67); bib.343, 351
Vigiliis, S. H. de, 263
Villanovanus, M. *see* Servetus, M.
villi *see* intestinal villi
Vimont, J., 181

enr
n